Cardiac Puzzles

Cardiac Puzzles

J. Willis Hurst, MD

Consultant to the Division of Cardiology

Professor and Chairman Department of Medicine (1957-1986)

Emory University School of Medicine

Atlanta, Georgia

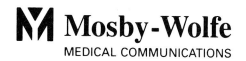

Mosby-Wolfe

MEDICAL COMMUNICATIONS

London   Baltimore   Bogota   Boston   Buenos Aires   Caracas   Carlsbad   Chicago   Madrid   Mexico City   Milan
Naples   New York   Philadelphia   St. Louis   Singapore   Sydney   Tokyo   Toronto   Wiesbaden

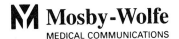

**Times Mirror
International Publishers**

For full details of all Times Mirror International Publishers Limited titles, please write to Times Mirror International Publishers Limited, Lynton House, 7-12 Tavistock Square, London WC1H 9LB, England.

A CIP catalogue record for this book is available from the British Library.

Library of Congress Cataloging-in-Publication Data
Hurst, J. Willis (John Willis), 1920-
  Cardiac puzzles / J. Willis Hurst.
      p.   cm.
    Includes bibliographical references and index.
    ISBN 0-7234-2469-1 (alk. paper)
    1. Cardiovascular system—Diseases—Diagnosis—Case studies.
  I. Title.
    [DNLM: 1. Cardiovascular Diseases—diagnosis—case studies. WG.
141 H966c   1995]
RC670.H86   1995
616.1'2075—dc20
DNLM/DLC
for Library of Congress   95–32144
                                                                        CIP

95 96 97 / 9 8 7 6 5 4 3 2 1

DEDICATION

This book is dedicated to physician-detectives who accept the challenge of solving diagnostic puzzles.

PREFACE

A skilled writer of detective stories introduces the reader to subtle clues that can be used to solve an intriguing mystery. The reader can solve the mystery if he or she discovers the clues and understands the significance of the clues. The physician's diagnostic efforts are similar to those of a detective looking for clues, and the patient's disease is similar to a mysterious event.

Sometimes, only *one major clue* is sufficient to solve the mystery. A major clue can be defined as one that indicates the presence of a certain disease. No other clues are needed. This is similar to a witness seeing someone steal a wallet.

At times, a *minor clue* may be discovered, but its presence is not sufficient to indicate the nature of the disease; several possibilities may exist. This is similar to the scene in which four people enter the room where a man has left his coat. He later discovers his expensive pen is missing. He believes that one of the four people stole his pen, but he cannot determine which one did it. Also, perhaps he lost it. He needs more information to determine the location of his pen.

At other times, *several minor clues* may be present. When each of the clues points toward the same disease, then the cluster of clues, added together, becomes a major clue. This is similar to observing a man walking down a road. He goes to a service station and fills a large can with gasoline. He then walks back down the road. A few minutes later, you see the man driving up the road in an automobile. You deduce that his car ran out of gasoline and that he has poured the gasoline from the can into the gas tank of his car. You never actually see him pour the gasoline into the gas tank, but the predictive value of the minor clues, when added together, approaches 100%.

Now I want to explain how to use this book. Initially, the physician-detective looks for clues to cardiovascular disease in the patient's history, physical examination, chest x-ray film, and electrocardiogram. These techniques are used in an effort to find major and minor diagnostic clues that indicate the presence of heart disease. When the diagnosis is not revealed using these techniques, additional data may be needed. The physician may order a highly technologic test. This is similar to a detective who wants to question another witness to a crime in an effort to identify the guilty party.

Part I of this book is a brief review of the diagnostic clues that can be found in the history, physical examination, chest x-ray film, and electrocardiogram.

Part II is devoted to the presentation of 50 patients. The data used to describe each patient were derived from several sources including patients I have seen in the office, on teaching rounds, and in teaching conferences. Accordingly, each patient is a composite of several patients. This method of presentation has been used in order to make a teaching point and to establish some of the diagnostic principles of cardiovascular sleuthing. Patient number one is normal but the remaining 49 patients have some type of cardiovascular disease.

I have chosen to display the abnormalities of each patient by (1) brief statements regarding the patient's symptoms, (2) terse descriptions or diagrams of the physical abnormalities, (3) a diagram of the chest x-ray film, and (4) as Robert Grant would have us do, diagrams of the cardiac vectors that represent the electrocardiograms. Diagrams are used because the abnormalities can be exaggerated, cartoon style, for teaching purposes.

The diagnostic *Clues and Questions* are placed on the right-hand pages of the book and the *Discussion and Answers*, including a discussion of the diagnostic clues and the diagnostic principles, are placed on the back of the same pages (and for one or two additional pages).

Do not turn the page to discover the answer before you think about the puzzle. That would be like reading the last chapter of a mystery novel before trying to discover the clues.

I wish to thank the medical students, house officers, and cardiology fellows at Emory University for their help in creating the "puzzles" in this book. For many years now, I have drawn these puzzles on the board and asked them to solve them. In solving these exercises, the trainees have taught me much medicine and, I hope, enjoyed the learning process as much as I have.

I thank David Marshall and Beth Adams of Mosby-Year Book for their continued optimism regarding the potential value of this book. They are experts in their fields—it is a pleasure to work with them. I also thank the Mosby production and manufacturing staff, including David Orzechowski, Chris Baumle, Nancy McDonald and Theresa Fuchs for their hard work under tight deadlines.

I wish to thank Carol Miller and Mary Cotton for preparing the manuscript. I thank Jan Mulder for the use of her artistic talent in creating the artwork that accompanies the puzzles. Finally, as always, I thank my wife Nelie. No Nelie—no book.

J. Willis Hurst, MD
Emory University

ACKNOWLEDGMENTS

I thank Mosby-Year Book, Inc. for permitting me to use illustrations that appeared in the following publications:

- Hurst JW: The examination of the heart: The importance of initial screening. *Dis-a-Month* 35(5):135-165, 1990. This is a Mosby–Year Book, Inc. publication.

- Hurst JW: *Cardiovascular diagnosis: The initial examination.* St. Louis, Mo, 1993, Mosby-Year Book, Inc.

- The copyright for Ventricular Electrocardiography, originally published by Gower in 1991, is now owned by Mosby–Year Book, Inc.

The source of each illustration is indicated in the legend of the illustration.

I also thank other publishers for permitting me to use certain illustrations. The exact sources are identified in the legend.

I am grateful to Dr. Steven Sigman, cardiology fellow at Emory University School of Medicine, for his review and suggestions regarding this manuscript.

CONTENTS

CONTENTS

PART II
Patient Puzzles

PART I

CLUES TO CARDIOVASCULAR DISEASE

INTRODUCTION

This part of this book discusses briefly the information (clues) that should be collected from the patient during the *initial examination* of the cardiovascular system.

The techniques employed by the physician-detective in his or her effort to discover diagnostic clues from the initial examination are:

1. The patient's *history* of symptoms and other subjective information related to the cardiovascular system

2. The *physical examination* of the cardiovascular system

3. The information related to the cardiovascular system that may be detected in the posteroanterior and/or left lateral *chest x-ray film*

4. The information that can be obtained from the *electrocardiogram*

CAVEAT

It is *always* necessary to interrelate the data discovered in the history, physical examination, chest x-ray film, and electrocardiogram. The diagnostic clues (or pieces) must fit together to create a picture that might not be perceived by studying each individual clue (or piece). The clues must fit together just as one fits the pieces of a jigsaw puzzle together. *Accordingly, the purpose of this book is to offer cardiovascular clues and to challenge the reader to fit them together in an effort to create different cardiovascular diagnoses.*

1 The History[1,2]

The history-taking period should be used for two important but different purposes: (1) to collect scientific data and (2) to create a trusting relationship with the patient. The history may be divided into three parts:

1. The *analysis of current and past symptoms* is one of the most important acts performed by the physician.
2. The *past history* may be important because a past history of rheumatic fever or chorea, for example, makes it more likely that the patient has rheumatic heart disease. Recent dental work increases the chances of endocarditis in a patient with a valve disease. The date a heart murmur was first heard or when elevated blood pressure was first discovered is extremely important.
3. The patient's *family history* may be important. Patients whose parents had coronary heart disease at a young age are more likely to have coronary heart disease. A family history of cardiomyopathy and congenital heart disease makes it more likely that the patient has a similar disease.

TYPES OF SYMPTOMS

Cardiovascular disease may cause chest discomfort, intermittent claudication, dyspnea, palpitation, syncope, and various less specific complaints.

CHEST DISCOMFORT

Myocardial Ischemia

The discomfort associated with myocardial ischemia that is described by the patient is usually located in the retrosternal area. The area of discomfort is about the size of the fist or larger. It may radiate to the left or right shoulder, left or right arm, throat, jaw, or back. Patients use their own descriptive words to explain the feeling to the physician. They may complain of tightness, indigestion, aches, pain, and so on. The main point is that it is an unpleasant feeling that has not been felt previously. The discomfort lasts for varying periods and is precipitated by effort or emotional stress or may occur without provoking events (see following discussion). However, the discomfort always lasts longer than it takes to snap one's fingers.

Coronary atherosclerosis is the usual cause of myocardial ischemia, including stable and unstable angina pectoris and myocardial infarction, as well as the other syndromes described next. Coronary atherosclerosis, however, is not the only cause of myocardial ischemia. For example, coronary artery spasm, coronary arteritis, coronary embolism, congenital anomalies of the coronary arteries, coronary ostial disease as occurs with syphilis or coronary ostial trauma, aortic dissection, coronary disease that occurs in transplanted hearts (which is unassociated with chest discomfort), and Kawasaki's disease may produce myocardial ischemia. Also, myocardial ischemia may be caused by noncoronary disease such as aortic valve stenosis, aortic valve regurgitation, hypertrophic cardiomyopathy, dilated cardiomyopathy, systemic hypertension, and pulmonary hypertension.

Stable Angina Pectoris. When the discomfort of myocardial ischemia lasts a brief period, such as 1 to 10 minutes, it is called angina pectoris. It is precipitated by effort or emotional stress. It is labeled as *stable* angina pectoris when no change has occurred in the frequency of the episodes or provoking causes within the previous 60 days.

Stable angina pectoris is caused by an increase in myocardial oxygen (O_2) demand rather than an abrupt decrease in myocardial O_2 supply.

Unstable Angina Pectoris. The discomfort of myocardial ischemia lasts a brief period, usually 1 to 10 minutes. It is precipitated by effort or emotional stress but often occurs at rest. It is labeled *unstable* when it occurs for the first time, or at rest, or when previously recognized angina pectoris increases in frequency, lasts longer than usual, or is precipitated with less effort during the last 60 days.

The pathophysiology responsible for unstable angina pectoris is very different to that of stable angina pectoris. Unstable angina pectoris is caused by a rather abrupt change in myocardial oxygen (O_2) supply rather than an increase in myocardial oxygen (O_2) demand. In other words, it is usually caused by a change in the caliber of diseased coronary arteries. In many patients it results from coronary thrombosis, which is precipitated by a "crack in an atheromatous plaque" located in the coronary artery.

It is vital to recognize the difference in stable and unstable angina pectoris because the prognosis and treatment are very different for each of the syndromes.

Angina Equivalents. At times, transient myocardial ischemia is manifested as transient dyspnea or weakness. These unpleasant symptoms are usually precipitated by effort. Chronic exhaustion can be caused by many conditions, but persistent myocardial ischemia is one possibility.

When the myocardium is becoming ischemic, left ventricular diastolic myocardial dysfunction may occur, followed by myocardial systolic dysfunction, followed by electrocardiographic (ECG) changes, which may be followed by angina. Diastolic and systolic dysfunction may produce transient pulmonary congestion and dyspnea; a transient decrease in cardiac output (CO) may cause transient weakness; or a persistent decrease in CO may cause persistent exhaustion.

Variant Angina (Prinzmetal's Angina Pectoris). Prinzmetal described a variation in the pattern of ordinary angina pectoris. Variant angina pectoris is located in the same area of the chest as usual angina and may last about the same length of time. Variant angina is not usually precipitated by effort and tends to occur when the patient is resting. It may be precipitated by smoking tobacco or alcohol withdrawal. It tends to occur the same time each day or occurs early in the morning. Coronary artery spasm caused by cocaine is a special type of problem and not usually classified as Prinzmetal's angina.

Variant angina pectoris is caused by coronary artery spasm. Usually, the coronary artery spasm occurs in a coronary artery that is diseased with atherosclerosis. A small percentage of patients with variant angina pectoris have no recognizable additional coronary artery disease.

Syndrome X. This poorly understood condition occurs more frequently in women. The chest discomfort may occur when the patient is at rest or with exercise. It tends to occur more frequently during the second half of the menstrual cycle. The exercise ECG may be abnormal, but the coronary arteriogram is normal. The condition is caused by an inability of the coronary arteries, including the resistance vessels, to dilate normally.

Prolonged Myocardial Ischemia. This term is used to designate the discomfort that is characteristic of myocardial ischemia but lasts longer than angina pectoris. The separation of this syndrome from ordinary angina is arbitrary, but when the discomfort lasts longer than 10 to 20 minutes, the physician must be concerned that the myocardial cell damage is not entirely reversible as it is with brief angina. One may wish to call this prolonged *angina* rather than prolonged myocardial ischemia. This is acceptable as long as the physician understands that the pathophysiology is different from ordinary angina and that the more prolonged the chest discomfort, the more likely it is that ventricular myocytes are being killed with hypoxia.

Prolonged myocardial ischemia can be further divided into (1) *prolonged myocardial ischemia without objective signs of myocardial infarction*; (2) *prolonged myocardial ischemia with ST segment and T wave changes in the ECG and elevation of the serum MB fraction of creatine phosphokinase (CPK) (non-Q wave infarction)*; and (3) *prolonged myocardial ischemia with QRS complex, ST segment, and T wave changes in the ECG plus elevation of the MB fraction of CPK (Q wave infarction).*

Symptomless Myocardial Ischemia. Patients may have transient myocardial ischemia and may experience no chest discomfort. This condition is usually referred to as *silent myocardial ischemia*. Even myocardial infarction may occur, and the patient may have no discomfort. These syndromes occur more often in elderly patients or in patients with diabetes mellitus.

Symptomless myocardial ischemia is usually discovered in the exercise ECG. Symptomless myocardial infarction is usually discovered on the resting ECG.

Dissecting Aortic Aneurysm
The chest pain from a dissecting aortic aneurysm is severe and usually reaches its peak intensity almost instantly. It is located in the interscapular area but may be felt to some degree in the chest's anterior portion. The pain is unrelenting and is poorly relieved with opiates. The pulsations normally felt in peripheral arteries may be eliminated. This type of pain, plus a simultaneous neurologic deficit, is diagnostic of dissection of the aorta.

Pulmonary Embolism and Infarction
Massive pulmonary embolism produces abrupt dyspnea and may cause syncope. Myocardial ischemia may also be precipitated by pulmonary embolism. Pulmonary infarction produces pleuritic chest pain that occurs at a varying period after the embolism. Pleuritic chest pain is located in the lateral or lower posterior portion of the thorax and is intensified by deep inspiration.

Pericarditis
The pain is located in the chest's anterior portion. It tends to be located slightly to the left of the sternum in the area typically referred to as the precordium. The pain may also be felt at the top of the shoulders. The characteristic feature of the pain of pericarditis is that it is aggravated by deep inspiration. The patient breathes shallowly in an effort to relieve the pain. The pain may be aggravated by leaning forward, twisting and turning the thorax, and swallowing.

Unpleasant Sensation Associated with Palpitation
Some patients "feel" every ectopic atrial or ventricular contractions, whereas others are oblivious to the presence of treacherous ventricular tachycardia.

Those who are sensitive to ectopic beats have a "sinking" feeling and dislike the tumultuous action, which is more frightening than painful.

Noncardiac Chest Pain that may be Misinterpreted as Being Caused by Heart Disease
Noncardiac chest pain has many causes, and some are often misinterpreted as resulting from myocardial ischemia, and vice versa.

Esophageal Reflux and Spasm. Esophageal reflux or esophageal spasm may mimic the chest discomfort of myocardial ischemia. However, more patients believe that angina pectoris, or the discomfort of prolonged myocardial ischemia, is caused by "indigestion" than assume that the discomfort of esophageal reflux or esophageal spasm is caused by angina pectoris.

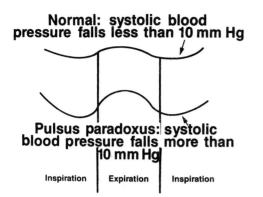

Fig. 2-6. Pulsus paradoxus. The effect of inspiration and expiration on the systolic blood pressure of a person without cardiopulmonary disease is shown in the upper diagram. The effect of inspiration and expiration on the systolic blood pressure of a patient with cardiac tamponade is shown in the lower diagram. Note that the systolic pressure falls more than 10 mm Hg during inspiration when pulsus paradoxus is present.

Reproduced with permission from Hurst JW: The examination of the heart: the importance of initial screening, *Dis Mon* 36(5):278, 1990.

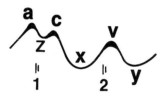

Fig. 2-7. Normal jugular venous pulse (see text for an explanation of the waves). The heart sounds are illustrated in the lower portion of the figure. NOTE: In the remainder of the figures in this chapter illustrating pulsations (with the exception of Fig. 2-9), the thicker portions of the lines or curves illustrating the pulsations indicate the parts that are actually felt or seen. The heart sounds illustrated in these figures should be used as reference points indicating the onset of systole and diastole.

Reproduced with permission from Hurst JW: The examination of the heart: the importance of initial screening, *Dis Mon* 36(5):280, 1990.

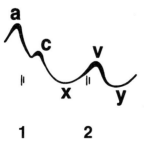

Fig. 2-8. Abnormal jugular venous pulse associated with a decreased right ventricular compliance or tricuspid stenosis. Note the abnormally large *a* wave (see text).

Reproduced with permission from Hurst JW: The examination of the heart: the importance of initial screening, *Dis Mon* 36(5):280, 1990.

A *cannon wave* occurs when the RA contracts against a closed tricuspid valve (Fig. 2-9). This occurs with complete heart block.

An early and prominent *v* wave is produced by tricuspid valve regurgitation (Fig. 2-10).

A *rapid y descent* suggests constrictive pericarditis (Fig. 2-11).

EXAMINATION OF PRECORDIUM

The physician should inspect and feel the movement of six areas of the chest's anterior portion (Fig. 2-12).

Area 1 (Second Right Intercostal Space)

Normally, no pulsation can be felt in this area. There may be a palpable systolic pulsation when the first part of the aorta is abnormally large, especially with associated aortic valve regurgitation. Such a pulsation may be present with an atherosclerotic or syphilitic aneurysm of the aorta's proximal portion and with dissection of the aorta (Fig. 2-13).

The systolic thrill of aortic valve stenosis may be felt in this area.

Area 2 (Second Left Intercostal Space)

Normally, no pulsation can be felt in this area. There may be a palpable systolic pulsation of the main pulmonary artery when the pulmonary artery pressure is elevated or when there is an increase in pulmonary artery blood flow. The abnormal pulsation that results from elevated pulmonary artery pressure is generally less abrupt and is shown in Fig. 2-14. The abnormal pulsation caused by an increase in blood flow, as occurs with an ostium secundum atrial septal defect, is more dynamic with a rapid upstroke.

A systolic thrill caused by pulmonary valve stenosis may be felt in this area, as may the prominent pulmonary valve closure sound caused by pulmonary artery hypertension.

Area 3 (Anterior Precordium)

The normal movement felt in area 3 is shown in Fig. 2-15.

The abnormal pulsation caused by RV hypertrophy and dilatation that results from an elevation of RV pressure is shown in Fig. 2-16. This causes a forceful and prolonged systolic movement. This may be the result of pulmonary valve stenosis, tetralogy of Fallot, mitral stenosis, Eisenmenger physiology, and primary pulmonary artery hypertension.

The abnormal pulsation caused by RV hypertrophy and dilatation related to a left-to-right shunt, as occurs with an ostium secundum atrial septal defect, is shown in Fig. 2-17. When the pulsation results from volume overload of the RV, the systolic movement is hyperdynamic.

Mitral regurgitation may produce an abrupt expansion of the left atrium (LA), which is located posteriorly. Such an expansion forces the heart anteriorly because the expansion posteriorly is limited by the vertebral column.

The precordial movement associated with an RA gallop sound may be felt in this area (Fig. 2-16). The RA gallop movement indicates poor compliance of the RV. An RV gallop movement may be felt; it implies the presence of RV dysfunction (Fig. 2-16).

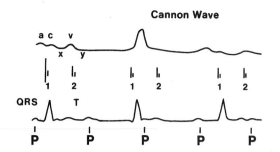

Cannon Wave

Fig. 2-9. Abnormal jugular venous pulse associated with a complete heart block in a patient with normal atrial activity. When the atrium contracts against a closed tricuspid valve, which exists during right ventricular systole, the venous pulse becomes a large cannon wave. Note the regular appearance of the *P* waves in the electrocardiogram and the *a* waves in the jugular pulse. The third *P* wave occurs during ventricular systole in this illustration. When the atrium contracts against a closed tricuspid valve, a large cannon wave occurs in the neck.

Reproduced with permission form Hurst JW: *Cardiovascular diagnosis: the initial examination.* St Louis, 1993, Mosby, p137.

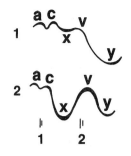

Fig. 2-11. Abnormal jugular venous pulse associated with constrictive pericarditis. The upper diagram illustrates the abnormal jugular venous pulse associated with chronic constrictive pericarditis. The *a*, *c*, and *v* waves may be seen, but it is the large negative *y* wave that is abnormal. The lower diagram illustrates the abnormal jugular venous pulse that is sometimes associated with subacute constrictive pericarditis in which pericardial effusion is still present. Note the prominent *x* descent and prominent *y* wave.

Reproduced with permission from Hurst JW: The examination of the heart: the importance of initial screening, *Dis Mon* 36(5):280, 1990.

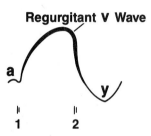

Regurgitant V Wave

Fig. 2-10. Abnormal jugular venous pulse associated with tricuspid valve regurgitation. The *v* wave becomes so prominent that it may be misinterpreted as an arterial pulse.

Reproduced with permission from Hurst JW: The examination of the heart: the importance of initial screening, *Dis Mon* 36(5):280, 1990.

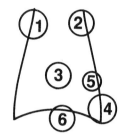

Fig. 2-12. The six areas of the chest's anterior portion that should be inspected and palpated. Area 1 is examined in an effort to detect abnormalities of the aorta. Area 2 is examined in an effort to detect abnormalities of the main pulmonary artery. Area 3 is examined in an effort to detect abnormalities of the right ventricle. Area 4 is examined in an effort to detect abnormalities of the left ventricle. Area 5 is examined in an effort to detect an ectopic pulsation of the left ventricle. Area 6 is examined for evidence of right ventricular hypertrophy in patients with pulmonary emphysema.

Reproduced with permission from Hurst JW: The examination of the heart: the importance of initial screening, *Dis Mon* 36(5):282, 1990.

Area 4 (Apical Area)

The pulsation of area 4 is caused by the movement of the apex of the left ventricle (LV). The normal pulsation is shown in Fig. 2-15. The normal pulsation should be located to the right of the midclavicular line in the fifth left intercostal space and should be about 2 cm in diameter.

The pulsation caused by a pressure overload of the LV lasts longer than normal, and the area of pulsation may be larger than normal (Fig. 2-16). Such a pulsation may be caused by systemic hypertension, aortic valve stenosis, or primary hypertrophy of the heart. A bifid systolic movement may occur when there is idiopathic hypertrophic subaortic stenosis.

The pulsation caused by volume overload of the LV is shown in Fig. 2-17. It is more dynamic than the pulsation produced by pressure overload of the LV. A rapid upstroke occurs. Such a pulsation may be caused by aortic valve regurgitation or mitral valve regurgitation.

Some diseases, such as multivalvular disease and dilated cardiomyopathy, produce a pulsation that is a mixture of pressure overload and volume overload of the LV.

The movements associated with an LA gallop sound and an LV gallop sound can be felt in area 4 (Fig. 2-16). The former is caused by poor compliance of the LV, as occurs with LV hypertrophy, and the latter is associated with LV dysfunction.

The systolic thrill associated with mitral regurgitation may be felt and the diastolic thrill associated with mitral stenosis palpated in area 4.

Area 5 (Ectopic Area)

Area 5 designates the usual area for an "ectopic" pulsation. Such a pulsation is usually caused by a myocardial infarction (Fig. 2-18). An actual ventricular aneurysm is not required to produce such a pulsation. An ectopic pulsation can also be produced by dilated cardiomyopathy.

Area 6 (Epigastric Area)

Area 6 is located in the infraxiphoid area. Occasionally, a prominent systolic pulsation is felt here in patients with cor pulmonale caused by pulmonary emphysema.

EXAMINATION OF HEART SOUNDS

Normally, in adults, it is often stated that two heart sounds exist. Actually, each of the two sounds is produced by the closure of two heart valves. The first sound is composed of the mitral valve closure sound followed by the tricuspid valve closure sound. The second sound is composed of the aortic valve closure sound followed by the pulmonary valve closure sound (Fig. 2-19). An additional sound, the normal third sound, can be heard at the cardiac apex in early diastole in children. Under abnormal circumstances, however, several additional heart sounds may be heard (Fig. 2-20). These include a LA or RA gallop sound, a LV or RV gallop sound, an aortic or pulmonary ejection sound, a mitral valve systolic click, an opening snap of the mitral valve, a LA tumor plop, a pericardial knock caused by constrictive pericarditis, a pericardial friction rub, and a mediastinal "crunch" caused by mediastinal emphysema.

NORMAL HEART SOUNDS

The two components of the normal first and second heart sounds are high pitched; they are heard best by using the stethoscope's diaphragm. The normal third sound heard at the cardiac apex of the child is low pitched and is heard best by using the stethoscope's bell.

The *first heart sound* should be studied at the cardiac apex. Normally, it may be equal to, fainter than, or louder than the second heart sound (Fig. 2-19). Mitral valve closure produces most of the sound, and the tricuspid valve closure sound is seldom heard. The loudness of the first sound is determined by three factors (see later discussion).

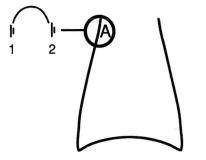

Fig. 2-13. No pulsation should be felt in this area in normal patients. An abnormally prolonged systolic pulsation may be felt in the second right intercostal space when there is an aneurysm of the ascending aorta, such as occurs with atherosclerosis, syphilis, and dissection of the aorta, or when the aortic arch is on the right side. The pulsation may be felt in the sternoclavicular joint.

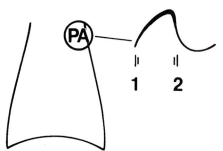

Fig. 2-14. No pulsation should be felt in this area in normal patients. Abnormal systolic pulsation in the second intercostal space, which is characteristic of an increase in pulmonary artery *(PA)* pressure; the onset and offset of the pulsation are gradual. Note that the second component of the second heart sound is depicted as being louder than normal. This also indicates pulmonary artery hypertension.

Reproduced with permission from Hurst JW: The examination of the heart: the importance of initial screening, *Dis Mon* 36(5):282, 1990.

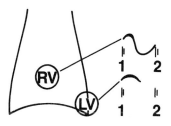

Fig. 2-15. Pulsations of the normal right ventricle *(RV)* and left ventricle *(LV)*. The normal pulsation of the RV is illustrated in the upper curve. Note that the brief outward pulsation is followed by a longer inward pulsation. The normal apex impulse of the LV is illustrated in the lower curve. Note that the outward pulsation occupies about one third of systole.

Reproduced with permission from Hurst JW: The examination of the heart: the importance of initial screening, *Dis Mon* 36(5):282, 1990.

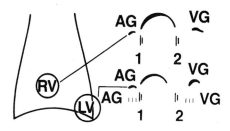

Fig. 2-16. Pulsations caused by systolic pressure overload of the right *(RV)* and left *(LV)* ventricles. Right and left atrial gallop movements and RV and LV gallop movements are shown. *Upper curve:* The long, outward systolic pulsation is caused by pressure overload of the RV. The right atrial gallop movement *(AG)* is caused by a decrease in RV compliance. The RV gallop movement *(VG)* indicates RV dysfunction. *Lower curve:* The long, outward systolic pulsation is caused by pressure overload of the LV. In addition, the apex impulse is larger than a 25-cent piece. A bifid systolic pulsation may be produced by idiopathic hypertrophic subaortic stenosis. The left atrial gallop movement *(AG)* is caused by a decrease in LV compliance. The LV gallop movement *(VG)* indicates LV dysfunction. *Bottom portion of figure:* This diagram shows the first and second heart sounds, the right and left atrial gallop sounds *(AG)*, and the RV and LV gallop sounds *(VG)*.

Reproduced with permission from Hurst JW: The examination of the heart: the importance of initial screening, *Dis Mon* 36(5):262, 1990.

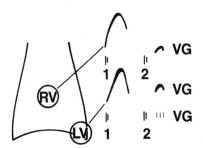

Fig. 2-17. Abnormal pulsations caused by volume overload of the right *(RV)* and left *(LV)* ventricles. RV and LV gallop movements are shown. *Upper curve:* The prominent systolic pulsation with its abrupt onset is characteristic of volume overload of the RV. This type of pulsation may be produced by an ostium secundum atrial septal defect. An RV gallop *(VG)* movement may be felt. *Lower curve:* The prominent pulsation with its abrupt onset is characteristic of volume overload of the LV. This type of pulsation may be produced by aortic regurgitation or mitral regurgitation. An LV gallop movement *(VG)* may be felt. *Bottom portion of figure:* This diagram shows the first and second heart sounds and the RV and LV gallop sounds *(VG)*.

Reproduced with permission from Hurst JW: The examination of the heart: the importance of initial screening, *Dis Mon* 36(5):282, 1990.

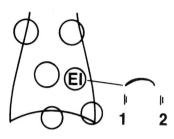

Fig. 2-18. Abnormal systolic ectopic impulse *(EI)*. No pulsation should be felt in this area in normal patients.

Reproduced with permission from Hurst JW: The examination of the heart: the importance of initial screening, *Dis Mon* 36(5):262, 1990.

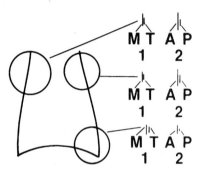

Fig. 2-19. The normal heart sounds. The first sound *(1)* is produced by mitral valve closure *(M)* followed by tricuspid valve closure *(T)*. The second heart sound *(2)* is produced by aortic valve closure *(A)* followed by pulmonary valve closure *(P)*. Note that the second sound is louder than the first sound when one is listening in the second intercoastal space adjacent to the sternum. This results from loudness of the aortic valve closure *(A)*. Also, note that the pulmonary valve closure sound *(P)* is louder in the second intercostal space adjacent to the sternum than it is at the cardiac apex. In normal subjects the pulmonary closure is not heard at the apex, or it is only barely heard.

Reproduced with permission from Hurst JW: The examination of the heart: the importance of initial screening, *Dis Mon* 36(5):294, 1990.

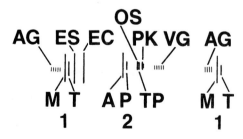

Fig. 2-20. The four normal and six abnormal heart sounds. *AG,* Atrial gallop; *M,* mitral valve closure; *T,* tricuspid valve closure; *ES,* ejection sound; *EC,* ejection click; *A,* aortic valve closure; *P,* pulmonary valve closure; *OS,* opening snap of the mitral valve; *PK,* pericardial knock; *VG,* ventricular gallop. A pericardial friction rub (not shown here) may have three components that coincide with heart movements: a rub when the atria contract, a rub associated with ventricular systole, and a rub associated with ventricular diastole. (See text for a discussion of normal and abnormal heart sounds.)

Reproduced with permission from Hurst JW: The examination of the heart: the importance of initial screening, *Dis Mon* 36(5):284, 1990.

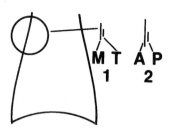

Fig. 2-21. The normal heart sounds in the second right intercostal space adjacent to the sternum. Note that the aortic valve closure sound *(A)* is the loudest component of the heart sounds. *M,* Mitral valve closure; *I,* tricuspid valve closure; *P,* pulmonary valve closure.

Reproduced with permission from Hurst JW: The examination of the heart: the importance of initial screening, *Dis Mon* 36(5):264, 1990.

The observer should listen initially in the second right intercostal space near the sternum. Normally, the second heart sound is always louder than the first sound in this area (Fig. 2-21). This is because the aortic valve closure sound in this area is louder than the other closure sounds. When the first sound is as loud or louder than the second sound in the second right intercostal area, one must deduce a condition is present that makes the first sound abnormally loud or a condition is present that makes the second sound abnormally faint.

The observer should study the *second heart sound* in the second left intercostal space near the sternum. The main purpose should be to estimate the amount of separation of aortic valve closure sound from the pulmonary valve closure sound and to determine the intensity (loudness) of the pulmonary valve closure sound. Normally, at the end of expiration, the pulmonary valve closure sound and aortic valve closure sound almost coincide, and the interval between the aortic valve closure sound and pulmonary valve closure sound is barely detectable (Fig. 2-22). During inspiration the sounds made by the aortic closure sound and the pulmonary closure sound separate. This is primarily caused by a delay in pulmonary valve closure because RV systole is prolonged as a result of the inspiratory increase of RV blood volume. The normal "splitting" of the second sound is just barely detectable, similiar to saying a letter of the alphabet twice as rapidly as possible.

ABNORMAL HEART SOUNDS

Auscultation of Sounds in Second Right Intercostal Space Near the Sternum

When the *intensity of the first heart sound,* which is produced mainly by the mitral valve closure sound, is as loud as or louder than the second heart sound, which is produced mainly by closure of the aortic valve, it should be recognized as being abnormal. One should consider that mitral stenosis is causing the first sound to be loud, that aortic stenosis is causing the second sound to become fainter than normal (Fig. 2-23), or that aortic valve closure is not possible because of a destroyed aortic valve, as occurs with moderate aortic valve regurgitation (Fig. 2-24). The absence of a systolic murmur excludes aortic valve stenosis as the cause, and the absence of a diastolic murmur excludes aortic valve regurgitation. In the absence of aortic stenosis and regurgitation, a first heart sound that is louder than the second sound in the second right intercostal space is usually caused by mitral stenosis. Although the diastolic rumbling murmur of mitral stenosis is almost never heard in this area, the abnormal heart sounds associated with mitral stenosis are typically transmitted to this area.

An *aortic systolic ejection sound* may be heard in this area but it is usually louder at the apex (Fig. 2-20). This suggests aortic valve stenosis caused by a congenital bicuspid aortic valve.

The *opening snap of the mitral valve* associated with mitral stenosis may be heard in this area (Fig. 2-25).

Gallop sounds are rarely heard in the second right intercostal space near the sternum.

Auscultation of Sounds in Second Left Intercostal Space Near Sternum

Abnormal Splitting of the Second Sound. When the second sound is more widely split than normal during expiration but the split becomes even wider during inspiration, it is usually caused by right bundle branch block (Fig. 2-26). When the splitting of the second sound is wider during expiration than during inspiration, it is usually caused by left bundle branch block and is referred to as *paroxysmal splitting* of the second heart sound (Fig. 2-27). When the second sound is widely split on expiration and remains widely split on inspiration, it is called *fixed splitting* of the second heart sound (Fig. 2-28). Fixed splitting of the second sound is usually caused by an ostium secundum atrial septal defect.

Intensity of Pulmonary Valve Closure Sound. The intensity (loudness) of the pulmonary valve closure sound must be determined while listening in the second left intercostal space near the sternum. Normally, it is not as loud as the aortic valve closure sound. When the pulmonary valve closure sound is louder than the aortic valve closure sound and is transmitted to the cardiac apex, it usually denotes an abnormal intensity of the sound and suggests pulmonary artery hypertension (Fig. 2-29).

The pulmonary valve closure sound is diminished in intensity when there is pulmonary valve stenosis.

Other Heart Sounds. A *systolic pulmonary ejection sound* may be heard in the second left intercostal space near the sternum and suggests pulmonary valve stenosis (see Fig. 2-20). *Gallop sounds* are rarely heard in this area.

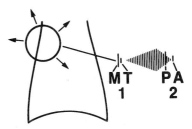

Fig. 2-23. Murmur of *severe aortic valve stenosis.* The aortic valve closure sound (A) is delayed and is faint or inaudible. In this illustration, it is so delayed that it follows the sound created by the closure of the pulmonary valve. The pulmonary valve closure sound (P) may be masked by the end of the murmur, even when it is louder than normal as a result of heart failure and mild pulmonary artery hypertension. Usually, neither component of the second heart sound is heard when there is extremely severe aortic valve stenosis. If both components of the second sound are heard, there may be paradoxical splitting of the second heart sound. That is, the second heart sound may become single on inspiration and split on expiration, which is opposite to normal. The peak of the coarse systolic murmur appears late in systole, and the murmur is transmitted into the neck, right shoulder, and upper part of the right arm.

Reproduced with permission from Hurst JW: The examination of the heart: the importance of initial screening, *Dis Mon* 36(5):285, 1990.

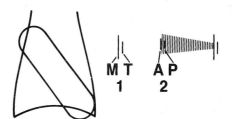

Fig. 2-24. High-pitched diastolic murmur of aortic valve regurgitation. The aortic valve closure sound (A) may be diminished in intensity because the valve leaflets may be damaged to such a degree that they cannot coapt. The murmur is heard with maximum intensity along the left sternal border when the patient is sitting and leaning forward. *M,* Mitral; *T,* tricuspid; *P,* pulmonary valve closure.

Reproduced with permission from Hurst JW: The examination of the heart: the importance of initial screening, *Dis Mon* 36(5):285, 1990.

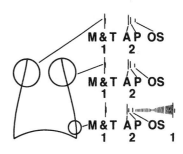

Fig. 2-25. Opening snap (OS), as well as other auscultatory features, of mitral stenosis. *Upper diagram:* Note the abnormally loud mitral (M) component of the first heart sound (1) when one is listening in the second right intercostal space. It is louder than the second sound (2). The pulmonary valve closure sound (P) may be heard. The OS of the mitral valve is also heard in this area. *Middle diagram:* The first heart sound is louder than normal, and an OS is heard when one is listening in the second left intercostal space. The pulmonary valve closure sound (P) is often heard. *Lower diagram:* The first sound is loud. An OS is heard, as well as a low-pitched, rumbling murmur of mitral stenosis. Note that the diastolic rumble of mitral stenosis is heard only at the cardiac apex, whereas the loud first sound and OS are widely transmitted.

Reproduced with permission from Hurst JW: The examination of the heart: the importance of initial screening, *Dis Mon* 36(5):284, 1990.

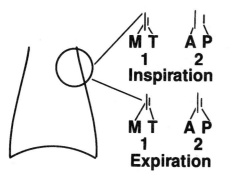

Fig. 2-22. Effect of inspiration and expiration on the splitting of the normal second heart sound (2), which is heard by placing the stethoscope's diaphragm in the second intercostal space near the sternum. *Upper diagram:* Note the degree of splitting of the second heart sound during inspiration. *Lower diagram:* Note that the duration of the gap between the sound made by aortic valve closure (A) and the sound made by pulmonary valve closure (P) is less than it is during inspiration. In fact, the second sound typically becomes single during expiration in most normal subjects.

Reproduced with permission from Hurst JW: The examination of the heart: the importance of initial screening, *Dis Mon* 36(5):284, 1990.

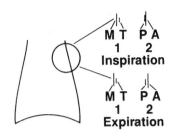

Fig. 2-26. Splitting of the second heart sound *(2)* in patients with right bundle branch block. *Lower diagram:* During expiration the aortic valve closure sound *(A)* and the pulmonary valve closure sound *(P)* are separated from each other by an interval greater than normal. *Upper diagram:* During inspiration the interval between the aortic valve closure sound *(A)* and the pulmonary valve closure sound *(P)* is increased beyond that observed during expiration.

Reproduced with permission from Hurst JW: The examination of the heart: the importance of initial screening, *Dis Mon* 36(5):294, 1990.

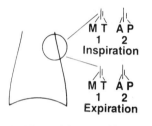

Fig. 2-27. Paradoxical splitting of the second heart sound *(2)* caused by left bundle branch block. *Lower diagram:* During expiration the aortic valve closure sound *(A)* is delayed because of left bundle branch block. Accordingly, the aortic valve closure sound may appear after the pulmonary valve closure sound *(P).* *Upper diagram:* During inspiration the pulmonary closure sound *(P)* is delayed, as it is normally, until it almost coincides with the aortic valve closure sound *(A).*

Reproduced with permission from Hurst JW: The examination of the heart: the importance of initial screening, *Dis Mon* 36(5):284, 1990.

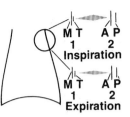

Fig. 2-28. Fixed, wide splitting of the second heart sound *(2)* during inspiration and expiration, characteristic of an ostium secundum atrial septal defect. The abnormally large lapse of time between the aortic *(A)* and pulmonary *(P)* valve closure sounds remains constant during inspiration and expiration. Note the systolic diamond-shaped pulmonary artery murmur that is caused by a large right ventricular stroke volume and becomes louder during inspiration. Also note that the pulmonary valve closure sound is louder than normal in the second left intercoastal space and at the apex because the pulmonary artery pressure may be slightly or moderately elevated.

Reproduced with permission from Hurst JW: The examination of the heart: the importance of initial screening, *Dis Mon* 36(5):284, 1990.

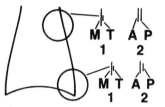

Fig. 2-29. Abnormally loud pulmonary valve closure *(P)* sound caused by pulmonary artery hypertension. *Upper diagram:* The pulmonary valve closure sound *(P)* is as loud as the aortic valve closure sound *(A);* this is abnormal and suggests pulmonary artery hypertension. *Lower diagram:* The pulmonary valve closure sound *(P)* is easily heard at the apex and is louder than usual; this is virtually diagnostic of pulmonary artery hypertension.

Reproduced with permission from Hurst JW: The examination of the heart: the importance of initial screening, *Dis Mon* 36(5):284, 1990.

Auscultation of Sounds Just to Left of Midportion of Sternum (Anterior Precordium)

A low-pitched *RA gallop sound* may be heard just before the first heart sound in this area. It increases in intensity during inspiration (Fig. 2-30). An RA gallop sound indicates poor compliance of the RV and is usually associated with RV hypertrophy.

An *RV gallop sound* may be heard in this area. It increases in intensity during inspiration (Fig. 2-31). An RV gallop sound indicates RV dysfunction.

Many of the abnormal heart sounds described earlier may be heard in this area, but this is not the ideal location to study them.

Auscultation of Sounds at Apex

The loudness of the first heart sound at the cardiac apex is determined by three variables:

- The interval that occurs between atrial and ventricular contraction is a major factor determining the loudness of the first heart sound. (This is related to the length of the PR interval in the electrocardiogram.) When the PR interval is long, about 0.18 to 0.22 second or longer, the first sound at the apex is faint (Fig. 2-32). When the PR interval is short, about 0.14 to 0.16 second, the first sound is loud. When complete heart block exists, the first sound varies in loudness (Fig. 2-33).

- The structural status of the mitral valve is an important factor in determining the loudness of the first heart sound. When the mitral valve is destroyed, resulting in severe mitral regurgitation, there may be inadequate valve tissue for valve coaptation. This may result in a faint first sound (Fig. 2-34). When the mitral valve leaflets are stiffer than normal but not calcified to the point they are immobile, as they are when there is rheumatic mitral valve stenosis, the first sound is louder than normal (see Fig. 2-25).

- The force of LV contraction also determines the loudness of the first heart sound. The first sound may be louder than normal in patients with thyrotoxicosis and may be fainter than normal in patients with dilated cardiomyopathy.

The pulmonary valve closure sound is rarely heard normally at the cardiac apex. When it is easily heard, it indicates the presence of *pulmonary artery hypertension* (see Fig. 2-29).

A high-pitched *systolic ejection sound* may be heard at the apex in patients with a bicuspid aortic valve. A similar sound may be heard in patients with aortic regurgitation. In such patients the sound probably results from rapid distention of the aorta.

A high-pitched, *midsystolic click (or clicks)* may be heard in patients with mitral valve prolapse (Fig. 2-35).

The high-pitched *opening snap of the mitral valve* may be heard in early diastole in patients with mitral stenosis (see Fig. 2-25).

The interval between the aortic valve closure sound and the opening snap is related to the degree of mitral stenosis. A long interval is associated with mild mitral stenosis, whereas a short interval is associated with severe mitral stenosis.

A *pericardial knock* occurs in early ventricular diastole. It is higher pitched than a gallop sound and occurs a little later than an opening snap of the mitral valve (see Fig. 2-20). It is caused by constrictive pericarditis.

Low-pitched atrial and ventricular *gallop sounds* may be heard at the apex. These sounds do not become louder during inspiration (Figs. 2-36 and 2-37). An LA gallop sound signifies poor LV compliance, as occurs with LV hypertrophy. An LV gallop sound signifies LV dysfunction.

A *pericardial friction rub* is usually heard in the precordial area. The rub may consist of three components, two components, or only one component (Fig. 2-38).

HEART MURMURS

Heart murmurs are produced when blood flows through heart valves or orifices. More often, murmurs result from abnormal valves or abnormal orifices. The variables that control the intensity, pitch, and shape of murmurs are (1) the velocity of blood flow, (2) the size of the openings of the valves or orifices, (3) the blood pressure on each side of the valvular openings or orifices, and (4) the force of ventricular contraction. The observer should create a mental image of the murmur's "shape." The physician should diagram the shape, intensity, and pitch (frequency of vibrations) of the murmur and heart sounds. The diagram should

be part of the medical record. The rule should be, if you cannot diagram the murmurs and heart sounds, you must return to the patient and listen again. The image created should reflect the physiologic derangement that produced the murmur and abnormal heart sounds. The physician should then think in terms of the possible pathologic conditions that could produce such a physiologic abnormality.

Grading of Murmurs

The intensity (loudness) of murmurs should be graded according to the method of Freeman and Levine:[2]

Grade 1: It is necessary to listen to several heart cycles to hear murmur.

Grade 2: Murmur is louder than grade 1; it is heard immediately.

Grade 3: Murmur is moderately loud.

Grade 4: Murmur is moderately loud. It is not heard when only a part of the stethoscope's rim is applied to the skin.

Grade 5: Murmur is heard when only a part of the stethoscope's rim is applied to the skin but is not heard when none of the rim touches the skin.

Grade 6: Murmur is heard when the stethoscope is not touching the skin.

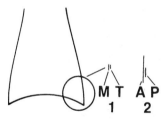

Fig. 2-32. Faint first heart sound (*1*) heard at the cardiac apex. The most common cause of a faint first heart sound is an abnormal period elapsing between atrial contraction and ventricular contraction in association with a long PR interval in the electrocardiogram.

One should visualize the mitral valve closing and the left ventricle contracting when listening to the first component of the second sound (*2*).

Reproduced with permission from Hurst JW: The examination of the heart: the importance of initial screening, *Dis Mon* 36(5):284, 1990.

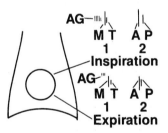

Fig. 2-30. Right atrial gallop sound. *Lower diagram:* During expiration the low-pitched atrial gallop sound *(AG)* is heard just before the mitral valve closure sound *(M)*. *Upper diagram:* During inspiration the atrial gallop sound *(AG)* increases in intensity.

Reproduced with permission from Hurst JW: The examination of the heart: the importance of initial screening, *Dis Mon* 36(5):284, 1990.

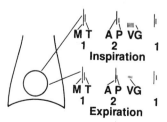

Fig. 2-31. Right ventricular gallop sound. *Lower diagram:* During expiration the low-pitched ventricular gallop sound *(VG)* occurs at about the one-third point in ventricular diastole. *Upper diagram:* During inspiration the ventricular gallop sound *(VG)* increases in intensity as compared with its loudness during expiration.

Reproduced with permission from Hurst JW: The examination of the heart: the importance of initial screening, *Dis Mon* 36(5):294, 1990.

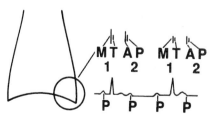

Fig. 2-33. Varying intensity of the first heart sound (*1*)—varying relationship of atrial contraction to ventricular contraction—associated with complete atrioventricular heart block. Note that the first component of the first heart sound is loud in the first heart cycle and that it is faint in the second heart cycle, since the *P* wave and atrial contraction occur nearer the QRS complex and ventricular systole in the first cycle than they do in the second heart cycle.

Reproduced with permission from Hurst JW: The examination of the heart: the importance of initial screening, *Dis Mon* 36(5):284, 1990.

Murmurs Heard in Second Right Intercostal Space Near Sternum

Systolic Murmur of Aortic Valve Sclerosis. This murmur is caused by sclerosis of the aortic valve, without significant aortic valve stenosis. The murmur is moderately high pitched, and the heart sounds are normal. This murmur occurs often in elderly patients.

Systolic Murmur of Aortic Valve Stenosis. Several different images of the murmur and heart sounds may be created, depending on the severity of the aortic valve stenosis:

- Aortic stenosis caused by a congenital bicuspid aortic valve (Fig. 2-39) (note systolic ejection sound)
- Moderately severe aortic stenosis (Fig. 2-40)
- Severe aortic stenosis (see Fig. 2-23)

Aortic valve stenosis may result from rheumatic heart disease, calcific disease of elderly patients, or a congenital bicuspid aortic valve (Fig. 2-39).

Systolic Murmur of Moderately Severe Aortic Valve Regurgitation. This murmur is caused by the increased velocity of blood flow associated with the rapid systolic ejection of a larger than normal volume of blood from the LV.

Diastolic Murmur of Aortic Valve Regurgitation. This murmur is high pitched and heard best with the stethoscope's diaphragm. It is usually heard more easily along the left sternal border when the patient is leaning forward and the breath has been exhaled (see Fig. 2-24). It may be heard at the cardiac apex. When the murmur is louder on the right than on the left side of the sternum, it is often caused by aortic root disease rather than aortic valve leaflet disease (Fig. 2-41).

- Aortic valve regurgitation may be caused by rheumatic heart disease, myxomatous degeneration of the aortic valve, endocarditis, dissection of the aorta, annuloaortic ectasia, and trauma. In such patients the second sound may be normal or diminished in intensity because the leaflets are either destroyed or do not coapt normally (see Fig. 2-24).
- Slight aortic regurgitation may be present in patients with severe aortic valve stenosis. An analogy might be that it is similar to the leak caused by a small hole in a saucer's center.
- Aortic valve regurgitation may result from severe systemic hypertension. The aortic valve closure sound may be louder than normal or have tambour quality in such patients.

Continuous Murmur of Aortic Septal Defect. The continuous murmur of an aortopulmonary communication may be heard in the second right intercostal space near the sternum, but the continuous murmur of patent ductus arteriosus is almost always louder in the second left intercostal space beneath the midportion of the left clavicle.

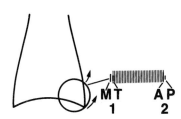

Fig. 2-34. Systolic murmur of mitral regurgitation caused by rheumatic fever. Note that the mitral valve closure sound *(M)* is decreased in intensity because the mitral valve leaflets are damaged and do not coapt properly, and that the murmur lasts throughout systole. This murmur may have several different configurations; the first heart sound *(1)* may be normal or even increased in intensity if the remaining leaflets of the mitral valve are sufficiently scarred by the rheumatic process.

Reproduced with permission from Hurst JW: The examination of the heart: the importance of initial screening, *Dis Mon* 36(5):285, 1990.

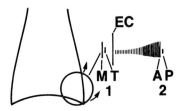

Fig. 2-35. Systolic murmur and ejection click *(EC)* of mitral valve prolapse. Many systolic ECs may occur, and the murmur may vary in configuration from the one illustrated here. The increase in intensity of the murmur illustrated here may be more apparent than real.

Reproduced with permission from Hurst JW: The examination of the heart: the importance of initial screening, *Dis Mon* 36(5):285, 1990.

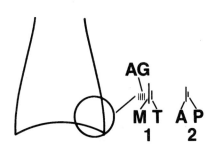

Fig. 2-36. Left atrial *(LA)* gallop sound. Heard at the cardiac apex, the LA gallop sound *(AG)* is low-pitched and immediately precedes the high-pitched first heart sound *(1)*. With a few exceptions, it is a sign of decreased left ventricular compliance.

Reproduced with permission from Hurst JW: The examination of the heart: the importance of initial screening, *Dis Mon* 36(5):284, 1990.

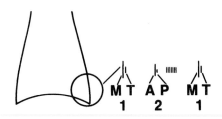

Fig. 2-37. Left ventricular *(LV)* gallop sound. Heard in ventricular diastole, the LV gallop sound is low-pitched and occurs at about the one-third point in diastole. With a few exceptions, it is a sign of LV dysfunction.

Reproduced with permission from Hurst JW: The examination of the heart: the importance of initial screening, *Dis Mon* 36(5):284, 1990.

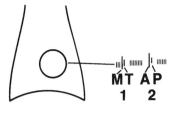

Fig. 2-38. Pericardial friction rub. Three components of the pericardial friction rub, usually heard over the precordial area, are shown here. The high-pitched, scratchy sounds are usually heard when the heart moves during atrial systole, ventricular systole, and ventricular diastole.

Reproduced with permission from Hurst JW: The examination of the heart: the importance of initial screening, *Dis Mon* 36(5):284, 1990.

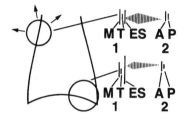

Fig. 2-39. Aortic valve stenosis caused by congenital bicuspid valve. *Upper diagram:* When one is listening in the second right intercostal space near the sternum, the first heart sound *(1)* may be louder than the second sound *(2)* because the second sound may be fainter than usual. A high-pitched ejection sound *(ES)* may be heard immediately after the first sound. The aortic valve closure sound *(A)* remains normal unless the stenosis is severe. With mild stenosis, the peak of the systolic murmur occurs early in systole. *Lower diagram:* The ejection sound *(ES)* may be louder at the apex than it is in the second right intercostal space.

Reproduced with permission from Hurst JW: The examination of the heart: the importance of initial screening, *Dis Mon* 36(5):285, 1990.

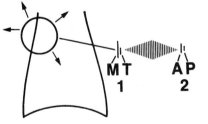

Fig. 2-40. Murmur of moderately severe aortic valve stenosis. Note that the first heart sound *(1)* is louder than the second sound *(2)*, because the normal mitral valve closure sound *(M)* is louder than the aortic valve closure sound *(A)*, which is diminished in intensity. The peak of the systolic diamond-shaped murmur occurs in midsystole.

Reproduced with permission from Hurst JW: The examination of the heart: the importance of initial screening, *Dis Mon* 36(5):285, 1990.

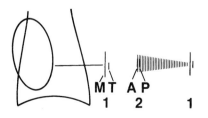

Fig. 2-41. The diastolic murmur of aortic valve regurgitation caused by aortic root disease may be heard with maximum intensity along the right sternal border.

Reproduced with permission from Hurst JW: The examination of the heart: the importance of initial screening, *Dis Mon* 36(5):285, 1990.

Murmurs Heard in Second Left Intercostal Space Near Sternum

Normal Systolic Murmur. Young subjects with a dynamic circulation may have a grade 1 systolic murmur in this area. The heart sounds are normal in such patients. The main pulmonary artery is near the anterior chest wall, whereas the aortic root is located deep inside the chest. Accordingly, a normal murmur is more likely to be heard in the second left intercostal space than in the second right intercostal space near the sternum.

Systolic Murmur Associated with Left-to-Right Shunt at Atrial Level. The systolic murmur is caused by a larger than normal quantity of blood ejected by the RV into the pulmonary artery.

The murmur usually results from an ostium secundum atrial septal defect but may be caused by an ostium primum defect, anomalous venous drainage, or a sinus venosus defect. Fixed splitting of the second sound always occurs, except with a sinus venosus defect, in which fixed splitting of the second sound occurs in about 80% of patients.

Systolic Murmur of Pulmonary Valve Stenosis. A systolic ejection sound may be present, and the pulmonary valve closure sound may be diminished in intensity. The image of moderately severe pulmonary valve stenosis is shown in Fig. 2-42.

Pulmonary valve stenosis is usually congenital in origin, but carcinoid disease may also produce thick pulmonary valve leaflets and a low-pitched systolic murmur.

Pulmonary Valve Regurgitation. This high-pitched murmur may also be heard a short distance down the left sternal border (Fig. 2-43). It is usually caused by pulmonary artery hypertension. The pulmonary valve closure sound is louder than normal and may be heard at the cardiac apex. Pulmonary artery hypertension may result from Eisenmenger physiology, primary pulmonary hypertension, repeated pulmonary emboli, and mitral stenosis with pulmonary hypertension (Graham Steell murmur).

The murmur of pulmonary valve regurgitation may be heard in patients with an ostium secundum atrial septal defect (or other left-to-right shunts at the "atrial" level); the murmur is caused by dilatation of the pulmonary valve annulus with or without an elevation of pulmonary artery pressure. Fixed splitting of the second heart sound occurs, and the pulmonary valve closure sound may be louder than normal.

Continuous Murmur of Patent Ductus Arteriosus. At birth, no murmur or only a systolic murmur is heard in the second left intercostal space near the sternum or beneath the midportion of the clavicle. Later in life the murmur of patent ductus is continuous. This implies that the murmur encompasses the second heart sound (Fig. 2-44).

Murmurs Heard Along Left Sternal Border

Diamond-Shaped Systolic Murmur of Aortic Valve Stenosis. The characteristics of the murmur and the aortic valve closure sounds are determined by the severity of the aortic stenosis (see earlier discussion of aortic valve stenosis).

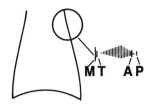

Fig. 2-42. Murmur of moderately severe pulmonary valve stenosis. The pulmonary valve closure sound (P) is delayed and is fainter than normal. The aortic valve closure sound (A) may be masked by the end of the diamond-shaped systolic murmur because tight ventricular ejection is prolonged. Therefore the second sound may be fainter than the normal first sound. The peak of the diamond-shaped murmur appears in midsystole or a little later. An early systolic sound (not shown here) may be present.

Reproduced with permission from Hurst JW: The examination of the heart: the importance of initial screening, *Dis Mon* 36(5):285, 1990.

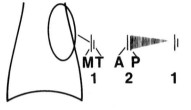

Fig. 2-43. Pulmonary valve regurgitation caused by pulmonary hypertension. Note the increase in intensity of the pulmonary valve closure sound (P).

Reproduced with permission from Hurst JW: The examination of the heart: the importance of initial screening, *Dis Mon* 36(5):285, 1990.

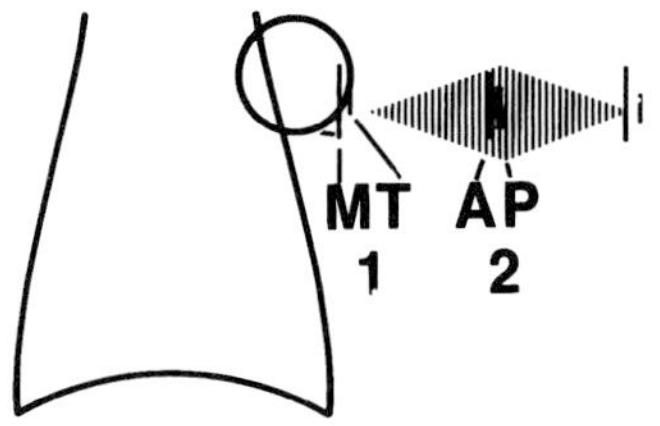

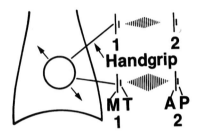

Fig. 2-44. Continuous murmur of patent ductus arteriosus. Note that the murmur builds up in intensity at the end of ventricular systole, envelops the second heart sound, and then continues into ventricular diastole. It is almost always louder in the second left intercostal space near the sternum or beneath the midportion of the clavicle.

Reproduced with permission from Hurst JW: The examination of the heart: the importance of initial screening, *Dis Mon* 36(5):286, 1990.

Fig. 2-45. Systolic murmur associated with idiopathic hypertrophic subaortic stenosis. The intensity of the murmur decreases with handgrip isometric exercise. It becomes louder when the patient stands from a squatting position.

Reproduced with permission from Hurst JW: The examination of the heart: the importance of initial screening, *Dis Mon* 36(5):285, 1990.

Systolic Murmur of Idiopathic Hypertrophic Subaortic Stenosis. The observer initially has difficulty determining if the murmur is caused by aortic valve stenosis or mitral valve regurgitation. The murmur begins after an easily identified clear period following the first heart sound. The aortic closure sound is usually heard. The murmur is uncommonly transmitted to the neck. The murmur becomes louder when the patient stands from a squatting position and during a Valsalva maneuver and becomes fainter with isometic exercise (handgrip) (Fig. 2-45). The systolic murmur of mitral regurgitation may be heard at the apex.

Systolic Murmur of Interventricular Septal Defect. This murmur, which may be heard in the midsternum, is pansystolic (Fig. 2-46). It may result from a congenital defect, a ruptured septum caused by a myocardial infarct, or trauma.

Diastolic Murmur of Aortic Regurgitation. This murmur is typically heard to the left of the sternum. It is enhanced by having the patient lean forward (Fig. 2-24). (See earlier discussion for a list of causes.)

Continuous Murmur. This murmur may be caused by a coronary arteriovenous fistula or a ruptured sinus of Valsalva (Fig. 2-47). The murmurs associated with these abnormalities are usually heard best to the right of the midsternum.

Murmurs Heard at Cardiac Apex

Systolic Murmur of Mitral Valve Regurgitation. This murmur may be faint or loud and radiates laterally around the chest and to the left lung base. It may be caused by several different diseases:

- Mitral valve prolapse is a common cause of mitral valve regurgitation. The systolic murmur is initiated by a midsystolic click or clicks (see Fig. 2-35). It is caused by myxomatous degeneration of the mitral valve. Its significance ranges from benign to malignant.
- Mitral valve regurgitation may occur in patients with an ostium primum atrial septal defect with a cleft mitral valve.
- Mitral valve regurgitation may result from rheumatic heart disease. The murmur may be faint or loud. The mitral component of the first heart sound may be faint because the leaflets of the mitral valve may be destroyed to the point they cannot coapt (see Fig. 2-34).
- Mitral valve regurgitation may be caused by papillary muscle dysfunction from myocardial infarct. As a rule, the base of the papillary muscle is infarcted, along with a portion of the LV wall.
- Mitral valve regurgitation may be caused by papillary muscle rupture that usually results from myocardial infarction. This catastrophe can occur from inferior infarction caused by isolated right coronary artery obstruction. The systolic murmur may not be loud because the mitral valve orifice may be wide open and the patient may be in cardiogenic shock.

- Mitral valve regurgitation may be caused by endocarditis of the mitral valve leaflets. Generally, endocarditis occurs on a valve that is abnormal because of mitral valve prolapse or rheumatic heart disease.
- Rupture of the chordae tendineae of the mitral valve produces unique murmurs. The most common such murmur has the following characteristics. A loud systolic murmur is heard at the cardiac apex, and it radiates laterally around the chest. Its unique feature, however, is that it is heard over the thoracic and cervical spine, top of the head, and sacrum.

  The less common type of murmur produced by rupture of the chordae tendineae is a systolic murmur, heard with maximum intensity at the apex. It radiates to the second intercostal space on the right near the sternum and simulates aortic valve stenosis.
- Patients with idiopathic hypertrophic cardiomyopathy may have mitral regurgitation. The systolic murmur of mitral regurgitation may be heard at the cardiac apex.

A left atrial gallop sound and an LV gallop sound may be produced by mitral regurgitation of any cause. Under these circumstances, a ventricular gallop sound may not signify LV dysfunction.

Diastolic Murmurs. Diastolic murmurs heard at the cardiac apex may result from several different causes and mechanisms:

- The high-pitched murmur of aortic valve regurgitation may be heard at the cardiac apex (see earlier discussion). The high-pitched murmur of pulmonary valve regurgitation is rarely, if ever, heard at the cardiac apex.
- The low-pitched rumbling diastolic murmur of mitral stenosis is heard in a small area at the cardiac apex. The opening snap of mitral stenosis and the loud first heart sound, however, are heard over the front of the chest (see Fig. 2-25).
- An Austin Flint diastolic rumble may be heard at the cardiac apex in patients with aortic regurgitation. The anterior leaflet of the mitral valve is depressed by the aortic regurgitation, which produces an impediment to the blood flow entering the LV from the LA. The first heart sound is usually normal, and an opening snap of mitral stenosis is not heard.
- A diastolic rumble may be heard at the cardiac apex secondary to mitral regurgitation. This occurs because a large volume of blood enters the LV through a normal-sized mitral valve orifice. This is probably the most common cause of a low-pitched diastolic rumble heard at the apex.

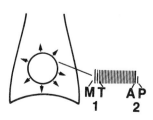

Fig. 2-46. Systolic murmur of interventricular septal defect. The murmur usually lasts throughout systole; it may taper a little at its end as the right ventricle becomes filled with blood.

Reproduced with permission from Hurst JW: The examination of the heart: the importance of initial screening, *Dis Mon* 36(5):285, 1990.

Murmurs Heard at End of Sternum

Systolic Murmur of Tricuspid Regurgitation. This murmur is increased in intensity by inspiration (Fig. 2-48). The tricuspid valve leaflets may be abnormal, as with Ebstein anomaly, or diseased, as with infective endocarditis or carcinoid heart disease. More often, however, the poorly structured tricuspid valve annulus dilates as a result of disease on the heart's left side, pulmonary arteriolar disease, pulmonary disease, pulmonary valve disease, or RV disease.

Tricuspid regurgitation may produce no murmur; it is more readily recognized by identifying a prominent *v* wave in the internal jugular venous pulse (see earlier discussion).

Diastolic Rumbles in Tricuspid Area. A tricuspid valve diastolic rumble has several causes:

- The low-pitched diastolic rumble of tricuspid stenosis is heard at the sternum's lower end. It may be associated with an opening snap of the tricuspid valve. The murmur's intensity is augmented on inspiration. Rheumatic heart disease may rarely cause tricuspid stenosis, and when it does, it is almost always associated with aortic and mitral valve disease. Carcinoid heart disease may be the cause of tricuspid stenosis, and Ebstein anomaly may rarely be responsible for tricuspid stenosis rather than regurgitation.

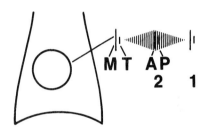

Fig. 2-47. Continuous murmur produced by the rupture of a sinus of Valsalva. Note that the murmur builds up in intensity and envelops the second heart sound (2).

Reproduced with permission from Hurst JW: The examination of the heart: the importance of initial screening, *Dis Mon* 36(5):286, 1990.

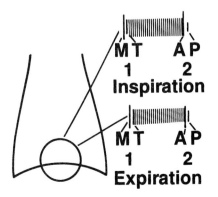

Fig. 2-48. Systolic murmur of tricuspid valve regurgitation. The murmur may increase in intensity during inspiration (*upper diagram*).

Reproduced with permission from Hurst JW: The examination of the heart: the importance of initial screening, *Dis Mon* 36(5):285, 1990.

- Patients with a moderately large *left-to-right shunt* at the atrial level, such as occurs with an ostium secundum atrial septal defect, an ostium primum defect, or anomalous venous drainage, may exhibit a diastolic rumble heard at the end of the sternum. The rumble results from the larger than normal amount of blood that traverses the tricuspid valve during diastole. An opening snap of the tricuspid valve may also be heard in these conditions.
- Patients with moderately severe tricuspid *valve regurgitation* may exhibit an associated tricuspid valve diastolic rumble. This latter murmur is the result of the large volume of blood flow that traverses the valve during diastole.

Murmurs and Bruits Heard in Noncardiac Areas

- A normal continuous murmur may be heard in the neck of children. It is a venous hum. It is heard when the child sits up but not when he or she lies down. It is easily obliterated by light pressure above the listening site on the neck.
- An arterial bruit may be heard over the carotid arteries. Such a bruit may indicate atheromatous lesions in the artery. A less common cause is fibromuscular hyperplasia.
- Systolic bruits may be heard over the kidney areas (anteriorly or posteriorly) when obstruction of the renal arteries occurs with atherosclerosis or fibromuscular hyperplasia.
- The systolic murmur of coarctation of the aorta may be heard in the back's interscapular area. Arterial bruits may be heard over the ribs of such patient's backs. They are caused by the large, tortuous, intercostal arteries.
- Patients with coarctation of the pulmonary artery branches may have arterial bruits heard over the rib cage posteriorly. Rarely, patients with a large pulmonary blood flow, such as occurs with an ostium secundum atrial septal defect, may exhibit abnormal bruits over the posterior region of the thorax when there are no localized constrictions of the pulmonary artery branches.
- The continuous murmur of a peripheral arteriovenous fistula may be heard over a scar resulting from trauma, surgery, or insertion of an arterial catheter. *Remember: do not look so very far until you listen over every scar.*
- The systolic murmur of a ruptured chordae tendineae of the mitral valve is often heard over the thoracic and cervical spine, top of the head, and sacrum.

A Precordial "Crunch"

Mediastinal Emphysema. A mediastinal "crunch" is produced when the heart moves against pockets of trapped air. The noise is easily identified, even though the observer may be hearing it for the first time. When alveoli rupture, the air dissects along the pulmonary arterioles and arteries to enter the mediastinum. This condition may occur in patients with pneumonia or pneumothorax.

REFERENCES

1. Hurst JW: Physical examination. In *Cardiovascular diagnosis: the initial examination*, St Louis, 1993, Mosby.

2. Freeman AR, Levine SA: Clinical significance of systolic murmurs: study of 1000 consecutive "non-cardiac" cases, *Ann Intern Med* 6:1371, 1933.

3 Examination of Chest X-Ray Film[1]

When the patient is asymptomatic and has a normal physical examination and electrocardiogram (ECG), ordering only a posteroanterior (PA) chest roentgenogram is sufficient. However, if heart disease is suspected, it is useful to obtain a left lateral x-ray view of the chest[1] as well as a PA view.

SIZE OF CARDIAC SILHOUETTE

The size of the cardiac silhouette is determined by inspecting the PA x-ray film of the chest (a portable x-ray film cannot be used). The intrathoracic diameter is determined by measuring the width of the inside of the rib cage at the level of the diaphragm's right leaf. This line may be referred to as T (Fig. 3-1). A vertical line (V) is then drawn down the middle of the chest film. The line's location is determined by locating the spine of the vertebrae. A horizontal line is then drawn from the vertical line (located in the chest's center) to the heart's right border. The most rightward portion of the heart's right side is used to make the measurement. This line may be referred to as R. A horizontal line is then drawn from the vertical line (located in the heart's center) to the heart's left border. The heart's most leftward portion is used to make the measurement. This line may be referred to as L (see Fig. 3-1). The formula $R + L = 1/2\ T$ is used to indicate the measurement of the normal cardiac silhouette. In other words, the width of the normal cardiac silhouette in the frontal view should be equal to less than one-half the width of the intrathoracic diameter. There are exceptions to this general rule. For example, patients with aortic valve stenosis or idiopathic hypertrophy may have a thick ventricle that is not dilated, and the heart size may be normal. The same is true for right ventricular (RV) hypertrophy because the frontal x-ray view may not reveal the size of the RV because it is located anteriorly. Also, the heart size, may have been on the small side of the normal range at one point in time and could have increased in size, but still be less than one-half the intrathoracic diameter. In such a case the increase in heart size would be abnormal.

PERICARDIAL EFFUSION

A small amount of pericardial fluid may not alter the size and shape of the cardiac silhouette. Pericardial fluid may "iron out" the upper portion of the heart's left border and increase the size of the cardiac silhouette (Fig. 3-2, A). The epicardial fat stripe may be seen in the left lateral view (Fig. 3-2, B). The lung fields may remain clear.

INDIVIDUAL CHAMBER ENLARGEMENT

The size of each cardiac chamber must be determined because the overall measurement of heart size may be normal but one or more of the individual chambers may be larger than normal.

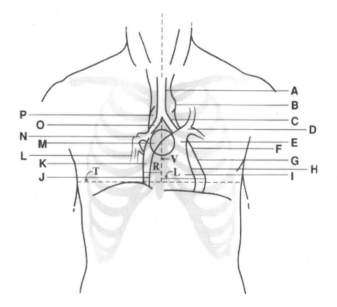

Fig. 3-1. Diagram of the heart as seen in posteroanterior x-ray film of the chest. Readers should pay close attention to the heart's border-forming structures because they are often used to identify abnormalities. **A**, trachea; **B**, aortic "knob"; **C**, left bronchus; **D**, left branch of the pulmonary artery; **E**, main pulmonary artery; **F**, region of left atrial appendage; **G**, left ventricle; **H**, interventricular groove; **I**, right ventricle; **J**, junction of the right atrium and right ventricle; **K**, right atrium; **L**, branches of right branch of pulmonary artery; **M**, left atrium; **N**, right branch of the pulmonary artery; **O**, right bronchus; **P**, ascending portion of the aorta; **T**, intrathoracic diameter; **V**, vertical line in center of chest; **R**, distance from **V** to farthest border of heart's right side; **L**, distance from **V** to farthest border of heart's left side.

Modified with permission from the Criteria Committee of the New York Heart Association: *Nomenclature and criteria for diagnosis of diseases of the heart and great vessels,* ed 8, Boston, 1979, Little, Brown, p 294.

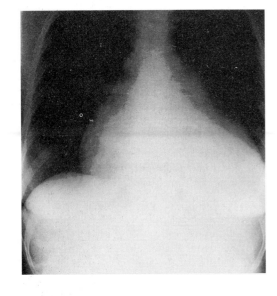

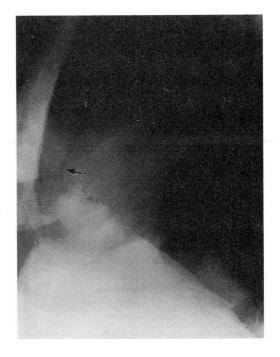

A

B

Fig. 3-2. A, Pericardial effusion. The cardiac silhouette is enlarged without specific chamber enlargement. Note that the contour produced by the main pulmonary artery is "ironed out." The pulmonary vascularity is normal or diminished in size. **B,** Pericardial effusion. An arrow points to a radiolucent line (epicardial fat stripe) that is displaced inward by fluid in the pericardial sac.

Courtesy Wade Shuford, MD, Professor of Radiology, Emory University School of Medicine; and Radiology Service at Grady Memorial Hospital, Atlanta.

Reproduced with permission from Hurst JW: *Cardiovascular diagnosis: the initial examination*, St Louis, 1993, Mosby, pp 429, 430.

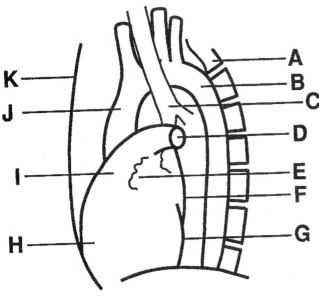

Fig. 3-3. Diagram of the normal heart as seen in left lateral x-ray film of the chest. **A,** Vertebral column; **B,** aorta; **C,** trachea; **D,** left branch of pulmonary artery; **E,** left atrial appendage; **F,** left atrium; **G,** left ventricle; **H,** right ventricle; **I,** main pulmonary artery; **J,** ascending aorta; **K,** sternum.

Modified with permission from the Criteria Committee of the New York Heart Association: *Nomenclature and criteria for diagnosis of diseases of the heart and great vessels,* ed 8, Boston, 1979, Little, Brown, p 295.

Left Atrial Size

The normal left atrium (LA) is located posteriorly in the chest's center. It is not located on the left as its name implies. The upper portion of the LA abuts the right and left bronchi. The normal LA is shown in Figs. 3-1 and 3-3. A large LA is shown in Figs. 3-4 and 3-5. At times, especially with rheumatic mitral stenosis or regurgitation, the LA appendage may become prominent. This produces the "four-bump" heart (Fig. 3-4).

Left Ventricular Size

When the left ventricle (LV) becomes abnormally dilated as well as hypertrophied, it extends abnormally to the left and seems to descend below the left leaf of the diaphragm (Fig. 3-6). In the left lateral chest film, it may or may not be more posteriorly located than normal. In fact, the long axis of the LV is directed anteriorly and toward the observer in this view. Accordingly, the LV must be moderately enlarged to project an abnormal degree posteriorly.

A bulge caused by an LV aneurysm may be noted in the lateral portion of the LV.

Right Atrial Size

It is difficult to determine the size of the right atrium (RA). It composes the heart's right border and, when it becomes larger than normal, simply extends farther to the right than normal, and its outer border assumes the shape of a semicircle (Fig. 3-7).

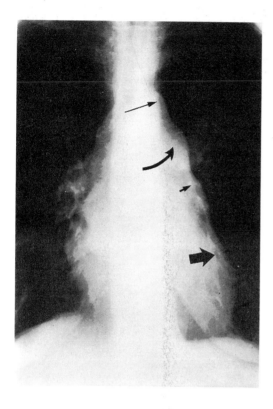

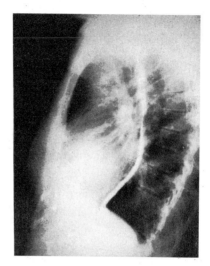

Fig. 3-5. Mitral valve stenosis. Posterior deviation of the barium-filled esophagus caused by a large left atrium.

Reproduced with permission from Cobbs BW Jr: Clinical recognition and medical management of rheumatic fever and valvular heart disease. In Hurst JW, Logue RB, editors: *The heart,* ed 1, New York, 1966, McGraw-Hill, p 540.

Fig. 3-4. Left atrial enlargement in a patient with mitral stenosis. A large double contour can be seen in the heart's central portion. This is a so-called four-bump heart. The four "bumps" are produced on the heart's left border by the aortic knob *(long narrow arrow),* main pulmonary artery *(curved arrow),* left atrial appendage *(short arrow),* and left ventricle *(broad arrow).* The right pulmonary artery is larger than normal and tapers promptly, suggesting pulmonary hypertension. The right atrium is large.

Courtesy Wade Shuford, MD, Professor of Radiology, Emory University School of Medicine; and Radiology Service at Grady Memorial Hospital, Atlanta.

Reproduced with permission from Hurst JW: *Cardiovascular diagnosis: the initial examination,* St Louis, 1993, Mosby, p 438.

Right Ventricular Size

The left lateral chest film is required to identify a larger than normal RV. This is true because the RV is not located on the right as the name implies, but is located more anteriorly. The normal-sized RV is shown in Fig. 3-3, and a large RV is shown in Fig. 3-8.

SIZE AND SHAPE OF PULMONARY ARTERIES

The size and shape of the normal main pulmonary artery and its left and right branches are shown in Figs. 3-1 and 3-9. Normally, the diameter of the right branch of the pulmonary artery is about the same diameter as the trachea. Note that the subdivisions of the left branch of the pulmonary artery are not seen in the PA film because the left branch passes posteriorly, whereas the right branch extends laterally and its branches are easily seen.

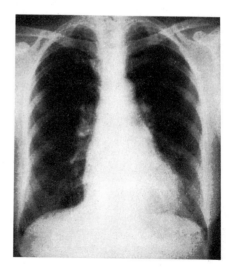

Fig. 3-6. Aortic valvular regurgitation. The left ventricle is dilated. There is downward and lateral displacement of the cardiac apex. The proximal portion of the aorta is dilated, and the pulmonary artery vasculature is normal.

Courtesy Wade Shuford, MD, Professor of Radiology, Emory University School of Medicine; and Radiology Service at Grady Memorial Hospital, Atlanta.

Reproduced with permission from Hurst JW: *Cardiovascular diagnosis: the initial examination,* St Louis, 1993, Mosby, p 440.

ASSESSING PULMONARY ARTERY BLOOD FLOW AND PRESSURE

Increased Pulmonary Blood Flow

When pulmonary blood flow is increased, the main pulmonary artery and its right branch become larger than normal when viewed in the PA x-ray film of the chest (Fig. 3-10). The left branch of the pulmonary artery is also dilated and may be seen in the left lateral view. When pulmonary blood flow increases and pulmonary blood pressure is elevated only slightly, the smaller branches of the right pulmonary artery can be seen to extend inferiorly for a moderate distance in the PA chest film.

An increase in pulmonary artery blood flow occurs in patients with a left-to-right shunt caused by an ostium secundum atrial septal defect, an ostium primum defect, anomalous pulmonary venous drainage, a sinus venosus defect, an interventricular septal defect, a patent ductus arteriosus, or an aortic septal defect.

Decreased Pulmonary Blood Flow

The main pulmonary artery may be smaller than normal or not identifiable, and the right and right pulmonary artery branches appear smaller than normal when pulmonary blood flow decreases. The smaller branches of the right branch of the pulmonary artery do not extend deeply into the lung fields (Fig. 3-11).

A decrease in pulmonary blood flow occurs in patients with tetralogy of Fallot, pulmonary atresia, tricuspid atresia, and type 4 truncus arteriosus.

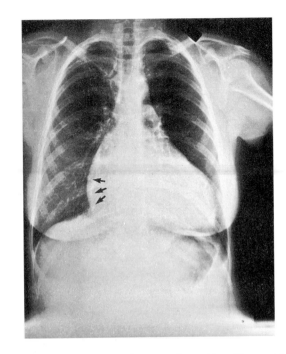

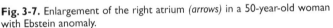

Fig. 3-7. Enlargement of the right atrium *(arrows)* in a 50-year-old woman with Ebstein anomaly.

Courtesy Paul Robinson, MD, Professor of Medicine (Cardiology); William Casarella, MD, Professor and Chairman, Department of Radiology, Emory University School of Medicine; and Radiology Service of Emory University Hospital, Atlanta.

Reproduced with permission from Hurst JW: *Cardiovascular diagnosis: the initial examination,* St Louis, 1993, Mosby, p 441.

A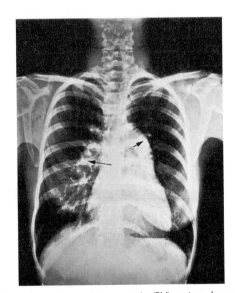

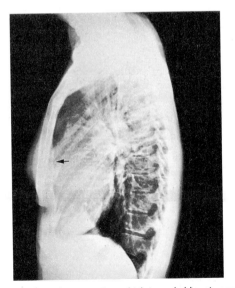 **B**

Fig. 3-8. Enlargement of the right ventricle (RV), main pulmonary artery, and right pulmonary artery. **A,** The PA view of the chest shows a large main pulmonary artery *(short arrow).* The left branch of the pulmonary artery is not seen. The right branch of the pulmonary artery is large and tapers abruptly, suggesting severe pulmonary artery hypertension *(long arrow).* **B,** The left lateral view reveals RV enlargement. Note how the RV crowds out the retrosternal space *(arrow).* Compare the size of the RV with the size of the normal RV illustrated in Fig. 3-3. The patient had surgical repair of an ostium secundum atrial septal defect as a child; she is shown here at age 39

with severe pulmonary hypertension, which is probably primary pulmonary hypertension, because the pulmonary artery pressure was only slightly elevated at the time of the surgical repair of the atrial septal defect. She has since had a successful lung transplant.

Courtesy William Casarella, MD, Professor and Chairman, Department of Radiology, Emory University School of Medicine; and Radiology Service of Emory University Hospital, Atlanta.

Reproduced with permission from Hurst JW: *Cardiovascular diagnosis: the initial examination,* St Louis, 1993, Mosby, p 442.

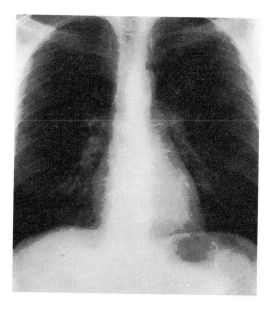

Fig. 3-9. Normal pulmonary blood flow. Note the size and shape of the pulmonary arteries.

Courtesy Wade Shuford, MD, Professor of Radiology, Emory University School of Medicine; and Radiology Service at Grady Memorial Hospital, Atlanta.

Reproduced with permission from Hurst JW: *Cardiovascular diagnosis: the initial examination,* St Louis, 1993, Mosby, p 446.

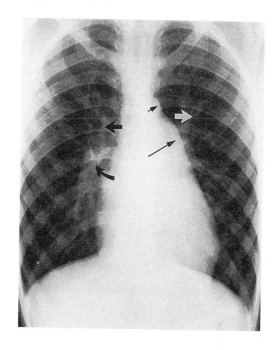

Fig. 3-10. Increased pulmonary blood flow in a patient with an ostium secundum atrial septal defect. Note the large main pulmonary artery *(long arrow),* large right pulmonary artery *(curved arrow),* large pulmonary veins *(broad arrows),* and small aortic knob *(short arrow).* The heart is slightly enlarged as a result of right ventricular and right atrial enlargement.

Courtesy Wade Shuford, MD, Professor of Radiology, Emory University School of Medicine; and Radiology Service at Grady Memorial Hospital, Atlanta.

Reproduced with permission from Hurst JW: *Cardiovascular diagnosis: the initial examination,* St Louis, 1993, Mosby, p 448.

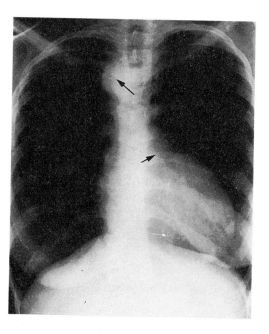

Fig. 3-11. Decreased pulmonary blood flow in a patient with tetralogy of Fallot. Note the right aortic arch *(long arrow).* The main pulmonary artery is not visible *(short arrow).* The shadows of the pulmonary arteries and veins are barely visible. The cardiac apex is elevated. These findings are characteristic of marked right ventricular hypertrophy rather than left ventricular hypertrophy.

Courtesy Wade Shuford, MD, Professor of Radiology, Emory University School of Medicine; and Radiology Service at Grady Memorial Hospital, Atlanta.

Reproduced with permission from Hurst JW: *Cardiovascular diagnosis: the initial examination,* St Louis, 1993, Mosby, p 447.

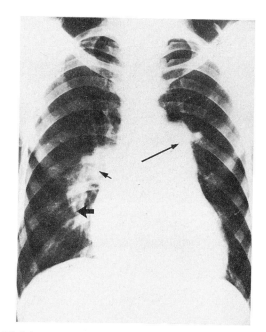

Fig. 3-12. Pulmonary artery hypertension. The main pulmonary artery is large *(long arrow).* The left pulmonary artery is not seen because it courses posteriorly. The right pulmonary artery is large *(short arrow);* it tapers *(broad arrow)* abruptly, signifying pulmonary artery hypertension. The patient had primary pulmonary hypertension.

Reproduced with permission from Weens HS, Gay BB Jr: *Radiologic examination of the heart.* In Hurst JW, Logue RB, editors: *The heart,* ed 1, New York, 1966, McGraw-Hill, p 162.

Pulmonary Valve Stenosis (An Exception to the Rule)

The pulmonary blood flow is normal in patients with pulmonary valve stenosis, but the main pulmonary artery is larger than normal. This is caused by the physical laws that dictate that the artery will become larger just beyond the valvular obstruction. The left branch, when it is seen in the PA view, is also larger than normal because it is an extension of the main pulmonary artery. The right branch is normal in size and shape because it branches off from the main pulmonary artery at right angles.

Increased Pulmonary Artery Pressure

The main pulmonary artery and its right and left branches are usually dilated when pulmonary artery pressure increases. When pulmonary pressure increases, the larger than normal right branch of the pulmonary artery tapers rather quickly compared with normal or when there is only an increase in pulmonary artery blood flow (Fig. 3-12). The branches of the left pulmonary artery also taper quickly but they are difficult to observe in the PA view of the chest.

The pulmonary artery blood pressure becomes elevated in patients with primary pulmonary artery hypertension, repeated pulmonary emboli, some patients with cor pulmonale, and patients with Eisenmenger's syndrome caused by atrial septal defect, interventricular septal defect, or patent ductus arteriosus.

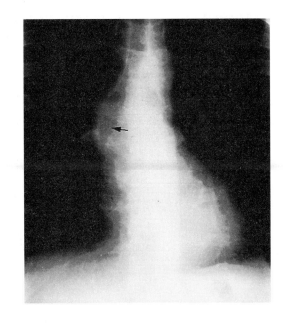

Fig. 3-13. Dilatation of the proximal portion of the aorta *(arrow)* caused by severe aortic valve stenosis (congenital bicuspid aortic valve). The enlargement of the proximal aorta in this example is almost aneurysmal in contour; the enlargement is usually more subtle. The left ventricle is large.

Courtesy Wade Shuford, MD, Professor of Radiology, Emory University School of Medicine; and Radiology Service at Grady Memorial Hospital, Atlanta.

Reproduced with permission from Hurst JW: *Cardiovascular diagnosis: the initial examination*, St Louis, 1993, Mosby, p 443.

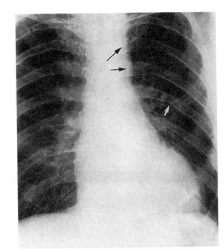

A

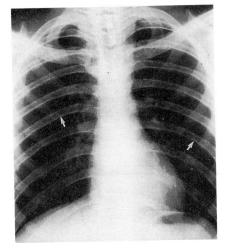

B

Fig. 3-14. A, Coarctation of the aorta. Note the notching of the inferior rib margins *(white arrow)* and the figure 3 sign *(black arrows)*. The upper segment is composed of dilated left subclavian artery *(long black arrow)*. The lower segment is produced by poststenotic dilation of the descending aorta *(short black arrow)*. **B,** Coarctation of the aorta. Note the slight notching of the inferior margins of the ribs *(arrows)*. Moderate cardiac enlargement results from left ventricular enlargement.

Courtesy Wade Shuford, MD, Professor of Radiology, Emory University School of Medicine; and Radiology Service at Grady Memorial Hospital, Atlanta.

Reproduced with permission from Hurst JW: *Cardiovascular diagnosis: the initial examination*, St Louis, 1993, Mosby, p 444.

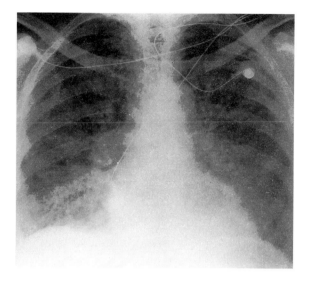

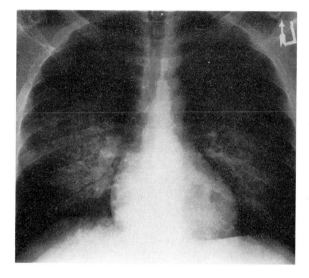

Fig. 3-15. Interstitial edema of the lungs caused by left ventricular dysfunction. Note the haziness and clouding of the lungs. The borders of the pulmonary arteries are indistinct (periarterial cuffing), and the pulmonary veins are prominent. The heart is enlarged.

Courtesy Wade Shuford, MD, Professor of Radiology, Emory University School of Medicine; and Radiology Service at Grady Memorial Hospital, Atlanta.

Reproduced with permission from Hurst JW: *Cardiovascular diagnosis: the initial examination*, St Louis, 1993, Mosby, p 459.

Fig. 3-16. Acute alveolar pulmonary edema as seen in the PA view of the chest. Diffuse alveolar bilateral infiltrates are noted in the central and posterior aspects of the lungs, forming a pattern of distribution that simulates butterfly wings. This type of pulmonary edema is caused by abrupt dysfunction of the left ventricle. It can also be caused by noncardiac conditions.

Courtesy Wade Shuford, MD, Professor of Radiology, Emory University School of Medicine; and Radiology Service at Grady Memorial Hospital, Atlanta.

Reproduced with permission from Hurst JW: *Cardiovascular diagnosis: the initial examination*, St Louis, 1993, Mosby, p 456.

A

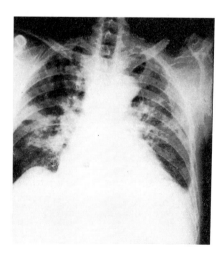

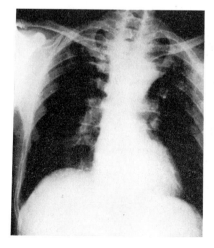

B

Fig. 3-17. Alveolar pulmonary edema caused by acute heart failure in a 64-year-old man with atherosclerotic heart disease and aortic regurgitation. **A,** Alveolar pulmonary edema of the lobular type that may be mistaken for pulmonary infection, pulmonary infarction, or pulmonary neoplasm. **B,** Clearing after 4 days of treatment for heart failure.

Reproduced with permission from Logue RB, Hurst JW: *Etiology and clinical recognition of heart failure*. In Hurst JW, Logue RB, editors: *The heart*, ed 1, New York, 1966, McGraw-Hill, p 263.

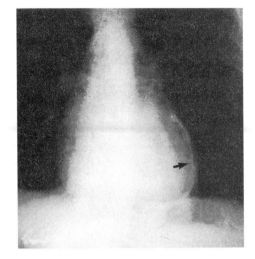

A

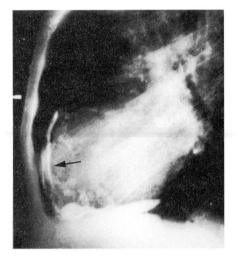

B

Fig. 3-18. Calcification of the pericardium is usually seen more easily in the left lateral view; in this patient it is seen in the PA **(A)** and left lateral **(B)** views *(arrows)*.

Reproduced with permission from Weens HS, Gay BB Jr: *Radiologic examination of the heart.* In Hurst JW, Logue RB, editors: *The heart,* ed 1, New York, 1966, McGraw-Hill, p 157.

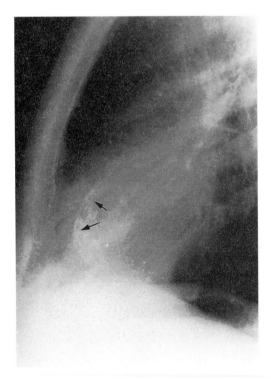

Fig. 3-19. Calcification at the site of an anteroseptal myocardial infarction *(arrows)*.

Courtesy Wade Shuford, MD, Professor of Radiology, Emory University School of Medicine; and Radiology Service at Grady Memorial Hospital, Atlanta.

Reproduced with permission from Hurst JW: *Cardiovascular diagnosis: the initial examination,* St Louis, 1993, Mosby, p 453.

SIZE AND SHAPE OF THORACIC AORTA

Aortic Root and Ascending Aorta

The root of the aorta is located within the cardiac shadow on the chest x-ray film. Accordingly, the aortic root can become large and may not be detected on the chest roentgenogram. The ascending portion of the aorta may become enlarged and can be easily detected (Fig. 3-13).

The aortic root and the ascending aorta may become larger than normal as a result of aortic valve stenosis, aortic valve regurgitation from rheumatic heart disease or myxomatous valve disease, annuloaortic ectasia, hypertension, syphilitic aortic disease, atherosclerotic aneurysm, or dissection of the aorta.

The aortic arch may be located on the right side in significant number of patients with tetralogy of Fallot (Fig. 3-11). A common trunk, associated with truncus arteriosus, may also be located on the right side.

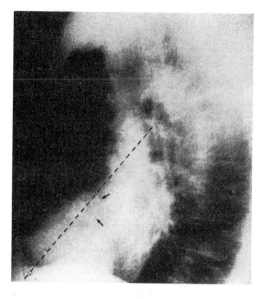

Fig. 3-20. Calcific aortic valve stenosis *(arrows)*. Note in the lateral view of the chest that the calcification straddles a line drawn from the carina to the anterior costophrenic angle.

Reproduced with permission from Rubens MB: *Chest x-ray in adult heart disease.* In Julian DG et al, editors: *Diseases of the heart,* London, 1989, Baillière Tindall, p 284.

Aortic Configuration Caused by Coarctation of Aorta

The "3 sign" of coarctation is caused by a dilated aorta, the coarcted segment of the aorta, and postcoarctation dilatation of the aorta (Fig. 3-14). Rib notching may be seen in patients older than 12 years.

CONGESTIVE HEART FAILURE

Congestive heart failure (CHF) can be recognized in the PA x-ray film of the chest by the presence of one or more of the following signs. The superior pulmonary veins may become more prominent than normal. The margins of the pulmonary arterial branches may become indistinct. This is known as periarterial cuffing. There may be obvious clouding of the midlung fields and interstitial or alveolar pulmonary edema (Figs. 3-15 to 3-17). Alveolar pulmonary edema may create a lobular pattern and may be mistaken for pulmonary infection, infarction, or neoplasm. Pleural fluid may be seen only on the right side, and when it is bilateral, it is more prominent on the right.

CALCIFICATION

Calcification may be noted in the following locations:
- *Pericardial calcification* is seen in patients with healed pericarditis. Cardiac constriction may or may not be present. The calcification is seen in the left lateral film of the heart (Fig. 3-18).

A

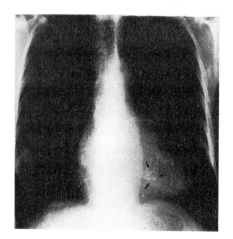

B

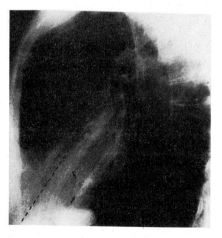

Fig. 3-21. Mitral valve calcification. **A,** On the frontal view the calcified valve *(arrows)* is lateral to the spine. **B,** On the lateral view the calcification *(arrows)* is posterior to a line drawn from the carina to the anterior costophrenic angle.

Reproduced with permission from Rubens MB: *Chest x-ray in adult heart disease.* In Julian DG et al, editors: *Diseases of the heart,* London, 1989, Baillière Tindall, p 285.

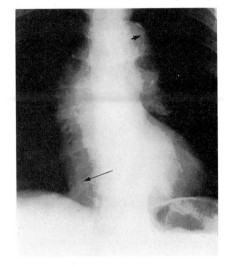

A

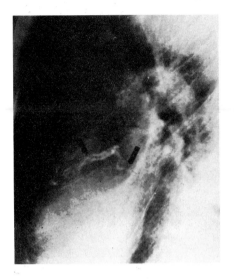

B

Fig. 3-22. A, PA view of the chest showing a calcified right coronary artery *(long arrow).* The aorta is dilated and tortuous. Note calcification of the interior of the aorta in the region of the aortic knob *(short arrow).* **B,** Calcification of the left anterior descending and circumflex coronary arteries *(arrows).*

A courtesy Wade Shuford, MD, Professor of Radiology, Emory University School of Medicine; and Radiology Service at Grady Memorial Hospital, Atlanta. **B** reproduced with permission from Weens HS, Gay BB Jr: *Radiologic examination of the heart.* In Hurst JW, Logue RB, editors: *The heart,* ed 1, New York, 1966, McGraw-Hill, p 156.

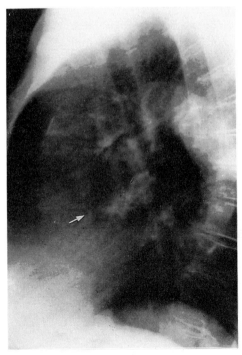

Fig. 3-23. Syphilitic aortitis. Note the calcification of the intima of the first portion of the aorta *(arrows)* in the left lateral chest film.

Courtesy Wade Shuford, MD, Professor Radiology, Emory University School of Medicine; and Radiology Service at Grady Memorial Hospital, Atlanta.

Reproduced with permission from Hurst JW: *Cardiovascular diagnosis: the initial examination,* St Louis, 1993, Mosby, p 445.

A

Fig. 3-24. A, Calcification of a left atrial myxoma *(arrows)* as seen in the PA view. **B,** Calcification of a left atrial myxoma as seen in the lateral view of the heart. (See top of next page for **B.**)

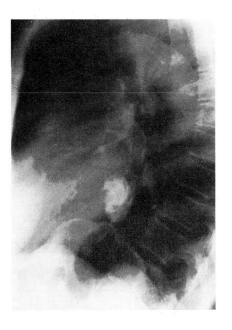

B

Fig. 3-24, Con't. Courtesy Wade Shuford, MD, Professor of Radiology, Emory University School of Medicine; and Radiology Service at Grady Memorial Hospital, Atlanta.

Reproduced with permission from Hurst JW: *Cardiovascular diagnosis: the initial examination*, St Louis, 1993, Mosby, p 452.

CALCIFICATION (con't.)

- *Calcification of a previous myocardial infarction* is occasionally seen in the PA or left lateral film of the chest (Fig. 3-19).
- *Calcification of the aortic and mitral valves* may be seen in the left lateral film of the chest (Figs. 3-20 and 3-21). Calcification of the aortic valve occurs in patients with a congenital bicuspid aortic valve, aortic stenosis from rheumatic heart disease, or calcific aortic valve disease in elderly persons. Mitral valve calcification is almost always caused by rheumatic heart disease.
- *Calcification of the coronary arteries* (Fig. 3-22) indicates severe coronary atherosclerosis.
- *Calcification of the early part of the aorta* (Fig. 3-23) may be caused by syphilis, Takayasu's disease, or giant cell arteritis.
- *Calcification of a left atrial myxoma* is shown in Fig. 3-24.
- *Calcification of the mitral valve annulus* is shown in Fig. 3-25.

REFERENCE

1. Hurst JW: Interpretation of the chest roentgenogram. In *Cardiovascular diagnosis: the initial examination*, St Louis, 1993, Mosby.

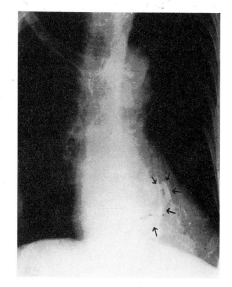

A

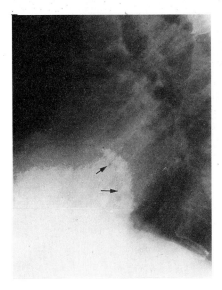

B

Fig. 3-25. Calcified mitral valve annulus. **A,** A large curved calcified structure *(arrows)* is seen in the PA view of the heart. **B,** A large curved calcified structure *(arrows)* is seen in the left lateral view of the heart.

Courtesy Wade Shuford, MD, Professor of Radiology, Emory University School of Medicine; and Radiology Service at Grady Memorial Hospital, Atlanta. Reproduced with permission from Hurst JW: *Cardiovascular diagnosis: the initial examination*, St Louis, 1993, Mosby, p 451.

4 Examination of the Electrocardiogram[1]

Normally, the heart's electrical activity originates in the sinus node and spreads through the atria and ventricles in an orderly manner. The spread of electrical activity is called the *depolarization process*. During this process the heart loses its electrical charges. The heart produces a different electrical field for each millisecond of depolarization of the atria and ventricles. It is important to understand that each of the electrical fields associated with depolarization extends to the body surface.

The loss of electrical charges is followed by the restoration of the electrical charges. This is called *repolarization*. The repolarization process also produces a series of electrical fields that extend to the body surface.

The heart is a three-dimensional structure, so the electrical fields are also three-dimensional "structures."

The electrocardiograph (ECG) machine and its attachments are used to record the ever-changing electrical fields created by depolarization and repolarization of the atria and ventricles. This series of electrical fields creates the ECG waves that are labeled P QRS T U (Fig. 4-1).

ECG interpretation demands a knowledge of cardiac anatomy; the specialized conduction system; the depolarization process; the repolarization process; how to visualize, measure, and diagram the electrical forces (vectors) by studying the 12-lead ECG; and the pathology of cardiac disease.

CARDIAC ANATOMY

Location of Atria and Ventricles

The *right atrium* (RA) is located on the right (Figs. 3-1 and 4-2, A). The *left atrium* (LA) is located posterior to the right atrium in the central portion of the chest and anterior to the spinal column and abuts the right and left bronchi superiorly (Figs. 3-1, 3-3, and 4-2, C).

The *left ventricle* (LV) is located on the left and inferiorly. The long anatomic axis of the LV is directed slightly anteriorly (Figs. 3-1, 4-2, B, and 4-2, C). The apex of the LV is thinner than its lateral walls.

The *interventricular septum* is a part of the LV and is located anteriorly (Fig. 4-2, C).

The *right ventricle* (RV) is located anteriorly (Figs. 3-1 and 4-2, B, and 4-2, C). The RV wall thickness in the newborn is normally about as thick as the LV. In the adult the LV wall is thicker than the RV wall.

Specialized Conduction System

The heart's electrical activity originates in the *sinus node* (Fig. 4-3). The depolarization process spreads anteriorly and inferiorly in the RA and then spreads inferiorly and posteriorly in the LA. No proven specialized atrial cells guide the process; the depolarization process spreads by preferential pathways created because so many orifices exist in the RA and LA walls (personal communication, Anton Becker, MD).

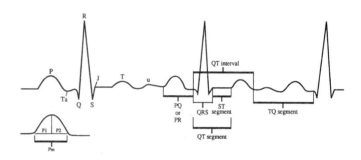

Fig. 4-1. Waves and intervals of the electrocardiogram (ECG). The waves are shown in the left-hand portion of the illustration. The *P wave (P)* is produced by depolarization of the atria and is divided into *P1* and *P2*. P1 is produced by depolarization of the right atrium, and P2 is produced by depolarization of the left atrium. The letters *Pm* (mean of the P) are used to represent the entire P wave. The letters *Ta* are used to designate the wave that is produced by repolarization of the atria. The *QRS complex* results from depolarization of the ventricles. The *Q wave* is the initial downward deflection of the QRS complex. The *R wave* is the initial upward deflection of the QRS complex. A second upward deflection of the QRS complex may be present and is designated as an *R prime (R')* wave. The *S wave* is the terminal downward deflection of the QRS complex. The *T wave (T)* results from repolarization of the ventricles. The cause of the *U wave* is controversial.

The intervals are shown in the right-hand portion of the illustration. The *PR interval*, or preferably the *PQ interval*, is measured from the beginning of the P wave to the beginning of ventricular depolarization (the beginning of the Q wave should be used when there is a Q wave; the beginning of the R wave should be used when there is no Q wave). The *duration of the QRS complex* is measured from the beginning to the end of the QRS complex. The *ST segment* is defined as the segment that begins with the end of the S wave and ends with the beginning of the T wave. The *QT interval* is measured from the beginning of the Q wave to the end of the T wave. The *QT segment* is measured from the beginning of the Q wave to the beginning of the T wave. The *TQ segment* is measured from the end of the T wave to the beginning of the QRS complex.

Redrawn with permission from Hurst JW: *Ventricular electrocardiography*, St. Louis, 1991, Mosby, fig 5.2.

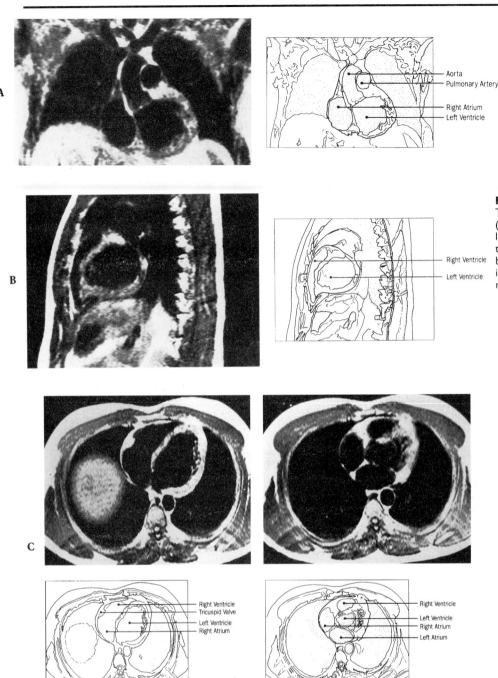

Aorta
Pulmonary Artery

Right Atrium
Left Ventricle

Right Ventricle
Left Ventricle

Right Ventricle
Tricuspid Valve
Left Ventricle
Right Atrium

Right Ventricle
Left Ventricle
Right Atrium
Left Atrium

Fig. 4-2. Location of the four heart chambers. The technique of magnetic resonance imaging (MRI) can be used to show the frontal view. **(A)**, left lateral view **(B)**, and transverse view **(C)** of the heart. The various cardiac chambers are labeled in the diagrams that accompany the MR images. These views of the heart must be kept in mind as one analyzes the heart's electrical forces.

Courtesy Mark Lowell, MD, Roderic I. Pettigrew, MD, and Radiology Department of Emory University School of Medicine and Hospital, Atlanta. Reproduced with permission from Hurst JW: *Ventricular electrocardiography*, St. Louis, 1991, Mosby, figs 4.5, 4.6, 4.7.

The *atrioventricular (A-V) node* is located in the lower portion of the RA (Fig. 4-3). The electrical activity is delayed by this structure.

The *common bundle of His* emerges out of the A-V node (Fig. 4-3). The conduction system then divides into the *left and right bundle* branches.

A *small branch of the left bundle* branch passes into the superior portion of the left side of the interventricular septum (Fig. 4-3).

The *left bundle branch* divides into three parts: *the left anterior superior division, the left posterior inferior division,* and an *intermediate part* that is, at this point in time, largely ignored or considered to be part of the anterior superior division (Fig. 4-3).

The *right bundle branch* spreads into the endocardium of the

RV without further subdivision (Fig. 4-3).

The *Purkinje fibers* are the final portion of the conduction system; they transmit the electrical impulses to the working myocytes.

The conduction system, as just described and as illustrated in Fig. 4-3, transmits electrical activity to specific parts of the heart. The long anatomic axis of the LV is directed to the left, inferiorly, and slightly anterior. However, the direction of the mean vector representing the direction of depolarization of a normal adult's ventricles is directed to the left, inferiorly, and posteriorly. The posterior direction is achieved because the left posterior inferior division of the left bundle directs the depolarization process posteriorly.

NORMAL ATRIAL DEPOLARIZATION AND ATRIOVENTRICULAR CONDUCTION

The depolarization of the atria produces the P wave in the ECG. The first half of the P wave is produced by depolarization of the RA and the second half of the P wave is produced by depolarization of the left atrium (see Fig. 4-4).

Normal Depolarization of Atria

The *direction* of RA depolarization is shown in Fig. 4-4, *A*, and the *direction* of the LA depolarization is shown in Fig. 4-4, *B*. The mean *direction* of atrial depolarization is visualized by adding 4-4, *A* to 4-4, *B* (Fig. 4-5).

The *duration* of the P waves is normally less than 0.12 second, and the amplitude of the P waves is normally less than 2.5 mm.

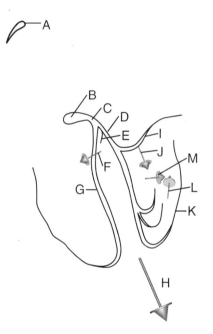

Fig. 4-3. Diagrammatic representation of the sinoatrial node, the atrioventricular node, and the left and right bundle branches. *A,* Sinoatrial node—responsible for the creation of electrical impulses that initiate depolarization of the atria. *B,* Atrioventricular node—slows and channels electrical activity to the bundle of His. *C,* Bundle of His—channels electrical activity to the right and left bundle branches. *D,* Left bundle branch. *E,* Twig of the left bundle branch—responsible for the early depolarization of the interventricular septum. *F,* Electrical force (represented by *arrow*) produced by depolarization of the first part of the septum. *G,* Right bundle branch. *H,* Electrical forces (represented by *arrow*) created by depolarization of the endocardial layer of the left and right ventricles. *I,* Left anterosuperior division (LASD) of the left bundle branch. *J,* Mean of the electrical forces (represented by *arrow*) created by the myocytes that are stimulated by the electrical impulse guided by the LASD of the left bundle branch. *K,* Left posteroinferior division (LPID) of the left bundle branch. *L,* Mean of the electrical forces (represented by *arrow*) created by the myocytes that are stimulated by the electrical impulse guided by the LPID of the left bundle. *M,* Vector sum of arrows *K* and *L;* the electrical forces responsible for *K* and *L* occur almost simultaneously, although the forces responsible for *L* may occur a little later than forces responsible for *K.*

This figure illustrates three consecutive electrical fields: the vector (*arrow*) *F* creates the first electrical field; the vector (*arrow*) *H* creates the second electrical field; and the vector (*arrow*) *M* creates the third electrical field. As discussed and illustrated later, the QRS complex is produced by a series of different electrical fields.

Reproduced with permission from Hurst JW: *Cardiovascular diagnosis: the initial examination,* St. Louis, 1993, Mosby, p 196.

Normal PR Interval

The PR interval is the measure of the time required for atrial depolarization, conduction through the A-V node, His bundle, bundle branches, and Purkinje fibers. It is measured from the beginning of the P wave to the beginning of the QRS complex. If a Q wave is present, the PQ interval is measured and one does not measure the PR interval. Convention dictates that the measurement is labeled as the PR interval even if the measurement is made using the Q wave. The normal PR interval is 0.20 second or less. An interval longer than 0.20 second is said to be first-degree A-V block. When the PR interval is less than 0.12 second, it may be caused by a bypass conduction tract that permits the electrical activity to circumvent the A-V node on its way to the ventricles. The length of the PR interval must always be assessed in relation to the heart rate (see Table 4-1 at the end of this chapter).

NORMAL VENTRICULAR DEPOLARIZATION AND CONDUCTION

Normal Depolarization of the Ventricles

The ventricular depolarization process spreads from endocardium to epicardium and produces electrical forces that are directed in the same direction. The first portion of the ventricular myocytes to depolarize is located in the left superior portion of the interventricular septum (Fig. 4-3). The depolarization process remains limited to the septum for 0.01 to 0.02 second. It produces electrical forces, the mean of which can be directed in any direction. However, it is usually directed as shown in Fig. 4-6, *A.*

The electrical activity travels at a rapid pace down the bundle branches to the endocardial myocytes of both ventricles. The depolarization process then proceeds from the endocardium of both ventricles toward the epicardium of both ventricles. So, during the next 0.02 to 0.04 second, the depolarization process spreads through the RV and LV of the newborn and young child, producing a mean electrical force that is directed to the right, inferiorly, and anteriorly. In the normal adult the depolarization process spreads through the RV and almost through the LV, producing a mean electrical force that is directed inferiorly, to the left, and parallel with the frontal plane (Fig. 4-6, *B*).

The last 0.2 second of ventricular depolarization in the adult is limited to the posterobasilar portion of the LV. This occurs because the posteroinferior division of the left bundle branch directs the electrical activity to the myocytes located in the posterobasilar portion of the LV. The mean of the electrical forces produced by this region of the LV is directed more to the left and posteriorly (Fig. 4-6, *C*).

Note that the electrical activity within the conduction system itself is not sufficiently large to be recorded in the surface ECG. The conduction is very slow in the A-V node, extremely rapid in the bundle branches, and is slowed again by the myocytes.

The direction of the electrical forces changes each millisecond of the depolarization process. This creates a QRS loop (Fig. 4-6, *D*). The contour of the QRS loop is produced because of the sequence in which the myocytes are stimulated, the location of the myocytes when they are stimulated, and the thickness of the ventricular myocardium. The QRS loop can be divided into three parts, as shown in Fig. 4-6. Note that an anatomic correlate exists for each of the parts. Each of the QRS complexes seen in the routine 12-lead ECG has a different shape because the electrodes are viewing the QRS loop from different vantage points.

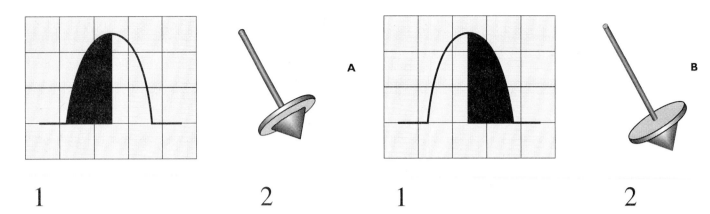

Fig. 4-4. A, First half of the P wave. *1*, The first half of the P wave is produced by depolarization of the right atrium. *2*, An arrow representing the mean of the electrical forces (vectors) responsible for the first half of the P wave is directed at about +60 to +70 degrees in the frontal plane; it is usually directed 10 to 15 degrees anteriorly. **B**, Last half of the P wave.

1, The last half of the P wave is produced by depolarization of the left atrium. *2*, An arrow representing the mean of the electrical forces (vectors) responsible for the last half of the P wave is directed at about +50 to +70 degrees in the frontal plane; it is usually directed 10 to 15 degrees posteriorly.

Reproduced with permission from Hurst JW: *Cardiovascular diagnosis: the initial examination*, St Louis, 1993, Mosby, p 241.

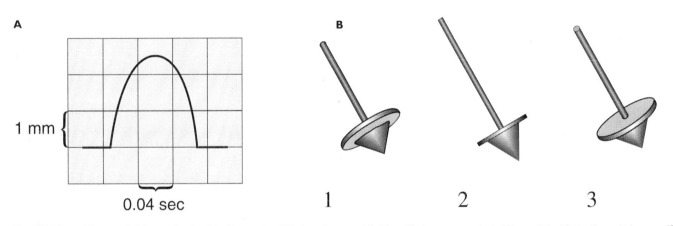

Fig. 4-5. Normal P wave. **A**, The amplitude of the P wave should be less than 2.5 mm; the duration should be less than 0.12 second. **B**, An arrow representing the mean of the electrical forces (vectors) responsible for the P wave may be directed at about +60 degrees in the frontal plane; it may be directed

(1) 10 to 15 degrees anteriorly, *(2)* parallel with the frontal plane, or *(3)* 10 to 15 degrees posteriorly.

Reproduced with permission from Hurst JW: *Cardiovascular diagnosis: the initial examination*, St Louis, 1993, Mosby, p 240.

Duration of Ventricular Depolarization

The normal duration of ventricular depolarization varies with the age of the subject. The duration of the QRS complex is 0.06 second in the infant and 0.08 second to 0.10 second in the normal adult.

The Ta wave may be seen more easily when the PR interval is long or when tachycardia is present, at which time the ST segment may be displaced by the Ta wave.

NORMAL ATRIAL REPOLARIZATION

Normal atrial repolarization occurs immediately after atrial depolarization. The process of repolarization apparently occurs in the same direction as the depolarization, but it produces electrical forces that are opposite to the direction of repolarization. Accordingly, the wave of repolarization of the atria, called the Ta wave, is often inverted in the deflection where the P wave is upright (Fig. 4-7). Presumably this electrical event occurs because the atrial wall is thin and the intraatrial pressure is low, which is quite different than the comparatively thick RV and LV walls and higher pressures within the RV and LV.

NORMAL VENTRICULAR REPOLARIZATION

Normal ventricular repolarization usually occurs after the ST segment. During the ST segment the ventricular myocytes are said to be excited or depolarized. The repolarization of the ventricular myocytes produces the T wave in the ECG.

One would expect the repolarization process to follow the same path as the depolarization process if each ventricular myocyte recharged itself after the same length of time. This does not occur in the adult ventricular myocardium. The repolarization process begins at the epicardium and spreads toward the endocardium. This produces electrical forces that are directed in the opposite direction.

Why does the wave of depolarization spread from endocardium to epicardium and the wave of repolarization spread from epicardium to endocardium? The true answer is unknown, but the current belief is that the transmyocardial pressure gradient is the cause. The depolarization process stimulates the myocytes to contract and produce mechanical ventricular systole. The T wave (repolarization) is produced late in mechanical ventricular systole. In other words, the physiologic environment associated with depolarization is quite different from the physiologic environment associated with repolarization. Accordingly, the direction of the repolarization process in the endocardium is delayed by the high endocardial pressure compared with the lower epicardial pressure.

There is a rather fixed relationship of the repolarization process with the depolarization process. That is, the direction of the mean of the repolarization process is predetermined by the direction of the mean of the depolarization process. The relationship of the QRS to T is different in the newborn, adolescent, and adult (Fig. 4-8).

THE DURATION OF VENTRICULAR DEPOLARIZATION PLUS VENTRICULAR REPOLARIZATION

This measurement is referred to as the Q-T interval. It is measured from the beginning of the Q wave to the end of the T wave. The interval varies with the heart rate (see Table 4-2 at the end of this chapter).

It is important to distinguish between a long Q-T interval caused by a longer than normal QRS duration and a long Q-T interval in which the QRS duration is normal. Obviously, too, this measurement includes the ST segment during which time the depolarized myocytes have not repolarized. Hypocalcemia may produce a long ST segment.

HOW TO VISUALIZE, MEASURE, AND DIAGRAM ELECTRICAL FORCES OF HEART

I prefer the Grant method of visualizing, measuring, and diagramming the heart's electrical forces because his method links the scientific basis for the wave form to the interpretation of each ECG.[2] In other words, his method encourages the use of one's knowledge of cardiac anatomy, the conduction system, the depolarization process, the repolarization process, and cardiac pathology. It is a method of thinking; it is different from memorizing wave forms.

The Machine

It is not necessary to discuss the details of the direct-writing ECG machine. It is sufficient to know that the machine can record the heart's electrical activity by sensing the electricity that is transmitted from the heart to the body surface. It is useful to view the machine as a galvanometer, or a volt-measuring device, that has a positive pole and a negative pole to which wires are attached. The wires are attached to electrodes, which are in turn attached to specific places on the patient's skin. It *is* necessary, however, to learn about ECG paper and electrode placement and leads (see subsequent discussion).

Electrocardiographic Paper

The modern direct-writing machine records the ECG tracing on special paper that moves at a speed of 25 mm each second. The paper is, in effect, a strip of moving graph paper (Fig. 4-9).

Note that the small squares are 1 mm wide and 1 mm high. A deflection that occupies 1 mm lasts 0.04 second. One tenth of a millivolt (mV) of electrical activity moves the stylus 1 mm up or down. The large squares are composed of five horizontal small squares and five vertical squares.

The machine is calibrated before each recording so that a 10 mm movement of the writing arm (stylus) equals 1 mV of electricity.

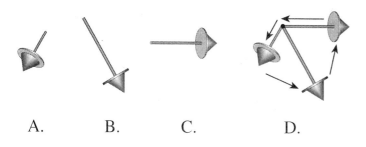

A.   B.   C.   D.

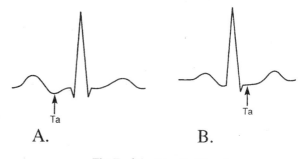

A.   B.

The T of the P (or Ta Wave)

Fig. 4-6. Diagrammatic representation of the depolarization sequence responsible for the QRS complex (see text). **A,** An arrow representing the electrical forces (vectors) produced by the initial depolarization of the septum is directed anteriorly and to the right. **B,** An arrow representing the electrical forces (vectors) produced by depolarization of the endocardial layer of the left and right ventricles (LV, RV) is directed inferiorly and slightly to the left and, in this illustration, is parallel with the frontal plane. **C,** An arrow representing the electrical forces (vectors) produced by depolarization of the posterolateral portion of the LV is directed to the left and posteriorly. **D,** A crude QRS loop is created when the origin of the electrical forces is assumed to arise from a common point and when a line (the loop) is drawn around the terminal of the electrical forces.

Reproduced with permission from Hurst JW: *Cardiovascular diagnosis: the initial examination*, St. Louis, 1993, Mosby, p 198.

Fig. 4-7. Repolarization of the atria (Ta wave). **A,** The Ta wave caused by atrial repolarization can be seen occasionally following the P wave. It is more likely to be seen when the PR interval is long or when P waves are unrelated to the QRS complex, as in patients with complete heart block. **B,** When the PR interval is short (in the range of 0.12 second), the Ta wave caused by atrial repolarization may displace the ST segment downward. Such a displacement may become evident with the tachycardia associated with exercise; it may be misinterpreted as being an "ischemic" response to exercise.

Redrawn with permission from Hurst JW: *Ventricular electrocardiography*, St. Louis, 1991, Mosby, fig 5.6.

Electrode Placement and Leads

Small metal plates (or small metal suction cups) are attached by wires to the two poles of ECG machine. The various combinations of attachments are called leads.

Bipolar Extremity Leads. Einthoven created the bipolar extremity lead system.[3] He immersed the right arm, left arm, and one leg of the subject into buckets of saline, which were the first primitive electrodes. He attached the "electrode" on the right arm to the galvanometer's negative pole and the "electrode" on the left area to the positive pole. He labeled this lead as lead I. He attached the electrode on the right arm to the galvanometer's negative pole and the electrode on one leg to the positive pole and labeled this lead lead II. He attached the electrode on the left arm to the galvanometer's negative pole and the electrode on the leg to the positive pole and labeled this lead III. Einthoven recognized that his "electrodes" were located a great distance from the heart. He knew the laws of physics that permitted him to consider them to be electrically "equidistant" from the origin of the heart's electrical activity. This permitted him to develop the Einthoven equilateral triangle (Fig. 4-10).

Einthoven's law, which follows the laws of physics, is that an ECG deflection noted on lead II equals the deflection noted on lead III plus the deflection on lead I.

The ECG machine measures the *difference of potential* that exists between the electrodes that are attached to the right arm, left arm, and leg.

These bipolar leads are often referred to as *frontal plane* leads because they are influenced mainly by electrical forces that are directed up or down and right or left but are not influenced greatly by the electrical forces directed toward the front or back.

Bayley created the *triaxial reference system*.[4] He developed a more usable bipolar extremity lead system by transposing the sides of Einthoven's equilateral triangle so that each side retained its orientation but passed through the area that was designated as the origin of electrical activity (Fig. 4-11). It is easier to visualize the extent an electrical force will project onto a lead axes when Bayley's triaxial display system is used than when Einthoven's equilateral triangle is used.

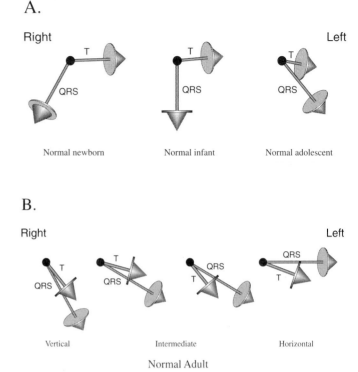

A.

Right — Left

Normal newborn   Normal infant   Normal adolescent

B.

Right — Left

Vertical   Intermediate   Horizontal

Normal Adult

Fig. 4-8. Directions of arrow representing the mean QRS vector and mean T vector in the normal newborn, normal infant, and normal adolescent **(A)**, and the normal adult **(B)**. When the mean QRS vector in the normal adult is directed vertically, the mean T vector should be located to its left. When the mean QRS vector is directed intermediately, the mean T vector can be located to its right or left. When the mean QRS vector is directed horizontally, the mean T vector should be directed inferior to it. The normal QRS-T angle may be 60 degrees but is usually 30 to 45 degrees or less. The mean T vector should always be anterior to the mean QRS vector.

Redrawn with permission from Hurst JW: *Ventricular electrocardiography*, St. Louis, 1991, Mosby, fig 5.9

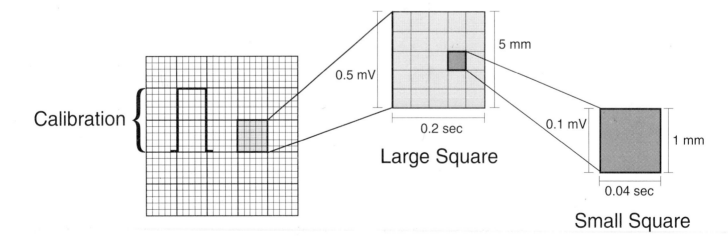

Calibration

0.5 mV
0.2 sec
Large Square

5 mm

0.1 mV
0.04 sec
1 mm
Small Square

Fig. 4-9. Paper used to record ECGs.

Reproduced with permission from Hurst JW: *Cardiovascular diagnosis: the initial examination*, St Louis, 1993, Mosby, p 203.

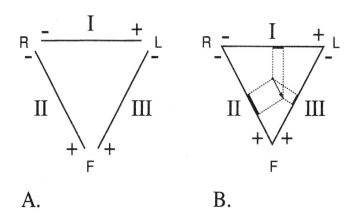

A.　　　B.

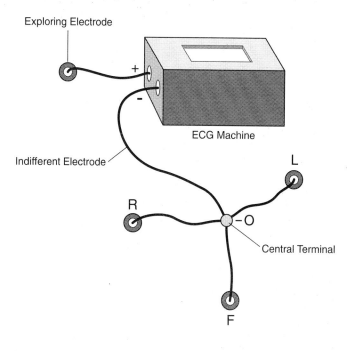

Fig. 4-10. Einthoven's bipolar extremity leads. **A,** Einthoven created lead I by attaching a wire from the right arm to the galvanometer's negative pole and a wire from the left arm to the positive pole. He created lead II by attaching a wire from the right arm to the galvanometer's negative pole and a wire from one leg to the positive pole. He created lead III by attaching a wire from the left arm to the galvanometer's negative pole and a wire from the leg to the positive pole. (He originally used buckets of saline for electrodes.) **B,** Einthoven viewed the bipolar extremity lead hookup between the patient and the ECG machine as an electrical equilateral triangle, since the "electrodes" recorded the electrical potential at points that were located a great distance from its origin. He pointed out that electrical forces were projected onto the lead axes as shown here. Note how the arrow "projects" its "shadow" onto each of the lead axes.

Reproduced with permission from Hurst JW: Cardiovascular diagnosis: the initial examination, St Louis, 1993, Mosby, p 204.

Fig. 4-12. Wilson's unipolar leads. Wilson connected the electrodes that were placed on the right arm, left arm, and one leg to a central terminal. He then connected the central terminal to the ECG machine's negative pole. This connection was referred to as the indifferent electrode. He connected the exploring electrode to the machine's positive pole. When the exploring electrode was placed on the chest, it was referred to as a V lead. When the exploring electrode was placed on the extremities, it was referred to as V_R, V_L, and V_F.

Slightly modified with permission from Hurst JW: Ventricular electrocardiography, St. Louis, 1991, Mosby, fig 4.20.

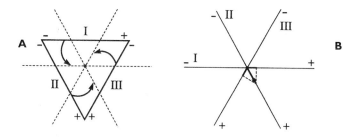

Fig. 4-11. Bayley's triaxial system. **A,** Bayley moved lead axes I, II, and III so that they pass through the same central point (considered the origin of the electrical forces). He maintained the same orientation of the lead axes as in Einthoven's electrical equilateral triangle (see Fig. 4-10, **B**). **B,** The same electrical force shown in Fig. 4-10 is reproduced in this figure. Note that the arrow projects the same amount on lead axes I, II, and III of Bayley's triaxial system as it did on the leads of Einthoven's electrical equilateral triangle.

Reproduced with permission from Hurst JW: Cardiovascular diagnosis: the initial examination, St Louis, 1993, Mosby, p 206.

Unipolar Extremity Leads. Wilson and his colleagues discovered a method of recording the electrical potential at a single electrode position.[5] With this discovery, it became possible to place an electrode anywhere on the body surface and measure the electrical activity produced by the heart at that particular spot. This can be accomplished by placing electrodes on the right arm, left arm, and one leg. Wires are then attached to each of these electrodes, and the ends of the three wires are then joined to form a *central terminal.* A wire leading from the central terminal is attached to the recording machine's negative pole. This electrode is labeled the *indifferent electrode.* An *exploring electrode* and wire are attached to the measuring device's positive pole. A unipolar lead measures the difference in electrical potential between that recorded by the exploring electrode and that recorded by a wire attached to the central terminal. However, because the electrical potential recorded from a wire attached to the central terminal is almost zero at all times, the exploring electrode records the true potential at any site it is placed (Fig. 4-12).

The Wilson unipolar extremity lead axes bisect the angles of the Bayley triaxial display system. The Wilson unipolar extremity leads recorded deflections that were smaller than those produced by the Einthoven bipolar system. Because of this, the amplitude of the deflections recorded by the Wilson unipolar lead system was originally boosted by amplifiers.

Goldberger discovered that by "breaking" the connection of the central terminal to the extremity where the exploring electrode was recording, he could increase the size of the deflection without changing its contour significantly.[6] Thus, we now use Goldberger's modification of Wilson's unipolar extremity leads. They are called aV_R, aV_L, and aV_F (Fig. 4-13).

A hexaxial display system is created when the Goldberger lead axes are superimposed on Bayley's triaxial system (Fig. 4-14). Note in Fig. 4-14 that a scale in degrees has been added. This enables those who interpret ECGs to identify the number of degrees an electrical force is directed away from the zero position in the frontal plane.

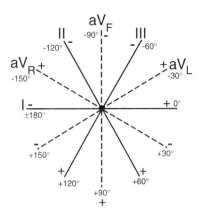

Fig. 4-14. Hexaxial reference system. The unipolar extremity lead axes bisect the angles produced by Bayley's triaxial system to create the hexaxial reference system. The direction of the vectors used to represent electrical forces can be designated as the number of degrees from the horizontal line created by lead I. Note that the 0-degree point is located at the left-hand end of lead axis I and the ±180-degree point is located at the right-hand end of lead axis I.

Reproduced with permission from Hurst JW: *Cardiovascular diagnosis: the initial examination*, St Louis, 1993, Mosby, p 209.

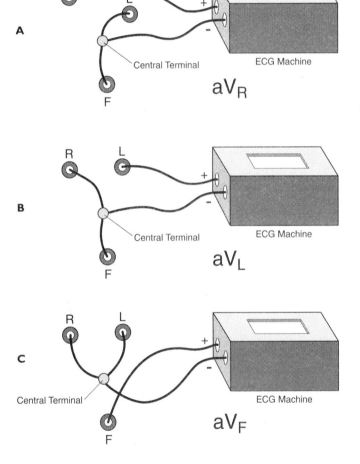

Fig. 4-13. Goldberger's augmented unipolar extremity leads. The letter *a* stands for the word *augmented*. **A**, Lead aV_R is created by disconnecting the wire from the right arm to Wilson's central terminal when the exploring electrode is placed on the right arm. **B**, aV_L is created by disconnecting the wire from the left arm to Wilson's central terminal when the exploring electrode is placed on the left arm. **C**, aV_F is created by disconnecting the wire from the leg to Wilson's central terminal when the exploring electrode is placed on the leg.

Slightly modified with permission from Hurst JW: *Ventricular electrocardiography*, St. Louis, 1991, Mosby, fig 4.24.

Unipolar Chest Leads. In the beginning, no chest leads were used because there were no "electrodes" except buckets of saline, which could not be applied to the chest. Later, a single bipolar chest lead was used. The electrode of one extremity was connected with a wire to the galvanometer's negative pole, and the exploring electrode was connected with a wire to the positive pole to create precordial lead C_R, C_L, or C_F in which R referred to the right arm, L referred to the left arm, and F referred to one leg. Later, six precordial electrode positions were developed, but bipolar connections were still used. Still later, the Wilson unipolar precordial leads were used. These leads require no augmentation because the electrodes are placed near the heart. They are often referred to as V leads (V stands for electrical potential). The precordial electrode positions are as follows:

V_1: Fourth right intercostal space near sternum
V_2: Fourth left intercostal space near sternum
V_3: Halfway between V_2 and V_4
V_4: Fifth left intercostal space at midclavicular line
V_5: On horizontal line at level of V_4 at anterior axillary line
V_6: On horizontal line at level of V_4 and V_5 at midaxillary line
V_{3R}, V_{4R}, V_{5R}: At the same position as V_3, V_4, V_5 but on chest's right side

Visualizing the Extremity and the Precordial Leads
The diagram shown in Fig. 4-15 illustrates the six extremity lead axes and the six precordial electrode positions and their relationship to the chest, the heart, and the "origin" of electrical activity.

Caveat
The electrodes of the 12 leads should be viewed as recording from various specified sample sites. All the leads record from the same series of electrical fields. As discussed next, Grant taught us how to determine the spatial orientation of the electrical forces and their electrical fields by inspecting the deflections or samples revealed in the 12-lead ECG.[2]

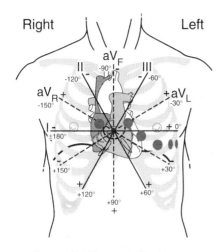

Precordial Electrode Positions

Fig. 4-15. Location of the chest electrodes. This figure also illustrates the relationship of the bipolar and unipolar extremity leads to the body and to each other. The heart is shown in its anatomically correct position. The semicircle indicates the location of the left atrium. The dot in the center of the heart represents the approximate location of the origin of the electrical forces.

Reproduced with permission from Hurst JW: *Cardiovascular diagnosis: the initial examination*, St Louis, 1993, Mosby, p 210.

Fig. 4-16. An arrow (the symbol for a vector) has three parts: the shaft, the arrowhead's base, and the arrowhead's rim. The base represents the zero potential plane. The rim represents the transitional pathway (see Fig. 4-17). The arrow's length represents the magnitude of the electrical force. The shaft's inclination represents the orientation of the electrical force in space. The arrowhead indicates the polarity (the sense) of the force, which, taken along with its inclination, indicates the direction of the force.

Reproduced with permission from Hurst JW: *Cardiovascular diagnosis: the initial examination*, St Louis, 1993, Mosby, p 199.

GRANT METHOD OF INTERPRETING ELECTROCARDIOGRAMS[2]

Grant recognized that the deflections recorded in the 12 leads of the ECG were samples of the series of electrical fields that reach the body surface. He developed a method of inspecting the 12 leads and visualizing the spatial orientation of the series of electrical forces that produce the electrical fields responsible for the shape and size of the P, QRS, and T waves. He reasoned that if

one knew the location of the cardiac chambers in the chest, visualized the conduction system, understood the sequence of depolarization and repolarization, and understood the pathology of cardiac disease, one should be able to interpret ECGs more scientifically than simply memorizing the shape of the deflections. Such an approach fulfilled Wilson's admonition[7]:

> The interpretation of the electrocardiogram is not merely a matter of memorizing a few characteristic pictures; there are many unusual variations and combinations of electrocardiographic phenomena which must be studied, analyzed, and correlated one with another and with other available data before any definite conclusion is possible. These situations demand some acquaintance with the electrical and physiologic principles by which they are determined....

Grant, who obviously heeded Wilson's warning, called his method "vector electrocardiography" to separate it from vector cardiography which depends on three-dimensional oscilliscopic recording of the P, QRS, and T loops.[2]

Vectors

The Grant method of interpretation uses two metaphors. The *vector concept* is used to visualize the heart's electrical forces, and an *arrow* is used to illustrate the vectors. It simplifies the process when these two metaphors are viewed as one and the arrow is called a vector.

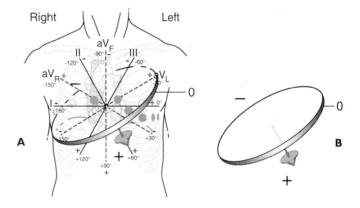

Fig. 4-17. Transmission of an electrical field to the body surface. **A,** An arrow representing the electrical force (vector) originating in the center of the heart is directed at +60 degrees in the frontal plane and 30 to 40 degrees posteriorly. The zero potential plane is perpendicular to the arrow's direction and divides the body into a negative area (in this example the negative portion of the electrical field is located superior to the zero potential plane) and a positive area (in this example the positive portion of the electrical field is located inferior to the zero potential plane). When the zero potential plane extends to the body surface (the skin), it creates the transitional pathway. In this example, the ECG machine will record a negative deflection superior to the transitional pathway, a positive deflection inferior to the transitional pathway, and zero potential along the transitional pathway. **B,** The arrow's length indicates the magnitude of the electrical force; the direction and sense of the electrical force is illustrated by the arrow's inclination and the arrowhead's location. The arrowhead itself has considerable meaning (see Fig. 4-16).

Reproduced with permission from Hurst JW: *Cardiovascular diagnosis: the initial examination*, St Louis, 1993, Mosby, p 201.

A vector (represented as an arrow) can be used to illustrate any force, whether mechanical or electrical. The arrow's length represents the force's *magnitude*. The arrow's inclination indicates its *direction*, and the arrowhead indicates its polarity or *sense* (Fig. 4-16).

MEASUREMENT OF ELECTRICAL FORCES OF HEART

The electrical forces produced by the atria and ventricles are "projected" onto all the lead axes. The deflections are, for the most part, different, only because each lead has a different relationship with the underlying series of electrical forces.

It is useful to illustrate how a single electrical force produces an electrical field and how it is projected onto the lead axes. A single electrical force is shown in Fig. 4-17. Note the electrical field that surrounds it. Observe that the chest's left side will record positive electrical charges when the machine is arranged so that the electrical force is directed toward the electrode that is connected to its positive pole. The entire chest is divided into two parts, a positive and a negative part. The chest's negative and positive parts are divided by the *zero potential plane*, which, when extended to the body surface, becomes the *transitional pathway*. The arrowhead's *rim* represents the transitional pathway, and the arrowhead's *base* represents the zero potential plane. The arrow's length indicates the *magnitude* of the electrical force.

Two steps are involved in determing the direction of an electrical force.[2] The two steps *must* be taken in sequence.

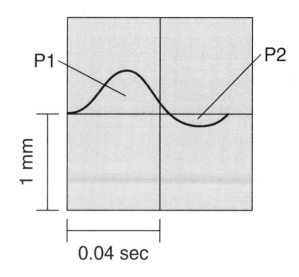

Fig. 4-19. Configuration of the P wave at electrode position V_1, according to Morris et al.[6] The first half of the P wave is usually upright (positive) when it is recorded at electrode position V_1. The last half of the P wave is usually recorded as a downward deflection (negative) when it is recorded at electrode position V_1. The normal size of the last half of the P wave can be determined by multiplying its duration by its depth. The normal measurement is about -0.03 mm·sec. In this illustration it is about 0.01 mm·sec.

Redrawn with permission from Hurst JW: *Ventricular electrocardiography*, St. Louis, 1991, Mosby, fig 5.5.

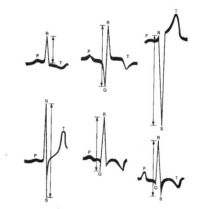

Fig. 4-20. Measurement of the total QRS amplitude. The total QRS amplitude is derived by adding the amplitude (positive and negative waves) of all the deflections recorded in all 12 leads of the ECG.

Redrawn with permission from Siegel RJ, Roberts WC: Electrocardiographic observations in severe aortic valve stenosis: correlative necropsy study to clinical, hemodynamic, and ECG variables demonstrating relation of 12-lead QRS amplitude to peak systolic transaortic pressure gradient, *Am Heart J* 103:212, 1982.

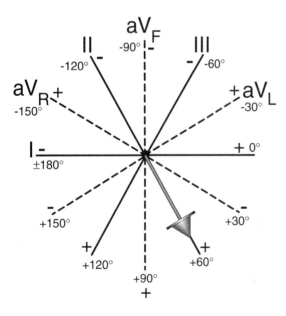

Fig. 4-18. Calculation of the direction of an electrical force (vector) in the frontal plane. When a deflection is largest in lead II, it can be represented by a vector (arrow) that is directed parallel with lead axis II. The deflection will simultaneously be smaller but equally large in leads I and III and smallest in lead aV_L, since the arrow will be perpendicular to lead axis aV_L. When the deflection is upright in lead II, the vector (arrow) will be directed toward the electrode of lead II that is attached to the positive pole of the ECG machine.

Reproduced with permission from Hurst JW: *Cardiovascular diagnosis: the initial examination*, St. Louis, 1993, Mosby, p 211.

Step One

The frontal plane direction of an electrical force can be determined by studying the deflections recorded in the extremity leads. *An electrical force that is relatively parallel to the extremity lead axis, in which the deflection is largest and relatively perpendicular to the lead axis in which the deflection is smallest* (Fig. 4-18). The polarity is determined by identifying if the force is upright in a certain lead. If it is, the electrical force will be directed relatively toward the electrode hooked to the measuring device's positive pole. Using this method, the direction of an electrical force can be identified with an error of about 5 degrees.

Step Two

(Never take step two without initially taking step one.) The precordial deflections are used to determine the anteroposterior direction of the electrical forces. *Do not use the largest deflection in the precordial leads* to draw a conclusion that the electrical force is parallel with the lead axis in which it is seen as one does when computing the frontal plane direction of an electrical force. This is not possible because the electrodes are much nearer to the heart than are the extremity electrodes and the electrode that is nearest the heart is likely to record the largest deflection. Accordingly, the largest precordial defection does not imply that the electrical force producing it is directed parallel with the lead axis in which it is found. In order to determine the anterior-posterior direction of an electrical force one must *identify the smallest precordial lead deflection and assume that the precordial lead axis in which it appears is recording from the transitional pathway. The transitional pathway is the body surface representation of the zero potential plane and the zero potential plane is perpendicular to the electrical force* (Fig. 4-17). Accordingly, the identification of the zero potential plane enables the observer to visualize the direction of the electrical force (vector) that produced it. The vector is then visualized as being perpendicular to the zero potential plane. The smallest deflection is identified by finding the deflection in which the area above the isoelectric line (baseline) of the electrocardiogram is equal to the area below the isoelectric line. This approach is valid because the location of the transitional pathway of an electrical force is not influenced greatly by the magnitude of the electrical force. The anterior or posterior direction of an electrical force can be determined with an accuracy of +/-15 degrees. When the mean vectors (that represent the

electrical forces) for the total P wave, total QRS complex, total ST segment, or total T wave are constructed, one should use the area under the wave, not the wave's amplitude, to determine the resultant size of the total wave. The same is true when only a part of a wave is studied; the area under the part, not its amplitude, is used to construct a mean vector to represent the part.

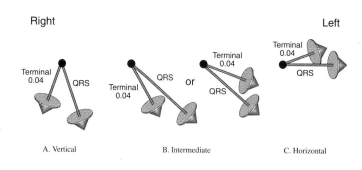

Fig. 4-22. Relationship of an arrow representing the mean of the electrical forces (vectors) responsible for the terminal 0.04 second of the normal QRS complex to an arrow representing the mean of the electrical forces (vectors) responsible for the entire QRS complex. **A,** An arrow representing the mean of the electrical forces (vectors) responsible for the terminal 0.04 second of the normal QRS complex should be located to the right of and posterior to a vertically directed arrow representing the mean of the electrical forces (vectors) responsible for the entire QRS complex. The angle between the two may be 60 degrees but is usually 30 to 45 degrees or less. **B,** An arrow representing the mean of the electrical forces (vectors) responsible for the terminal 0.04 second of the normal QRS complex may be located on either side of and posterior to an intermediately directed arrow representing the mean of the electrical forces (vectors) responsible for the entire QRS complex. The angle between the two may be 60 degrees but is usually 30 to 45 degrees or less. **C,** An arrow representing the mean of the electrical forces (vectors) responsible for the terminal 0.04 second of the normal QRS complex should be located superior and posterior to a horizontally directed arrow representing the mean of the electrical forces (vectors) responsible for the entire QRS complex. The angle between the two may be 60 degrees but is usually 30 to 45 degrees or less.

Redrawn with permission from Hurst JW: *Ventricular electrocardiography*, St. Louis, 1991, Mosby, fig 5.13.

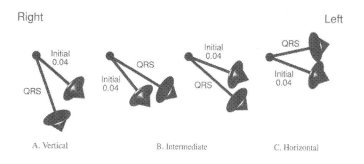

Fig. 4-21. Relationship of an arrow representing the mean of the electrical forces (vectors) responsible for the initial 0.04 second of the normal QRS complex to an arrow representing the mean of the electrical forces (vectors) responsible for the entire QRS complex. **A,** An arrow representing the mean of the electrical forces (vectors) responsible for the initial 0.04 second of the normal QRS complex should be located to the left of and anterior to a vertically directed arrow representing the mean of the electrical forces (vectors) responsible for the entire QRS complex. The angle between the two may be 60 degrees but is usually 30 to 45 degrees or less. **B,** An arrow representing the mean of the electrical forces (vectors) responsible for the initial 0.04 second of the normal QRS complex can be located to the right or left of and anterior to an intermediately directed arrow representing the mean of the electrical forces (vectors) responsible for the entire QRS complex. The angle between the two may be 60 degrees but is usually 30 to 45 degrees or less. **C,** An arrow representing the mean of the electrical forces (vectors) responsible for the initial 0.04 second of the normal QRS complex should be directed inferior and anterior to a horizontally directed arrow representing the mean of the electrical forces (vectors) responsible for the entire QRS complex. The angle between the two may be 60 degrees but is usually 30 to 45 degrees or less.

Redrawn with permission from Hurst JW: *Ventricular electrocardiography*, St. Louis, 1991, Mosby, fig. 5.12.

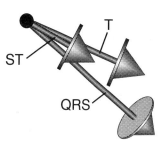

The Normal ST Vector

Fig. 4-23. Normal ST segment vector. An arrow representing the normal mean ST segment vector (when there is one) should be directed parallel, with an arrow representing the mean T vector. At times, when there is a large mean T vector, the mean ST segment vector may also be large. This is referred to as *normal early repolarization*. An arrow representing a prominent mean ST segment vector that is parallel with an arrow representing a normal or abnormal mean T vector is called a *secondary* ST segment vector because it is part of the repolarization process. Exceptions to this rule occur when the mean ST segment vector is due to epicardial injury as it is with early generalized pericarditis or early apical infarction.

Reproduced with permission from Hurst JW: *Cardiovascular diagnosis: the initial examination*, St Louis, 1993, Mosby, p 260.

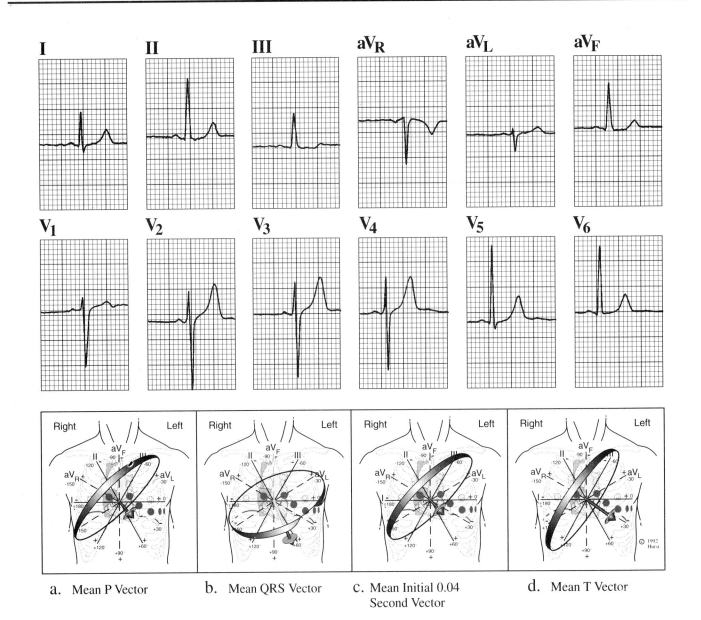

a. Mean P Vector

b. Mean QRS Vector

c. Mean Initial 0.04
Second Vector

d. Mean T Vector

Fig. 4-24. Normal intermediately directed mean QRS vector.
- *Rhythm:* Normal sinus rhythm
  Rate: Undetermined in short strip
  PR interval: 0.16 second
  QRS duration: 0.08 second
  QT interval: 0.34 second
- *Vector diagrams of electrical forces:* See *a, b, c,* and *d* below the ECG
- *Electrophysiologic considerations:*
  The mean QRS vector is directed about + 70 degrees inferiorly and about 50 degrees posteriorly.
  The mean initial 0.04-second QRS vector is directed to the left of and anterior to the mean QRS vector (it may normally be directed to the right or left or an intermediately directed mean QRS vector).
  The QRS-T angle is 60 degrees, and the mean T vector is directed to the left of and anterior to the mean QRS vector. (It may normally be directed to the right or left of an intermediately directed mean QRS vector.)

- The size and direction of the mean vectors representing depolarization of the atria and ventricles, the initial 0.04 second of the QRS complex, and repolarization of the ventricles are normal.
- *Clinical differential diagnosis:* The heart may be normal, or the patient could have coronary atherosclerotic heart disease, mild valvular disease, or systemic hypertension that has not as yet produced left ventricular hypertrophy. The patient could have a history of arrhythmias of past pericarditis. It is unlikely that the patient has hypertrophic, dilated, or restrictive cardiomyopathy. Other clinical data are needed to determine which diagnosis is correct.
- *Discussion:* This ECG was recorded from a 27-year-old normal male physician. He was of average body build and exhibited no evidence of heart disease.

ECG courtesy Mark Lowell, MD. Reproduced with permission from Hurst JW: *Ventricular electrocardiography,* St. Louis, 1991, Mosby, fig 5.26.

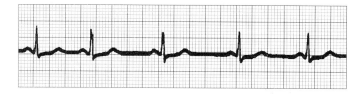

Fig. 4-25. Sinus arrhythmia. There is a normal sinus node mechanism of impulse formation, normal atrioventricular conduction, and normal ventricular response. In this tracing the rate of sinus node impulse formation varies more than 0.12 second between the longest and shortest cycles (longest cycle = 0.97 second; shortest cycle = 0.70 second; therefore the variation = 0.27 second). The lack of variation in P wave morphology and in the PR interval differentiates sinus arrhythmias from a wandering atrial pacemaker.

From Hurst JW, Myerburg RJ: *Introduction to electrocardiography,* ed 2, New York, 1932, McGraw-Hill, p 232. Reprinted with permission from the author.

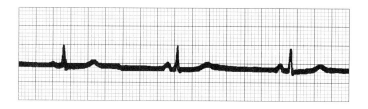

Fig. 4-26. Sinus bradycardia. The rhythm is regular, the mechanism is of normal sinus origin, and the rate is less than 60 ventricular depolarizations per minute. In this tracing the PP and RR intervals are 1.31 second; the rate therefore is 46 ventricular depolarizations per minute. The small "wave" after the first T wave is an artifact. An RR interval of 1 second represents a rate of exactly 60 depolarizations per minute; thus an interval greater than 1 second indicates a rate of less than 60 per minute.

From Hurst JW, Myerburg RJ: *Introduction to electrocardiography,* ed 2, New York, 1973, McGraw-Hill, p 236. Reprinted with permission from the author.

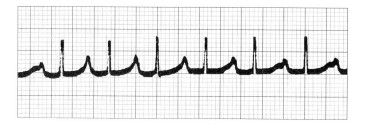

Fig. 4-27. Sinus tachycardia. The rhythm is usually regular, the mechanism is of normal sinus origin, and the rate is more than 90 depolarizations per minute. In this tracing the first, sixth, and seventh P waves can be distinguished from the preceding T waves. P waves are not ordinarily obscured by T waves at this rate (133 ventricular depolarizations per minute); however, in this case, first-degree heart block (prolonged PR interval) is responsible for the obscured P waves. Slight rhythmic variation in the rate of a supraventricular tachycardia tends to favor the diagnosis of sinus tachycardia rather than paroxysmal atrial tachycardia or atrial flutter. The rate variation in atrial fibrillation is usually erratic rather than rhythmic.

From Hurst JW, Myerburg RJ: *Introduction to electrocardiography,* ed 2, New York, 1973, McGraw-Hill, p 238. Reprinted with permission from the author.

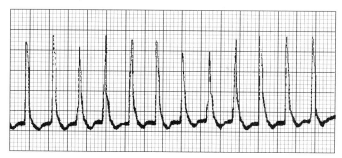

Fig. 4-28. Paroxysmal supraventricular tachycardia. A short strip of an ECG obtained during an attack of paroxysmal supraventricular tachycardia demonstrates a heart rate of 222 depolarizations per minute (RR interval = 0.27 second). The P waves cannot be discerned because of the extremely rapid rate. The duration of the QRS complex is normal.

From Hurst JW, Myerburg RJ: *Introduction to electrocardiography,* ed 2, New York, 1973, McGraw-Hill, p 239. Reprinted with permission from the author.

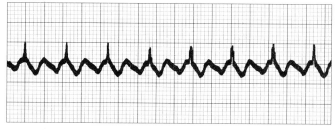

Fig. 4-29. Atrial flutter with 2:1 atrioventricular conduction. The duration of the QRS complex is normal. The atrial flutter rate is 272 per minute (PP interval = 0.22 second), and the ventricular rate is 136 ventricular depolarizations per minute (RR interval = 0.44 second). Sawtooth flutter waves may be less obvious in the presence of the more rapid ventricular response.

From Hurst JW, Myerburg RJ: *Introduction to electrocardiography,* ed 2, New York, 1973, McGraw-Hill, p 241. Reprinted with permission from the author.

NORMAL ELECTROCARDIOGRAM[1]

The ECG is said to be normal when:
- The rate and rhythm are normal. The normal rate is 60 to 90 complexes per minute.
- The P waves should be less than 0.12 second in duration, and the amplitude should be less than 2.5 mm.
- The PR interval (or PQ interval) should be less than 0.20 second. One should refer to reference tables, in which the normalcy of the PR interval is determined by relating it to the patient's heart rate and age (see Table 4-1 at the end of this chapter).
- The QRS duration in the normal child is 0.06 to 0.08 second. The normal QRS duration in adults is 0.08 to 0.10 second.
- The normal QT interval is 0.36 to 0.40 second when the heart rate is normal. One should refer to reference tables, in which the normalcy of the QT interval is determined by relating it to the heart rate (see Table 4-2 at the end of this chapter).

- The mean P vector is normally directed at about +60 degrees in the frontal plane and slightly anterior (Fig. 4-5).
- The mean vector for the first half of the P wave is produced by the depolarization of the RA. It is normally directed at about +65 degrees in the frontal plane and +20 to 30 degrees anteriorly (see Fig. 4-4).
- The mean vector for the second half of the P wave is produced by the depolarization of the LA. It is normally directed at about +55 degrees and is parallel or slightly posterior to the frontal plane (Fig. 4-4). The area of the second half of the P wave measured in lead V_1 is normally about -0.03 mm•sec or less (Fig. 4-19).
- The mean QRS vector is normally *directed* to the right and anteriorly in the neonate (Fig. 4-8). It is directed more vertically and less anteriorly in the young child and adolescent (Fig. 4-8). It may be directed *vertically* at about +80 degrees (rarely more than +90 degrees) and about 40 degrees posteriorly in normal adults (see Fig. 4-8). It is commonly directed in an *intermediate* position at +40 to +60 degrees in the frontal plane and about 40 degrees posteriorly in normal adults (see Fig. 4-8). It may be directed horizontally as far to the left as -20 degrees and 30 to 40 degrees posteriorly in normal adults (see Fig. 4-8). The 12-lead *amplitude* of the QRS complexes is normally 80 to 185 mm.[8] It is computed by adding, in arithmetic fashion, all the negative and positive portions of the QRS complexes of all 12 leads (Fig. 4-20).
- The mean vector for the initial 0.04 second of the QRS complex should be directed to the left of a vertically directed mean QRS vector, to the left or right of an intermediately directed mean QRS vector, and inferior to a horizontally directed mean QRS vector. It should always be directed anterior to the mean QRS vector. The initial 0.04-second-QRS angle should be less than 60 degrees and is commonly 30 to 45 degrees (Fig. 4-21).
- The mean vector for the terminal 0.04 second of the QRS complex is usually directed to the right of a vertically directed mean QRS vector, to the left or right of an intermediately directed QRS vector, and superior to a horizontally directed mean QRS vector. It is usually directed posterior to the mean QRS vector. The terminal 0.04-second-QRS angle is usually 45 to 60 degrees (Fig 4-22).
- The intrinsicoid deflection in lead V_5 or V_6 should normally be 0.04 second or less. The calculation is made by measuring the amount of time that elapses from the beginning of the QRS complex to its zenith.
- The normalcy of the direction of the mean T vector should always be judged by its distance from the mean QRS vector. The normal mean T vector in adults should be located to the left of a vertically directed mean QRS vector, to the right or left of an intermediately directed mean QRS vector, and inferior to a horizontally directed mean QRS vector. It is usually directed parallel with the frontal plane or about 10 to 15 degrees anteriorly. It should be directed anterior to the mean QRS vector. The QRS-T angle of the normal adult should be 45 to 60 degrees or less (see Fig. 4-8). The ventricular gradient, which is an indication of how nearly the sequence of repolarization follows the sequence of depolarization, can be determined by constructing a parallelogram in which the diagonal becomes the ventricular gradient. The gradient should be

directed toward the left lower quadrant of the hexaxial display system. It should be directed anterior to the mean QRS vector and posterior to the mean T vector.
- Normally, no ST segment displacement may occur. When it does occur in normal subjects, the vector representing the ST segment displacement in 12 leads will be directed relatively parallel with the mean T vector; it is rarely more than 45 degrees away from the larger than usual mean T vector. It is caused by early repolarization forces (Fig. 4-23).
- Small U waves are occasionally seen in normal subjects.

An example of a normal ECG is shown in Fig. 4-24. The mean QRS vector is directed in the intermediate zone.

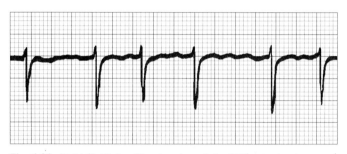

Fig. 4-30. Atrial fibrillation. The duration of the QRS complex is normal. There is a grossly irregular ventricular response, with RR intervals varying from 0.76 to 0.45 second. The baseline shows fibrillatory wave activity with some variation in the depth of the waves.

From Hurst JW, Myerburg RJ: *Introduction to electrocardiography*, ed 2, New York, 1973, McGraw-Hill, p 242. Reprinted with permission from the author.

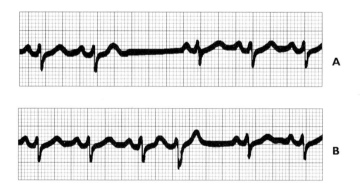

Fig. 4-31. Premature atrial depolarizations, conducted and nonconducted. **A,** The T wave of the second QRS complex on the tracing is slightly deformed by the P wave of the premature atrial depolarization. The premature atrial depolarization is not conducted to the ventricles; thus there is no QRS complex following it. **B,** The fourth atrial depolarization is premature and alters the shape of the T wave. It is conducted, but the QRS complex shows slight aberration of ventricular conduction. There is a P wave in the fourth T wave (note the difference in shape compared with the other T waves). This P wave is not conducted.

From Hurst JW, Myerburg RJ: *Introduction to electrocardiography*, ed 2, New York, 1973, McGraw-Hill, p 246. Reprinted with permission from the author.

ABNORMAL ELECTROCARDIOGRAM[1]

The ECG may be abnormal because of an abnormality of: the heart rate or rhythm, the PR interval, the QRS complex duration, the QT interval, the P waves, the QRS complexes or a part of the QRS complexes, the T waves, or the ST segments.

Abnormalities of Heart Rate and Rhythm

No attempt is made here to discuss and illustrate all the abnormal cardiac rate and rhythm disturbances. Only the common abnormalities are illustrated, and the discussion is limited to the legends (Figs. 4-25 to 4-49).

Abnormal Intervals

The *PR interval* varies with the heart rate: the faster the heart rate, the shorter the PR interval; the slower the heart rate, the longer the PR interval (see Table 4-1 at the end of the chapter). When the heart rate is normal, the PR interval should be 0.20 second or shorter. The PR interval may be longer than normal as the result of *A-V node disease*, such as occurs with myocarditis, digitalis medication, sclerosis from coronary disease, or infiltrative disease. The PR interval may be 0.12 second or less when there is a bypass tract, such as occurs with the Wolff-Parkinson-White syndrome.

The *QRS duration* in adults is normally less than 0.10 second. A QRS duration of 0.11 may develop when an intraventricular conduction defect is present. As a rule, the QRS duration is 0.12 second in patients with right or left bundle branch block. When the other features of right bundle branch block are present, the QRS duration may be only 0.11 second in young people. When the QRS duration is longer than 0.12 second, it is wise to consider a conduction defect in addition to the bundle branch block (see subsequent discussion). This is included as one of the types of complicated bundle branch block.

The normal *QT interval* varies with the heart rate (see Table 4-2 at the end of the chapter). A short QT interval may be caused by digitalis medication or hypercalcemia. A long QT interval may be caused by quinidine, procainamide, coronary disease, hypocalcemia, myocardial disease, or the Romano-Ward syndrome. Patients with a long QT interval are more likely to have ventricular arrhythmia and sudden death. The U wave may become prominent in patients with hypokalemia. When the U wave fuses with the T wave, it may be erroneously interpreted as a long QT interval.

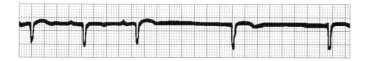

Fig. 4-32. Sinus pause or arrest with junctional escape. The first three complexes show normal sinus rhythm. The duration of the QRS complex is normal. A long pause (1.54 second) follows the third complex and is terminated by an escape beat. The junction escaped several times before a normal sinus mechanism returned. The escape QRS complexes have the same QRS configuration as the sinus beats.

From Hurst JW, Myerburg RJ: *Introduction to electrocardiography*, ed 2, New York, 1973, McGraw-Hill, p 249. Reprinted with permission from the author.

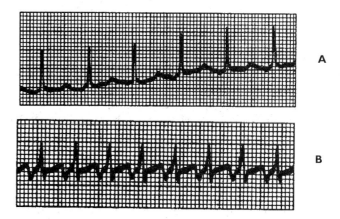

Fig. 4-33. Junctional tachycardia. **A,** The duration of the QRS complex is normal. A relatively slow junctional tachycardia is demonstrated, the rate being approximately 111 ventricular depolarizations per minute. The rhythm is perfectly regular. Since the lead is standard lead II and each QRS complex is preceded by an inverted P wave with a PR interval of 0.09 second, the assumption may be made that retrograde activation of the atria from the junctional pacemaker is occurring. **B,** A rapid junctional tachycardia is shown. The duration of the QRS complex is normal. The rhythm is perfectly regular, and the rate is about 182 ventricular depolarizations per minute. Lead II is shown here, and the QRS complexes are preceded by inverted P waves with a PR interval of 0.10 second, indicating retrograde atrial activation from the junctional pacemaker.

From Hurst JW, Myerburg RJ: *Introduction to electrocardiography*, ed 2, New York, 1973, McGraw-Hill, p 256. Reprinted with permission from the author.

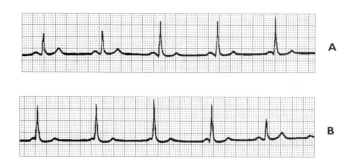

Fig. 4-34. Atrioventricular (A-V) dissociation caused by sinus bradycardia and junctional escape. **A,** The first two complexes are initiated in the sinus node. The A-V conduction is normal. The duration of the QRS complex is normal. The heart rate is just below 60 depolarizations per minute. The third depolarization is a junctional escape beat with a slightly different QRS morphology and shorter interval between the onset of the P wave and the onset of the QRS complex than the preceding depolarizations. **B,** The sinus node rate slows a little more during the next cycles, and the junctional escape rate remains relatively constant, perpetuating the A-V dissociation. As the sinus node rate increase, the P waves emerge from the QRS complexes and finally recapture the ventricles (last complex). The atrial (higher) pacemaker is slower than the junctional (lower) pacemaker during the period of dissociation, permitting the A-V dissociation to occur.

From Hurst JW, Myerburg RJ: *Introduction to electrocardiography*, ed 2, New York, 1973, McGraw-Hill, p 257. Reprinted with permission from the author.

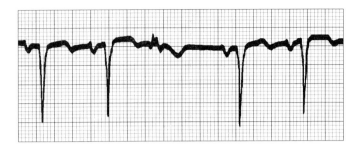

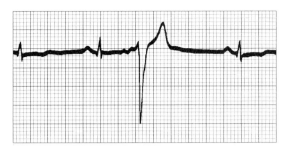

Fig. 4-35. Premature ventricular depolarizations. There is normal sinus rhythm. The third QRS complex occurs early and has a greatly different configuration from that of the normal QRS complexes. It has a QRS duration in excess of 0.12 second and is not preceded by a discernible P wave. It is followed by a full compensatory pause. These characteristics favor the diagnosis of a premature ventricular depolarization. Finally, it could be positively demonstrated in a longer rhythm strip that the sinus node cycle was not interrupted.

From Hurst JW, Myerburg RJ: Introduction to electrocardiography, ed 2, New York, 1973, McGraw-Hill, p 260. Reprinted with permission from the author.

Fig. 4-36. Premature atrial impulse with aberrant ventricular conduction. The first two complexes on the tracing are produced by normal sinus impulses. The P waves, QRS complexes, and PR intervals are normal, and the rate is 67 depolarizations per minute. The T wave of the second complex is deformed by an abnormal, biphasic, early P wave, which is followed by a QRS complex of a distinctly abnormal configuration. Because of the presence of the premature P wave coupled to the abnormal QRS complex by a normal PR interval, the diagnosis of a premature atrial impulse with aberration of ventricular conduction may be made. This occurs because of refractiveness of parts of the A-V junction at the time when the premature impulse arrives, causing an abnormal pathway of conduction. In the case of a premature A-V junctional depolarization with aberrant conduction, the differentiation from premature ventricular depolarization may be more difficult or impossible, depending on the P wave relationship.

From Hurst JW, Myerburg RJ: Introduction to electrocardiography, ed 2, New York, 1973, McGraw-Hill, p 263. Reprinted with permission from the author.

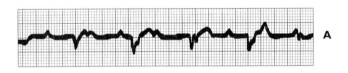

A

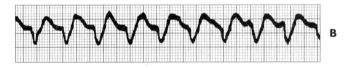

B

Fig. 4-37. Accelerated ventricular rhythm, ventricular tachycardia, and complete heart block. **A,** The duration of the QRS complex is 0.11 second. A-V dissociation is present, as manifested by the absence of any relationship between the P waves and QRS complexes and an idioventricular rhythm. The rate of the idioventricular rhythm, however, is much more rapid than the normal escape rate of a ventricular pacemaker (PR interval of basic rhythm = 0.86 second; rate = 70 depolarizations per minute). Therefore, even though the rate does not conform to the usual definition of tachycardia (rate = 100), it is abnormal for this pacemaker and is called an accelerated ventricular rhythm.

B, Ventricular tachycardia with a rate of 136 depolarizations per minute (recorded from the same patient as in A). Complete heart block is present, and some of the P waves are easily seen. Since the PP intervals are quite constant, the presence of the other P waves is inferred. The P waves and QRS complexes are completely independent of each other because of the complete heart block.

From Hurst JW, Myerburg RJ: Introduction to electrocardiography, ed 2, New York, 1973, McGraw-Hill, p 265. Reprinted with permission from the author.

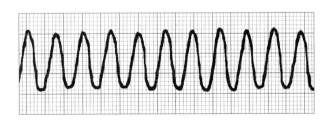

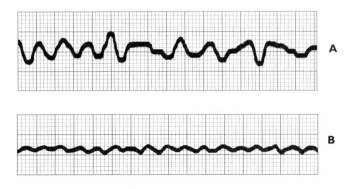

A

B

Fig. 4-38. Ventricular flutter. This rhythm forms a clinical bridge between ventricular tachycardia and ventricular fibrillation. There are very smooth, regular wave forms at a rate of 207 depolarizations per minute. The patient still had a cardiac output at the time of this event, but it was greatly reduced. This rhythm rarely lasts more than a few seconds to a minute, tending to progress rapidly to ventricular fibrillation or to revert to ventricular tachycardia or another rhythm.

From Hurst JW, Myerburg RJ: Introduction to electrocardiography, ed 2, New York, 1973, McGraw-Hill, p 267. Reprinted with permission from the author.

Fig. 4-39. Ventricular fibrillation. This rhythm is incompatible with life, since it represents uncoordinated ventricular activity with no cardiac output. It is, however, frequently treatable, with the success of treatment depending on the setting in which it occurs. **A,** Coarse ventricular fibrillation. Note the irregular wave form activity. **B,** Fine ventricular fibrillation. This type of pattern frequently precedes the complete cessation of electrical activity at the time of biologic death of the heart and is very difficult to defibrillate.

From Hurst JW, Myerburg RJ: Introduction to electrocardiography, ed 2, New York, 1973, McGraw-Hill, p 268. Reprinted with permission from the author.

Right, Left, and Biatrial Abnormalities

Right Atrial Abnormality. An RA abnormality usually signifies RV disease or tricuspid valve disease.

- An RA abnormality may be identified when the mean P vector is directed inferiorly at 50 to 80 degrees and anteriorly.
- The P waves may be more than 2.5 mm high, and their duration may be less than 0.12 second.
- A vector representing the first half of the P wave is directed anteriorly so that portion of the P wave is usually several millimeters high in lead V_1. Such P waves may be seen in patients with pulmonary valve stenosis, tetralogy of Fallot, tricuspid atresia, Ebstein anomaly, pulmonary hypertension caused by primary pulmonary hypertension, Eisenmenger's physiology, repeated pulmonary emboli, severe mitral stenosis or cor pulmonale from chronic lung disease of any cause.

The ECG shown in Fig. 4-50 illustrates an RA abnormality.

An exception exists to the rules just discussed. The ECG abnormality suggesting an LA abnormality may occasionally appear when the RA is greatly enlarged, as with Ebstein's anomaly or tricuspid atresia. This occurs because the wave of RA depolarization travels initially in an anteroinferior direction and then travels inferiorly and posteriorly before it enters the LA wall. In such cases the second half of the P wave may be negative in leads V_1 and V_2 but it is narrow and sharp rather than broad and blunt as it is when there is an LA abnormality.

Left Atrial Abnormality. An LA abnormality usually signifies LV disease or mitral valve disease. An LA abnormality is said to be present when the P wave is 0.12 second or longer in duration and less than 2.5 mm high. The P wave is typically notched at the halfway mark. The second half of the P wave, when represented as a mean vector, is directed inferiorly at about 30 to 60 degrees and 20 to 30 degrees posteriorly. The second half of the P wave is commonly negative in leads V_1, occasionally in lead V_2, and rarely in lead V_3. The size of the second half of the P wave in lead V_1 is greater than -0.03 mm•sec (see Fig. 4-19).[9] The abnormality becomes more likely as the size of this measurement increases.

An LA abnormality may be caused by mitral stenosis, mitral regurgitation, or LV disease from any cause, such as coronary artery disease, cardiomyopathy, hypertension, or aortic valve disease.

The electrocardiogram shown in Fig. 4.51 illustrates an LA abnormality.

Biatrial Abnormality. This abnormality can be occasionally recognized when there are clues to RA and LA abnormalities.

Left Ventricular Hypertrophy

The problem associated with the identification of LV hypertrophy in adults stems from the normal adult having normal LV dominance. Because of this, it is not always possible to separate the ECG features that indicate normal LV dominance from those that indicate abnormal LV hypertrophy.

- *LA abnormality.* A LA abnormality is typically present in patients with LV hypertrophy. Romhilt and Estes[10] give as much diagnostic value to an LA abnormality as they give to increased QRS amplitude in diagnosing LV hypertrophy.

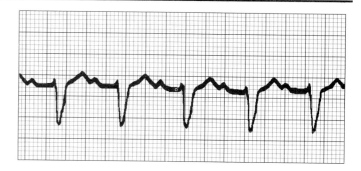

Fig. 4-40. First-degree A-V block. The PR interval is constant and prolonged to 0.27 second. When the heart rate is rapid in the presence of first-degree A-V heart block, the P waves may be buried in the T waves of the preceding complexes.

From Hurst JW, Myerburg RJ: *Introduction to electrocardiography*, ed 2, New York, 1973, McGraw-Hill, p 279. Reprinted with permission from the author.

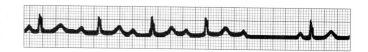

Fig. 4-41. Second-degree heart block, type I (Wenckebach phenomenon). The characteristics of the Wenckebach phenomenon are (1) progressively increasing PR intervals with (2) progressively decreasing RR intervals and (3) a pause caused by a dropped ventricular depolarization, the pause being less than twice the length of the last RR interval (usually the shortest) in the period. The greatest increment in the PR interval occurs between the first and second complexes of any period, and the increment progressively decreases through the period. Thus, in the first Wenckebach period in the ECG, the first PR interval is 0.20 second and the second PR interval is 0.30 second, giving an increment of 0.30 - 0.20 = 0.10 second; the next increment is 0.33 - 0.30 = 0.03 second; and the last increment is 0.35 - 0.33 = 0.02 second. The RR intervals decrease from 0.92 to 0.84 second. The last RR interval before the pause should also decrease but does not do so in this case because of the presence of the concomitant sinus rate variation. The duration of the pause caused by the dropped ventricular depolarization is 1.63 second, which is less than twice the RR interval of the last cycle of the period (0.85 x 2 = 1.70).

From Hurst JW, Myerburg RJ: *Introduction to electrocardiography*, ed 2, New York, 1973, McGraw-Hill, p 280. Reprinted with permission from the author.

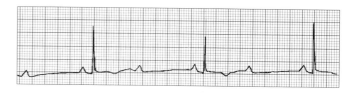

Fig. 4-42. Second-degree heart block, type II. The first, third, and fifth atrial depolarizations (P waves) are blocked. The second, fourth, and sixth atrial depolarizations are conducted with a normal PR interval. The patient has 2:1 A-V block.

From Hurst JW, Myerburg RJ: *Introduction to electrocardiography*, ed 2, New York, 1973, McGraw-Hill, p 281. Reprinted with permission from the author.

- *Duration of the QRS complex.* The QRS complex may be slightly prolonged but does not exceed 0.10 second.
- The *intrinsicoid deflection* measured in leads V_5 or V_6 may be longer than 0.04 second. This measurement is made by determining the duration of the QRS complex from its beginning to its zenith.
- *Direction of the mean QRS vector.* The mean QRS vector is usually directed inferiorly at about +45 degrees. It tends to be more leftward than it was before the development of LV hypertrophy, but is not directed as far as -30 degrees to the left. When the mean QRS vector is -30 degrees or more to the left, an associated conduction defect usually exists. The mean QRS vector is usually directed 40 to 60 degrees posteriorly. When the entire QRS loop is more posterior than normal, as it may be when systolic pressure overload of the LV exists, there may be no R wave in leads V_1, V_2, and V_3. Such an abnormality may be misdiagnosed as anterior myocardial infarction (Fig. 4-52).
- *Amplitude of the QRS complexes.* Numerous criteria are aimed at identifying a larger than normal QRS amplitude. I currently use the total QRS amplitude suggested by Odom et al.[8] The upright and downward deflections of the QRS complexes of all 12 leads are added together arithmetically to determine the 12-lead total QRS amplitude. Normally, the range is 80 to 185 mm. A 12-lead total amplitude of 200 mm in a patient of average body build would signify the *high probability* of LV hypertrophy. A 12-lead total amplitude of 170 mm in an obese patient *might* be caused by LV hypertrophy. This example is given to point out the difficulty or impossibility of the development of any criteria that will always separate normal LV dominance from abnormal LV hypertrophy.
- The *T waves and associated ST segments* become abnormal when LV hypertrophy exists. Systolic pressure overload of the LV tends to produce a type of T wave and ST segment abnormality that differs from the T wave and ST segment abnormality of diastolic pressure overload of the LV.
- *Systolic pressure overload of the LV.* The mean T vector may be directed normally in relation to the mean QRS vector. The mean T vector gradually shifts in direction, and the QRS-T angle gradually increases. The mean T vector can eventually be directed 180 degrees away from the mean QRS vector. Accordingly, it shifts rightward and anteriorly when the mean QRS vector is directed in the intermediate or horizontal position, and tends to shift anteriorly and become superior to a vertically directed mean QRS vector. The mean ST vector tends to be directed within 45 to 60 degrees of the mean T vector. The change in T wave direction is caused by the gradual elimination of the transventricular pressure gradient because of high systolic pressure in the LV.

Systolic pressure overload of the LV is produced by systemic hypertension, aortic valve stenosis, hypertrophic cardiomyopathy, and as discussed next, late in the course of diastolic pressure overload of the LV.

The ECG shown in Fig. 4-53 illustrates LV hypertrophy caused by systolic pressure overload of the LV.

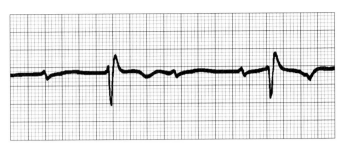

Fig. 4-43. Complete heart block. The duration of the QRS complex is 0.16 second. The ventricular rate is 32 depolarizations per minute, and the ventricular rhythm is regular. No fixed relationship exists between the P waves and QRS complexes. Some of the P waves fall within the QRS complexes or T waves and may be difficult to discern. A longer rhythm strip revealed some variation in the PP intervals. Note in this short strip that the P wave irregularity has a definite pattern; namely, the PP interval tends to be shorter when a QRS complex falls between the two P waves and tends to be longer when the two P waves fall between two QRS complexes. This phenomenon is called *ventricular sinus arrhythmia*, a common finding in complete heart block with normal atrial activity.

From Hurst JW, Myerburg RJ: *Introduction to electrocardiography,* ed 2, New York, 1973, McGraw-Hill, p 282. Reprinted with permission from the author.

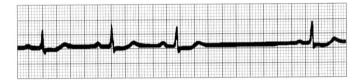

Fig. 4-44. Intermittent second-degree sinoatrial block (type II). The first three complexes on the tracing are normal sinus beats at a rate of approximately 60 ventricular depolarizations per minute. These are followed by a pause approximately equal to two cycle lengths. No P wave is seen during this pause. Since the pause is equal to two cycle lengths, it is inferred that the normal pacemaker function of the sinus node has not been interrupted and that the block therefore must have occurred between the sinus node and the atrial tissue (sinoatrial junction). A second pause was observed later in the rhythm strip. It was terminated by a junctional escape depolarization, since the pause was long enough to allow the escape of the intrinsic junctional pacemaker. The clue indicating the escape mechanism was the short PR interval of the escape depolarization, indicating that the A-V node escaped before the atrial impulse could be conducted through the A-V node.

From Hurst JW, Myerburg RJ: *Introduction to electrocardiography,* ed 2, New York, 1973, McGraw-Hill, p 287. Reprinted with permission from the author.

- *Diastolic pressure overload of the LV* produces a different type of T wave abnormality, than the abnormality just described. This abnormality is seen early in the course of diastolic pressure overload or when the condition causing it is mild. Later, the T wave abnormality may become similar to that described for systolic pressure overload of the LV. When early or mild diastolic pressure overload of the LV occurs, the mean T vector becomes larger than normal but may be directed normally. This probably occurs because the endocardial surface area is larger when diastolic pressure overload causes LV dilatation. The initial portion of the QRS complex also becomes larger than normal for the same reason. The mean ST vector tends to be directed parallel to the T wave.

The ECG shown in Fig. 4-54 illustrates LV hypertrophy caused by diastolic pressure overload of the LV.

Right Ventricular Hypertrophy

The normal newborn child has normal RV dominance. The mean QRS vector is normally directed to the right and anteriorly. Therefore, it is sometimes difficult to determine the presence of abnormal RV hypertrophy. One clue is that the mean T vector is directed anteriorly in the newborn when RV hypertrophy exists, whereas it is normally directed posteriorly.

As the normal child grows older, the mean QRS vector gradually shifts inferiorly, leftward, and posteriorly and the mean T vector gradually shifts to a position that is inferior, leftward, and parallel with the frontal plane (see Fig. 4-8). With the preceding as background, it is possible to identify two types of RV hypertrophy.

- *Systolic pressure overload of the RV.* This type of RV hypertrophy can be divided into two types of abnormalities. First, RV hypertrophy caused by conditions that are present at birth, such as pulmonary valve stenosis or tetralogy of Fallot, may produce a mean QRS vector that is directed to the right and anteriorly. The mean T vector is directed inferiorly to the left and posteriorly. In such cases the mean QRS vector never shifts to the left, inferiorly, and posteriorly as it does normally (Fig. 4-55). Second, when RV hypertrophy develops in a patient in whom the normal shift of the mean QRS vector to the left, inferiorly, and posteriorly has already occurred, the mean QRS vector may become directed inferiorly and slightly posteriorly. For example, patients with mitral stenosis may initially have a mean QRS vector that is directed normally, but as pulmonary hypertension develops, the mean QRS vector shifts inferiorly but may remain posteriorly directed. Later, the mean QRS vector is directed to the right and anteriorly. The direction of the mean T vector shifts from its normal position to be directed more leftward and posteriorly. This same sequence occurs in patients with primary pulmonary hypertension, repeated pulmonary emboli, the gradual development of Eisenmenger physiology, and chronic pulmonary disease.

The additional abnormalities include the presence of an RA abnormality and increase QRS amplitude. The latter is not as important as it is in identifying LV hypertrophy because the direction of the mean QRS vector in the adult with RV hypertrophy is so obviously abnormal that, as a rule, the amplitude is disregarded. Occasionally it is useful to measure the amplitude of the R wave in lead I when the mean QRS vector is directed inferiorly and parallel with the frontal plane. RV hypertrophy is likely when the R wave in lead V_1 is as tall or taller than the S wave is deep, when the R wave in lead V_1 is more than 3 mm high, and when the intrinsicoid deflection in lead V_1 is more than 0.03 second.

The QRS amplitude may be less than normal in patients with RV hypertrophy caused by obstructive lung disease and emphysema.

- *Diastolic pressure overload of the RV.* The most common cause of diastolic pressure overload of the RV is ostium secundum septal defect. This produces an RV conduction delay on the ECG, which masks the findings of diastolic overload of the RV that could theoretically develop. An RV conduction delay is characterized by a QRS duration of 0.08 to 0.10 second; mean QRS vector directed to the right and anteriorly; terminal 0.04 second of the QRS complexes, when represented as a mean vector, is directed

to the right and anteriorly (this produces an rSR¹ deflection in lead V_1), and a mean T vector directed to the left and posteriorly away from the RV. This type of tracing may evolve into right bundle branch block.

The ECG shown in Fig. 4-56 illustrates right ventricular conduction delay (RVCD). RVCD can mark diastolic overload of the RV.

QRS Conduction Abnormalities

Left Ventricular Conduction Delay. LV conduction delay is identified when the QRS duration is 0.10 or 0.11 second and all other features of uncomplicated left bundle branch block are present. The condition is often associated with LV hypertrophy but may also represent a conduction abnormality in the septum.

Uncomplicated Left Bundle Branch Block. This common conduction abnormality has the following features:

- The duration of the QRS complexes is 0.12 second.
- The mean QRS vector is directed to the left and posteriorly. It will shift only 45 to 60 degrees to the left of its preblock position and is never directed beyond -30 degrees in the frontal plane.
- The mean initial 0.04-second vector is directed to the left and posteriorly because the septum is depolarized from right to left. Therefore, no Q wave occurs in leads I and V_6, and the R wave is small or absent in lead V_1.
- The mean terminal 0.04-second vector is directed to the left and posteriorly and indicates the LV area that depolarizes last.
- The mean T vector is directed about 150 to 180 degrees away from the mean QRS vector. It is directed to the right and anteriorly.
- The mean ST segment vector is directed within 45 to 60 degrees of the mean T vector.
- The ventricular gradient is directed normally.

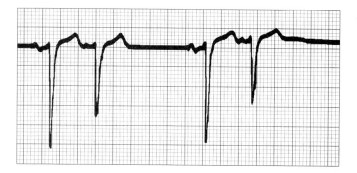

Fig. 4-45. Atrial bigeminy. The first and third P-QRS complexes on the tracing are normal sinus depolarizations. Each is followed by a premature atrial depolarization, which is followed by slightly aberrant ventricular conduction, and a pause occurs after each premature depolarization. Therefore the characteristic feature is groups of two depolarizations—one normal and one premature—followed by a pause. The coupling interval, the interval between the sinus P wave and the ectopic P wave, is constant at 0.55 second. The pattern is designated as atrial bigeminy because the coupled ectopic beats are atrial in origin.

From Hurst JW, Myerburg RJ: *Introduction to electrocardiography,* ed 2, New York, 1973, McGraw-Hill, p 289. Reprinted with permission from the author.

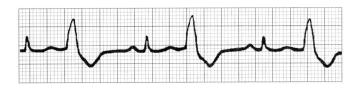

Fig. 4-46. Ventricular bigeminy. The first, third, and fifth complexes on the ECG are normal depolarizations. Each of these is followed by an ectopic ventricular depolarization of abnormal configuration and a QRS complex prolongation beyond 0.12 second. No P waves precede these ectopic complexes. (NOTE: The positive deflections preceding the ectopic complexes are the T waves of the preceding sinus depolarizations.) The ectopic depolarizations are coupled to the preceding depolarizations by a fixed coupling interval of 0.48 second, as measured from the onset of the sinus-induced QRS to the onset of the ectopic QRS. A pause then occurs; therefore the depolarizations are occurring in groups of two (bigeminy). Because the ectopic ventricular depolarizations fulfill the criteria for ventricular ectopic depolarizations, and because the pattern occurs in groups of two depolarizations, the rhythm is called ventricular bigeminy.

From Hurst JW, Myerburg RJ: *Introduction to electrocardiography*, ed 2, New York, 1973, McGraw-Hill, p 290. Reprinted with permission from the author.

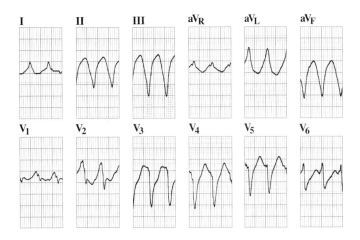

Fig. 4-47. Ventricular tachycardia (VT) proved with electrophysiologic studies; recorded from a patient with idiopathic dilated cardiomyopathy). It is not always possible to identify VT by examining a surface ECG, since there are many other causes of a wide–QRS complex tachycardia. For example, a patient with sinus tachycardia or supraventricular tachycardia (SVT) who has right bundle branch block, left bundle branch block, or preexcitation of the ventricles may have an ECG that simulates VT. In addition, a patient with SVT may develop aberrant ventricular conduction, and the abnormal QRS complexes may mimic VT. Most troublesome of all is that a narrow–QRS complex tachycardia may occasionally be ventricular in origin; the impulse originates in the upper portion of the septum. The following points should be made regarding VT:

- When the duration of the QRS complex is 0.14 second or more with a right bundle branch block pattern or greater than 0.16 second with a left bundle branch block pattern, the diagnosis is usually VT. When the QRS duration is 0.12 second during an episode of tachycardia in a patient whose QRS complex was normal before the episode, SVT with ventricular aberrancy or VT may be the cause. VT may be present when the QRS duration is only 0.11 second; this, however, occurs infrequently.
- The ventricular rate of VT is usually about 150 to 200 depolarizations per minute; however, it may be greater than 200. A ventricular rate less than 100 depolarizations per minute is called *accelerated ventricular rhythm*. The ventricular rate cannot be used to distinguish SVT with aberrancy from VT.
- The rhythm of VT is usually regular when the tachycardia is sustained. The rhythm may be slightly irregular when the VT is not sustained and may be difficult to distinguish from atrial fibrillation with aberrant ventricular conduction.

- When the P waves are easily seen and have no relationship to the abnormally wide QRS complexes, VT is present. When inverted P waves follow the QRS complexes. they are considered to be retrograde P waves; this may occur in VT. Unfortunately, it is not always possible to identify the P waves with certainty.
- Tachycardia that is preceded by a fusion beat is usually caused by VT.
- The shape of the QRS complex provides perhaps the most important means of distinguishing VT from SVT with aberrant ventricular conduction: the QRS complex recorded at electrode position V₁ has a larger R wave than the R′ wave when there is VT, whereas a small initial R wave followed by a larger R′ wave indicates SVT with aberrant conduction. When the QRS deflection recorded at each of the precordial electrode positions is negative or positive, the rhythm is usually VT.
- Physical signs of VT include a first heart sound that may vary in intensity from beat to beat because the relationship of atrial contraction to ventricular contraction varies from beat to beat. This sign is not present when atrial fibrillation occurs in conjunction with VT. Also, the pulsation of the internal jugular veins may be erratic, since the right atrium may occasionally contract against a close tricuspid valve in patients with VT.
- Based on the clinical setting, a patient with a fresh myocardial infarct is more likely to have VT than SVT with aberrant ventricular conduction, whereas a young woman who has no other apparent cardiac disease is more likely to have SVT with aberrant ventricular conduction than VT.
- Accelerated ventricular rhythm is usually not as serious as VT but is occasionally the forerunner of more serious ventricular arrhythmias.
- Bidirectional VT is usually caused by digitalis intoxication.
- When the rhythm cannot be identified with certainty, it should be managed as VT.
- If the rhythm is believed to be SVT with ventricular aberrancy, adenosine should be administered. Verapamil should be avoided for treatment of a wide-complex tachycardia.

Courtesy Sina Zaim, MD, Emory University School of Medicine, Atlanta.

Reproduced with permission from Hurst JW: *Cardiovascular diagnosis: the initial examination*, St Louis, 1993, Mosby, pp 234-235.

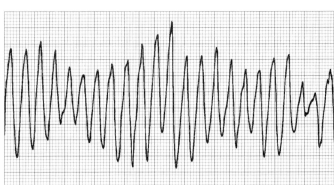

Fig. 4-48. Ventricular tachycardia showing torsades de pointes. The words *torsades de pointes* mean "turning on a point." This rhythm occurred in this 48-year-old man several days after coronary bypass surgery. He probably had an intraoperative myocardial infarction.

Courtesy Sina Zaim, MD, Emory University School of Medicine, Atlanta.

Reproduced with permission from Hurst JW: *Cardiovascular diagnosis: the initial examination*, St Louis, 1993, Mosby, p 236.

When the duration of the QRS complex is 0.12 second and the mean QRS vector, initial and terminal 0.04 vectors, mean T and ST vectors, and ventricular gradient are arranged as just described, the conduction of defects is labeled as being *uncomplicated left bundle branch block*.

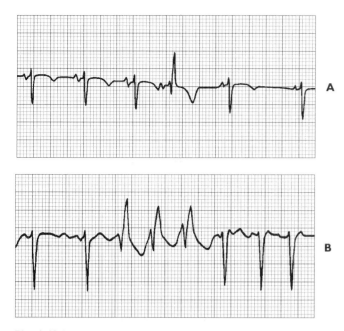

Fig. 4-49. Ventricular aberration. **A,** A premature atrial depolarization is followed by a ventricular depolarization that has a different shape than the preceding ventricular complexes. The shape is different because the electrical impulse occurs so early that a certain part of the ventricles is still refractory. Accordingly, the ventricles are depolarized in an aberrant manner. The altered QRS complex typically simulates the complexes that are characteristic of right bundle branch block. **B,** Ashman phenomenon is identified in patients with atrial fibrillation. It is a special type of aberrant conduction. The refractory period of the ventricles is determined by the length of the RR interval. Stated another way, the refractory period adjusts to the heart rate. When the rate is slow, the refractory period is long; when the rate is rapid, the refractory period is short. The varying RR interval associated with atrial fibrillation causes varying refractory periods. Accordingly, whenever an impulse arrives early and follows a complex with a preceding long RR interval, it sets the stage for aberrant ventricular depolarization. Note here that the RR interval preceding the first aberrant complex is short and that it follows the long RR interval of the previous ventricular depolarization. The shape of the third, fourth, and fifth QRS complexes is altered because of aberrant conduction in the ventricles.

A from Stein E: *Electrocardiographic interpretation: a self-study approach to clinical electrocardiography,* Philadelphia, 1991, Lea & Febiger, p 609. Reprinted with permission. **B** from Fox W, Stein E: *Cardiac rhythm disturbances: a step-by-step approach,* Philadelphia, 1983, Lea & Febiger, p 179. Reprinted with permission.

This abnormality may be caused by coronary artery disease, cardiomyopathy, severe aortic valve disease, cardiac surgery, extreme LV hypertrophy from any cause, and disease of the conduction system (Lenegre's disease, Lev's disease).

An example of uncomplicated left bundle branch block is shown in Fig. 4-57.

Complicated Left Bundle Branch Block. Complicated bundle branch block is said to be present when one or more of the following additional abnormalities are present:

- The duration of the QRS complex may be longer than 0.12 second. This occurs when the conduction defect also involves the more distal parts of the conduction system. It suggests a Purkinje-myocyte junction defect. It is caused by cardiomyopathy, including multiple large or small myocardial infarctions, myocarditis, severe aortic valve disease, hypothermia, cardiotoxic drugs, and primary disease of the conduction system.

- The mean QRS vector is 0.12 second or longer and is directed more than 30 degrees to the left. This indicates left bundle branch block and left anterosuperior division block (Fig. 4-58). This may be caused by the same conditions just listed.
- The mean T vector may be directed so that the ventricular gradient is not normal. This may be caused by coronary heart disease, including ischemia associated with myocardial infarction or cardiomyopathy. This is called a *primary T wave abnormality.*
- When the ST segment vector is more than 60 degrees from the mean T vector, it may be caused by epicardial injury of infarction.

Note that with left bundle branch block, it is difficult to identify an initial QRS force abnormality when a myocardial infarction exists, but the ST and T wave abnormalities of infarction may be identifiable (Fig. 4-59).

Left Anterosuperior Division Block. Note in Fig. 4-3 that the left bundle has two major divisions. When the anterosuperior division of the left bundle fails to conduct, the depolarization of the LV is initiated by the electrical impulse that is transmitted by the posteroinferior division of the left bundle. This shifts the entire LV depolarization process to the left and posteriorly. The following ECG characteristics are to be expected:

- The duration of the QRS complex may become slightly longer than normal but does not exceed 0.10 or 0.11 second.
- The mean QRS vector is directed at -30 degrees or more to the left and posteriorly.
- A secondary T wave abnormality may develop.

This abnormality may accompany LV hypertrophy and may be caused by coronary artery disease, cardiomyopathy, or primary disease of the conduction system. At times it is unexplained.

An example of left anterosuperior division block is shown in Fig. 4-60.

Left Posteroinferior Division Block. This conduction defect is often associated with right bundle branch block but may appear as an isolated abnormality.

- The QRS duration is no longer than 0.10 second.
- The mean QRS vector is directed +120 degrees to the right and slightly posterior.
- The terminal mean 0.04-second vector is directed far to the right. It may be directed posteriorly or may be parallel with the frontal plane.

It is difficult to identify posteroinferior division block without a previous tracing showing normal conduction. One must rule out RV conduction delay, RV hypertrophy, and lateral infarction as causes of the rightward shift of the QRS vector.

This conduction defect may be caused by coronary artery disease, cardiomyopathy, or primary disease of the conduction system.

Left posteroinferior division block is typically associated with right bundle branch block. It is suspected when the mean QRS vector is more than +120 degrees to the right (see Fig. 4-62).

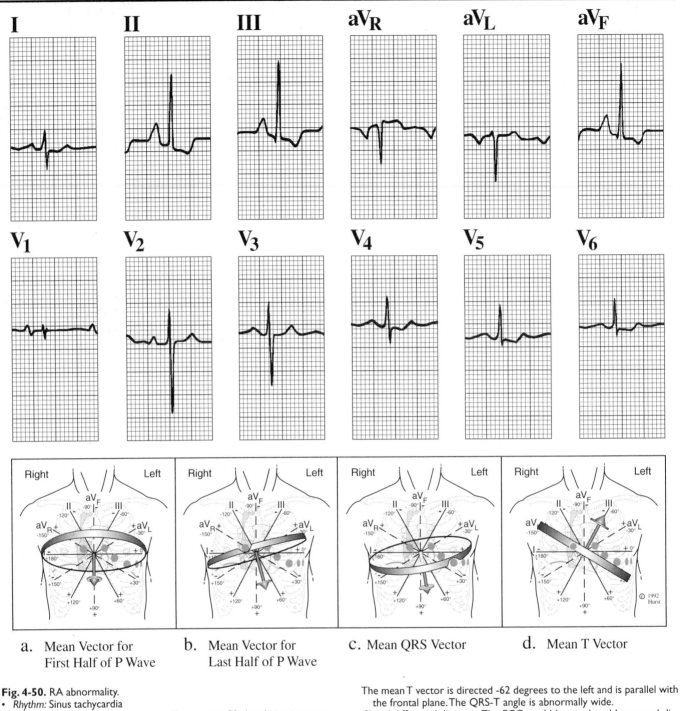

I II III aV_R aV_L aV_F

V₁ V₂ V₃ V₄ V₅ V₆

a. Mean Vector for First Half of P Wave

b. Mean Vector for Last Half of P Wave

c. Mean QRS Vector

d. Mean T Vector

Fig. 4-50. RA abnormality.

- *Rhythm:* Sinus tachycardia
  Rate: Undetermined in short strip. There were 99 depolarizations per minute in a longer strip.
  PR interval: 0.16 second in lead II. Note that the PR interval in lead I is 0.13 second; the first half of the P wave in this lead is isoelectric.
  QRS duration: 0.07 second
  QT interval: 0.28 second
- *Vector diagrams of electrical forces:* See *a, b, c,* and *d* under the ECG.
- *Electrophysiologic considerations:*
  The P waves are abnormal. The duration of the P wave in lead II is 0.09 second, and its amplitude is 4 mm. The vector representing the first half of the P wave is directed about +90 degrees inferiorly and is anteriorly directed. These abnormalities indicate an RA with a predictive value of 100%. The last half of the P wave is normal.
  The mean QRS vector is directed about +78 degrees inferiorly and about 30 degrees posteriorly. The direction of this QRS vector could be normal but is likely to be abnormal when a definite RA abnormality is present. The vertical but posterior direction of the vector suggests that it could be RV hypertrophy from acquired heart disease.

The mean T vector is directed -62 degrees to the left and is parallel with the frontal plane. The QRS-T angle is abnormally wide.

- *Clinical differential diagnosis:* The ECG could be produced by several diseases that can cause an RA abnormality and a vertically directed mean QRS vector that is posteriorly directed. These include repeated pulmonary emboli, Eisenmenger syndrome, and primary pulmonary hypertension. A mean QRS vector of this type is not caused by congenital heart disease such as tetralogy of Fallot or severe pulmonary valve stenosis. This type of QRS vector is typically seen during the early course of acquired RV hypertrophy, such as may occur from one of the conditions just listed.
- *Discussion:* This ECG was recorded from a 50-year-old woman with primary pulmonary hypertension. The systolic pressure in the pulmonary artery was 100 mm Hg.

Reproduced with permission from Hurst JW: *Cardiovascular diagnosis: the initial examination,* St Louis, 1993, Mosby, pp 271, 272.

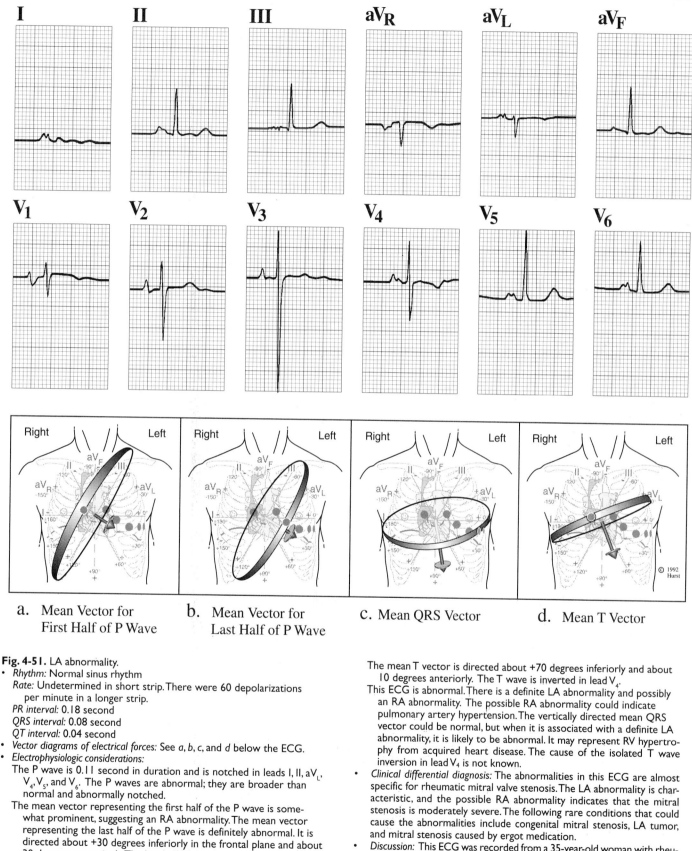

a. Mean Vector for
   First Half of P Wave

b. Mean Vector for
   Last Half of P Wave

c. Mean QRS Vector

d. Mean T Vector

Fig. 4-51. LA abnormality.

- *Rhythm:* Normal sinus rhythm
  Rate: Undetermined in short strip. There were 60 depolarizations per minute in a longer strip.
  PR interval: 0.18 second
  QRS interval: 0.08 second
  QT interval: 0.04 second
- *Vector diagrams of electrical forces:* See *a, b, c,* and *d* below the ECG.
- *Electrophysiologic considerations:*

  The P wave is 0.11 second in duration and is notched in leads I, II, aV$_L$, V$_4$, V$_5$, and V$_6$. The P waves are abnormal; they are broader than normal and abnormally notched.

  The mean vector representing the first half of the P wave is somewhat prominent, suggesting an RA abnormality. The mean vector representing the last half of the P wave is definitely abnormal. It is directed about +30 degrees inferiorly in the frontal plane and about 30 degrees posteriorly. The last half of the P wave in lead V$_1$ measures at least 0.08 mm·sec; this indicates an LA abnormality with a predictive value of 100%.

  The mean QRS vector is directed about +80 degrees inferiorly and about 50 degrees posteriorly.

  The mean T vector is directed about +70 degrees inferiorly and about 10 degrees anteriorly. The T wave is inverted in lead V$_4$.

  This ECG is abnormal. There is a definite LA abnormality and possibly an RA abnormality. The possible RA abnormality could indicate pulmonary artery hypertension. The vertically directed mean QRS vector could be normal, but when it is associated with a definite LA abnormality, it is likely to be abnormal. It may represent RV hypertrophy from acquired heart disease. The cause of the isolated T wave inversion in lead V$_4$ is not known.

- *Clinical differential diagnosis:* The abnormalities in this ECG are almost specific for rheumatic mitral valve stenosis. The LA abnormality is characteristic, and the possible RA abnormality indicates that the mitral stenosis is moderately severe. The following rare conditions that could cause the abnormalities include congenital mitral stenosis, LA tumor, and mitral stenosis caused by ergot medication.
- *Discussion:* This ECG was recorded from a 35-year-old woman with rheumatic mitral stenosis. The mitral valve area was 0.7 cm, and the resting pulmonary artery pressure was 38/18 mm Hg.

ECG courtesy Henry Hanley, MD, University of Louisiana at Shreveport.

Reproduced with permission from Hurst JW: *Cardiovascular diagnosis: the initial examination,* St Louis, 1993, Mosby, pp 268, 269.

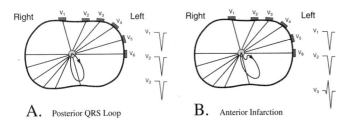

A. Posterior QRS Loop

B. Anterior Infarction

Fig. 4-52. Absent R waves in leads V$_1$, V$_2$, and V$_3$. **A,** When the QRS loop is located posteriorly, the initial portion of the loop may project negatively on leads V$_1$, V$_2$, and V$_3$. This may be produced by LV hypertrophy, septal infarction, or for unknown reasons. In an individual tracing, it cannot be declared that it is definitely caused by infarction (as is frequently done). **B,** Note the difference in this ECG compared with the one shown in **A.** Leads V$_1$ and V$_2$ show complexes, and lead V$_3$ shows a Q wave followed by an R wave and S wave. Compare the QRS loop shown here with the QRS loop shown in **A.** Here the initial electrical forces (vectors) are directed posterior to the subsequent electrical forces (vectors). This abnormality usually indicates the presence of a septal dead zone. Only the initial 0.01 to 0.02 second of the electrical forces (vectors) may be altered in this situation. This is an example of an initial QRS abnormality caused by a dead zone that does not occupy the initial 0.04 second of the QRS complex. It is usually caused by septal infarction but may be caused by any process that infiltrates the septum's superior portion.

Reproduced with permission from Hurst JW: *Cardiovascular diagnosis: the initial examination*, St Louis, 1993, Mosby, p 360.

Uncomplicated Right Bundle Branch Block. This common abnormality has the following features:

- The duration of the QRS complex is 0.12 second. In children it may be only 0.11 second.
- The mean QRS vector shifts to the right and anteriorly no more than 45 to 60 degrees from its preblock direction. The mean QRS vector is not directed more than 110 to 120 degrees to the right.
- The initial QRS forces change very little because the septum depolarizes normally from left to right. Accordingly, myocardial infarcts can be recognized when right bundle branch block occurs.
- The mean T vector is directed to the left and posteriorly away from the mean QRS vector.
- The ventricular gradient remains normal when only a secondary T wave change exists.
- The mean ST vector is directed relatively parallel with the mean T vector. It is usually directed less than 45 to 60 degrees away from the mean T vector.

The conduction defect can be caused by coronary artery disease, cardiomyopathy, cardiac surgery, and RV dilatation and hypertrophy such as occurs with pulmonary emboli or ostium secundum atrial septal defect.

An example of uncomplicated right bundle branch is shown in Fig. 4-61.

Complicated Right Bundle Branch Block. Complicated right bundle branch block can be identified when one or more of the following additional abnormalities are present:

- The duration of the QRS complexes may be more than 0.12 second. This suggests a conduction abnormality in the distal portion of the conduction system, as may occur with coronary artery disease, cardiomyopathy, or extreme dilatation of the RV, or primary disease of the conduction system.

- The mean QRS vector may be directed more than +120 degrees to the right. This is usually caused by additional left posteroinferior division block. The terminal mean 0.04 vector may be directed far to the right and anterior or parallel with the frontal plane. This unusual abnormality may be caused by coronary artery disease, cardiomyopathy, or primary disease of the conduction system.
- The mean initial 0.04-second vector may become abnormal because of myocardial infarction. This can occur because the ventricular septum and LV endocardium depolarize almost normally in patients with right bundle branch block.
- The mean T vector may be abnormal when an additional *primary repolarization* abnormality exists. This can be recognized when the ventricular gradient is abnormal. This may be caused by ischemia resulting from coronary artery disease.
- A *primary ST segment abnormality* may be identified when the ST segment vector is more than 45 to 60 degrees away from the mean T vector. It may be caused by epicardial injury of myocardial infarction.

An example of complicated right bundle branch block is shown in Fig. 4-62.

Right Bundle Branch Block Plus Left Anterosuperior Division Block. This combination of conduction defects has the following features:

- The QRS duration is 0.12 second or more.
- The mean QRS vector is directed more than -30 degrees to the left and anteriorly.

Such an abnormality may be caused by an ostium primum atrial septal defect, cardiomyopathy (including ischemic cardiomyopathy from coronary disease), or primary disease of the conduction system.

An example of this abnormality is shown in Fig. 4-63.

Right Bundle Branch Block Plus Left Posteroinferior Division Block. This combination of conduction abnormalities should be suspected when the QRS complex is 0.12 second or more in duration and the mean QRS vector is directed more than 120 degrees to the right and anteriorly. The terminal mean 0.04-second vector is directed far to the right and may be directed anteriorly or parallel with the frontal plane.

Such an abnormality may be caused by coronary artery disease, cardiomyopathy, or primary disease of the conduction system.

An example of this abnormality is shown in Fig. 4-62.

S$_1$, S$_2$, S$_3$ Type of Conduction Defect. This unusual conduction defect has the following characteristics:

- The duration of the QRS complex is normal.
- A mean vector for the QRS complexes is difficult to diagram because the basic QRS loop is rotund. The first half of the QRS complex is directed inferiorly, and the last half of the QRS complex is directed superiorly.
- The mean T vector is directed normally. It may be larger than usual.

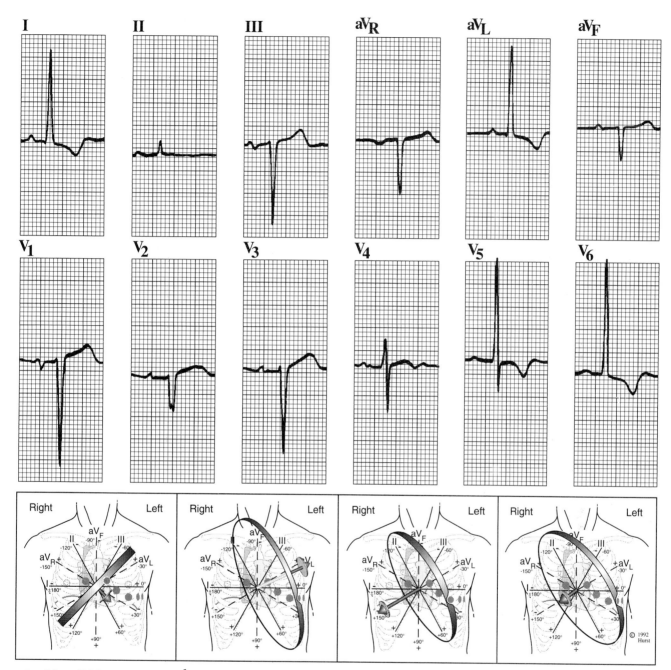

a. Mean P Vector b. Mean QRS Vector c. Mean T Vector d. Mean ST Vector

Fig. 4-53. LV hypertrophy caused by systolic pressure overload of the LV.
- *Rhythm:* Normal sinus rhythm
  Rate: Undetermined in short strip. There were 70 depolarizations per minute in a longer strip.
- *PR interval:* 0.20 second
  QRS duration: 0.09 second
  QT interval: 0.40 second
- *Vector diagrams of electrical forces:* See *a, b, c,* and *d* below the ECG.
- *Electrophysiologic considerations:*
  The PR interval is 0.20 second; this is at the upper limit of normal but is more likely to be abnormally long for this patient.
  The mean P vector is directed about +50 degrees inferiorly and is parallel with the frontal plane. The last half of the P wave in lead V_1 measures -0.08 mm·sec. This indicates a definite LA abnormality.
  The mean QRS vector is directed about -25 degrees to the left and 50 to 60 degrees posteriorly. The 12-lead QRS amplitude is 202 mm. This indicates LV hypertrophy.

The mean T vector is directed +150 degrees to the right and 30 to 40 degrees anteriorly. Note that it is directed opposite to the mean QRS vector.
The mean ST vector is parallel with the mean T vector.
These abnormalities are characteristic of LV hypertrophy caused by pressure overload of the LV.
- *Clinical differential diagnosis:* Systolic pressure overload of the LV may be caused by aortic valve stenosis, systemic hypertension of the heart or may occur in the late course of aortic regurgitation.
- *Discussion:* This ECG was recorded from a 66-year-old man with aortic valve stenosis. The systolic gradient across the aortic valve was 119 mm Hg.

Reproduced with permission from Hurst JW: *Cardiovascular diagnosis: the initial examination,* St. Louis, 1993, Mosby, pp 282, 283.

This type of defect may occur in otherwise normal hearts. It may represent a congenital anomaly of the conduction system. It may occur in patients with cor pulmonale or idiopathic hypertrophy of the heart.

Myocardial Infarction

Three potential abnormalities (see Fig. 4-66a) are associated with myocardial infarction:

- The abnormalities of the *initial portion of the QRS complex*. The dead zone of an infarct is usually largest in the endocardium and smallest at the epicardium. Infarcts are located in the LV, septum, and occasionally in the RV. The dead zone removes electrical forces and permits the electrical forces of the opposite wall of the myocardium to produce abnormally large electrical forces.

    Therefore, the initial 0.03 to 0.04 second of the QRS complex, when represented as a mean vector, is directed away from the area of dead tissue (Figs. 4-64 and 4-65).

- A new *ST segment displacement* develops and, when represented as a mean vector, is directed toward the area of predominant epicardial injury that surrounds the dead zone. The mean ST vector is directed toward a segment of the myocardium, rather than toward the centroid of the LV, as it does with pericarditis (Fig. 4-66). The ST segment displacement caused by epicardial injury usually decreases in magnitude during the days and weeks after a myocardial infarction. When it persists, it usually results from a ventricular aneurysm.

    The mean ST vector associated with subendocardial injury is directed away from the centroid of the subendocardial injury. Accordingly, it is typically directed opposite to the mean QRS vector.

- An area of predominant epicardial ischemia surrounds the area of predominant epicardial injury. A mean vector representing the T wave is directed away from the area of epicardial ischemia (Fig. 4-66).

Examples of ECGs illustrating myocardial infarction are shown in Figs. 4-62 and 4-67 to 4-73.

Myocardial infarction is usually caused by atherosclerotic coronary heart disease but may be caused by coronary embolus, coronary arteritis, coronary artery spasm, Kawasaki syndrome, dissection of the aorta, and trauma.

Pseudomyocardial "Infarction"

Some persons memorize that all large abnormal Q waves are caused by myocardial infarction from atherosclerotic coronary heart disease. Such an approach to the interpretation of ECGs leads to many diagnostic errors because abnormal Q waves have many causes other than myocardial infarction. For example, patients with preexcitation of the ventricles, idiopathic ventricular hypertrophy, systolic pressure overload of the LV, diastolic pressure overload of the LV, cardiomyopathy from infiltrative disease processes such as amyloid or neoplasia, pulmonary embolism, or complex congenital heart disease may have abnormal Q waves suggesting myocardial infarction.

Idiopathic Hypertrophy

Myocardial infarction does not usually produce increased QRS amplitude that suggests LV hypertrophy. Therefore, when signs of LV hypertrophy plus signs of myocardial infarction are present in the ECG, it is wise to consider the likelihood of idiopathic hypertrophy of the heart or two coexisting conditions, such as aortic valve stenosis or hypertension plus atherosclerotic coronary heart disease.

Idiopathic hypertrophy of the heart produces subaortic valve obstruction, predominant midventricular hypertrophy, or apical hypertrophy. The following ECG abnormalities may be seen:

- A left atrial abnormality
- An increase in amplitude of the QRS complexes
- Abnormal initial 0.04-second vector suggesting a septal, inferior, or anterior myocardial infarction
- An abnormal, persistent, mean ST vector suggesting epicardial injury
- The mean T wave vector may be directed more than 60 degrees away from the mean QRS vector. At times the T wave abnormality is huge. This, when appearing alone, favors apical hypertrophy

The ECG of a patient with idiopathic hypertrophy is shown in Fig. 4-74.

Pericarditis

The electrocardiographic abnormalities of three types of pericardial disease are listed below.

- *Acute pericarditis* produces damage to the epicardium. The damage is usually generalized when caused by a viral or bacterial infection. It may be localized occasionally when it is caused by cardiac surgery or trauma.

    A *PQ segment depression* develops but may not be seen in all leads.

    The QRS amplitude does not change unless sufficient pericardial fluid exists to produce low QRS amplitude.

    A new ST segment vector develops that, when represented as a vector, is directed toward the centroid of the LV when generalized epicardial damage exists. It is usually directed inferiorly, to the left, and parallel with the frontal plane. When, on rare occasions, there is localized pericarditis, the mean ST vector is directed toward the damaged segment of epicardium.

    The mean T vector is directed away from the centroid of epicardial damage. Accordingly, it is directed opposite to the mean ST vector. The T vector becomes larger as the ST vector becomes smaller.

- The QRS amplitude does not change unless sufficient pericardial fluid exists to produce low QRS amplitude.

The three stages of acute pericarditis are illustrated in Fig. 4-75. An example of an ECG illustrating acute pericarditis is shown in Fig. 4-76.

- *Pericardial effusion* produces low QRS amplitude. The other abnormalities of pericarditis may or may not be evident. Electrical alternans may be present. It may be recognized by the alternating amplitude of the QRS complexes (Fig. 4-77).
- *Constrictive pericarditis* may produce atrial fibrillation, low QRS amplitude, and ST and T vectors that are directed more than 45 to 60 degrees away from the mean QRS vector.

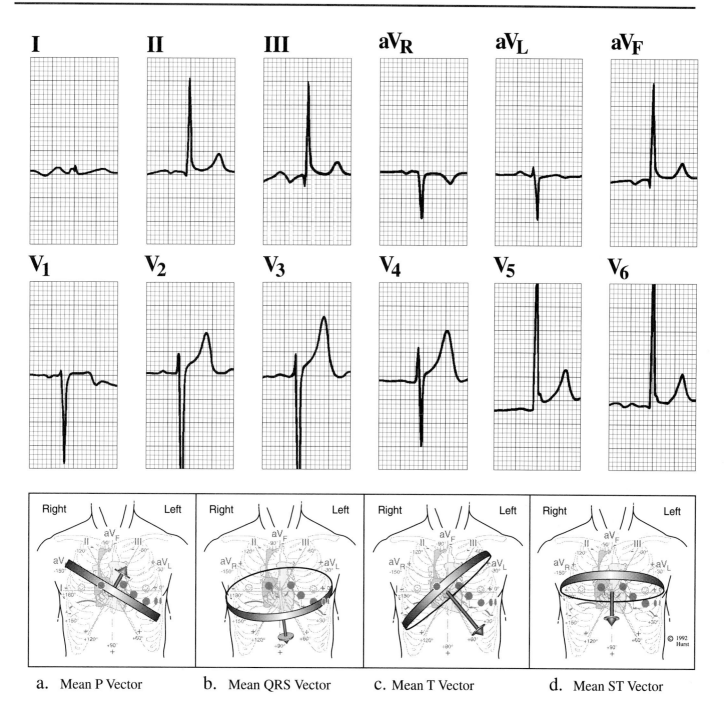

a. Mean P Vector b. Mean QRS Vector c. Mean T Vector d. Mean ST Vector

Fig. 4-54. LV hypertrophy caused by diastolic pressure overload.

- *Rhythm:* Lower atrial rhythm
  Rate: Undetermined in short strip
  PR interval: 0.15 second
  QRS duration: 0.08 second
  QT interval: 0.44 second
- *Vector diagrams of electrical forces:* See *a, b, c,* and *d* below the ECG.
- *Electrophysiologic considerations:*

  The mean P vector is directed about -60 degrees superiorly and is parallel with the frontal plane. This indicates retrograde depolarization of the atria. The PR interval is 0.15 second, which eliminates a junctional rhythm. The rhythm originates in an ectopic, lower atrial site.

  The mean QRS vector is directed about +80 degrees inferiorly and at least 60 to 70 degrees posteriorly. The posterior rotation is abnormal. The 12-lead amplitude of the QRS complexes is more than 230 mm; this indicates LV hypertrophy.

The mean T vector is large and is directed about +50 degrees inferiorly and about 10 degrees anteriorly. The QRS-T angle is abnormal and is about 80 degrees.

The mean ST vector is relatively parallel with the mean T vector.

The abnormalities can be caused by diastolic pressure overload of the LV.

- *Clinical differential diagnosis:* The combination of ECG abnormalities indicates LV hypertrophy. The size of the T waves and ST segment vectors suggests LV hypertrophy caused by diastolic pressure overload of the LV. These abnormalities can be caused by aortic valve regurgitation, mitral valve regurgitation, ventricular septal defect, or patent ductus arteriosus.
- *Discussion:* This ECG was recorded from a 24-year-old man with aortic valve regurgitation caused by a bicuspid aortic valve. The echocardiogram and Doppler study revealed aortic regurgitation and an LV diastolic diameter of 60 mm.

ECG reproduced with permission from Hurst JW: *Ventricular electrocardiography,* St. Louis, 1991, Mosby, fig 9.6.

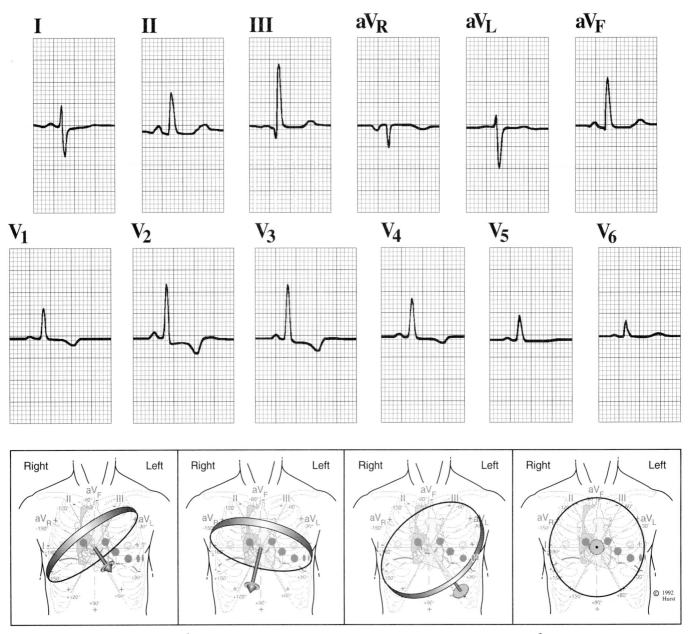

a. Mean P Vector b. Mean QRS Vector c. Mean T Vector d. Mean ST Vector

Fig. 4-55. RV hypertrophy caused by systolic pressure overload of the RV.
- *Rhythm:* Normal sinus rhythm
  Rate: Undetermined in short strip. There were 60 depolarizations per minute in a longer strip.
  PR interval: 0.14 second
  QRS interval: 0.08 second
  QT interval: 0.40 second
- *Vector diagrams of electrical forces:* See *a, b, c,* and *d* below the ECG.
- *Electrophysiologic considerations:*
  The mean P vector suggests an RA abnormality because it is directed slightly more anteriorly than usual.
  The mean QRS vector is directed to the right about +105 degrees. It is directed anteriorly at least 30 degrees (the exact number of degrees cannot be determined without recordings from additional electrode positions). The direction of the mean QRS vector indicates RV hypertrophy.
  The mean T vector is directed about +55 degrees inferiorly and about 80 degrees posteriorly. It is directed away from the RV. The spatial QRS-T angle is at least 110 degrees.

The mean ST vector is small; it is barely visible in the frontal plane; it is directed 90 degrees posteriorly and is relatively parallel with the mean T vector. The abnormalities are characteristic of systolic pressure overload of the RV, such as occurs with congenital pulmonary valve stenosis, congenital subpulmonary valve stenosis, tetralogy of Fallot, and late in the course of primary pulmonary hypertension, repeated pulmonary emboli, Eisenmenger's syndrome caused by interventricular septal defect, or patent ductus arteriosus. Conceivably, the abnormalities could occur in patients with longstanding severe mitral stenosis, but this is unlikely.
- *Discussion:* This ECG was recorded from a 36-year-old woman with congenital subpulmonic infundibular stenosis. The pulmonary artery pressure was 25/17 mm Hg, and the RV pressure was 229/6 mm Hg. The RA pressure was 18/10 mm Hg.

Reproduced with permission from Hurst JW: *Cardiovascular diagnosis: the initial examination,* St Louis, 1993, Mosby, pp 290, 291.

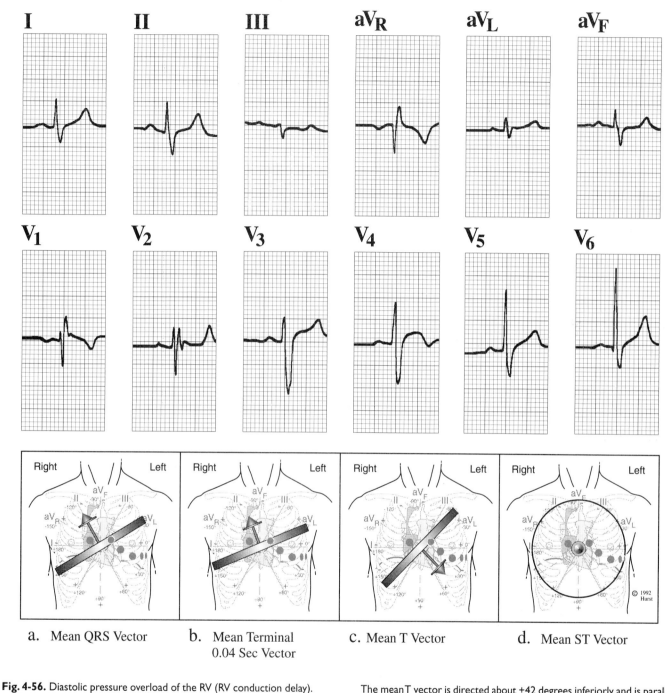

a. Mean QRS Vector

b. Mean Terminal 0.04 Sec Vector

c. Mean T Vector

d. Mean ST Vector

Fig. 4-56. Diastolic pressure overload of the RV (RV conduction delay).

- *Rhythm:* Sinus bradycardia

  Rate: Undetermined in short strip. There were 50 depolarizations per minute in a longer strip.

  PR interval: 0.16 second

  QRS duration: 0.10 second

  QT interval: 0.40 second

- *Vector diagrams of electrical forces:* See *a, b, c,* and *d* below the ECG.

- *Electrophysiologic considerations:*

  The mean QRS vector is directed -120 degrees superiorly and is parallel with the frontal plane. This abnormality is caused by the terminal 0.04-second QRS abnormality.

  The mean terminal 0.04 second QRS vector is directed -115 degrees superiorly and is parallel with the frontal plane. This abnormality is caused by RV conduction delay and is typically associated with diastolic volume overload of the LV. Actually, it masks the theoretic arrangements of vectors that would be predicted to be caused by diastolic pressure overload of the RV.

The mean T vector is directed about +42 degrees inferiorly and is parallel with the frontal plane.

The mean ST vector is barely visible in the frontal plane and is directed anteriorly. The cause of the isolated T wave negativity in lead V_4 is not known.

This type of ECG occurs in patients with diastolic volume overload of the RV, including secundum atrial septal defect and anomalous drainage of the pulmonary veins into the RA. RV conduction delay can also occur in otherwise normal subjects.

- *Discussion:* This ECG was recorded from a 26-year-old man with an ostium secundum atrial septal defect. The left-to-right shunt was 1.5:1, and the systolic pulmonary artery pressure was 55 mm Hg. This tracing illustrates how RV conduction delay masks, or overshadows, the theoretic arrangements of vectors that could be caused by diastolic volume overload of the RV.

Reproduced with permission from Hurst JW: *Cardiovascular diagnosis: the initial examination,* St Louis, 1993, Mosby, pp 294, 295.

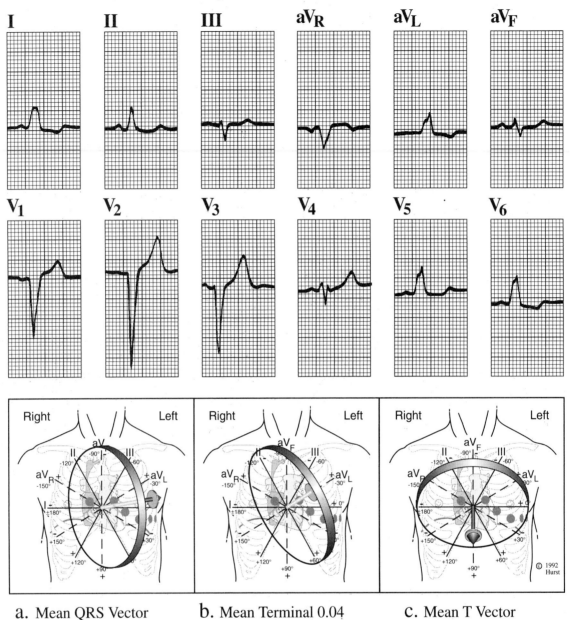

a. Mean QRS Vector

b. Mean Terminal 0.04 Second Vector

c. Mean T Vector

Fig. 4-57. Uncomplicated left bundle branch block (LBBB).
- *Rhythm:* Normal sinus rhythm
  Rate: Undetermined in short strip
  PR interval: 0.14 second
  QRS duration: 0.12 second
  QT interval: 0.42 second
- *Vector diagrams of electrical forces:* See *a*, *b*, and *c* below the ECG.
- *Electrophysiologic considerations:*
  The P waves are normal.
  The mean QRS vector is directed about -8 degrees to the left and about 50 degrees posteriorly. It shifted about 60 degrees to the left of its position before the development of LBBB and about 30 degrees posterior to its preblock direction.
  The mean terminal 0.04-second QRS vector is directed about -30 degrees to the left and about 40 degrees posteriorly. It points toward the basilar portion of the LV and is characteristic of LBBB. Previously it was

directed +60 degrees inferiorly and about 70 degrees posteriorly. Note how it has shifted to the left about 90 degrees.
  The mean T vector is directed about +90 degrees inferiorly and about 85 degrees anteriorly. It is directed about 115 degrees from the QRS vector. The ventricular gradient remains within the normal range.
  The abnormalities are consistent with the diagnosis of uncomplicated LBBB.
- *Clinical differential diagnosis:* Uncomplicated LBBB occurs in patients with atherosclerotic coronary heart disease, cardiomyopathy, or primary conduction system disease. It also occurs in patients with LV hypertrophy. The QRS gradually widens in such patients.
- *Discussion:* The cause of the uncomplicated LBBB in this patient is unknown. The tracing is shown to discuss the changes that occur in the postblock tracing with those in the preblock tracing.

ECG from Stein E: *Electrocardiographic interpretation: a self-study approach to clinical electrocardiology,* Philadelphia, 1991, Lea & Febiger, p 432. Reprinted with permission.

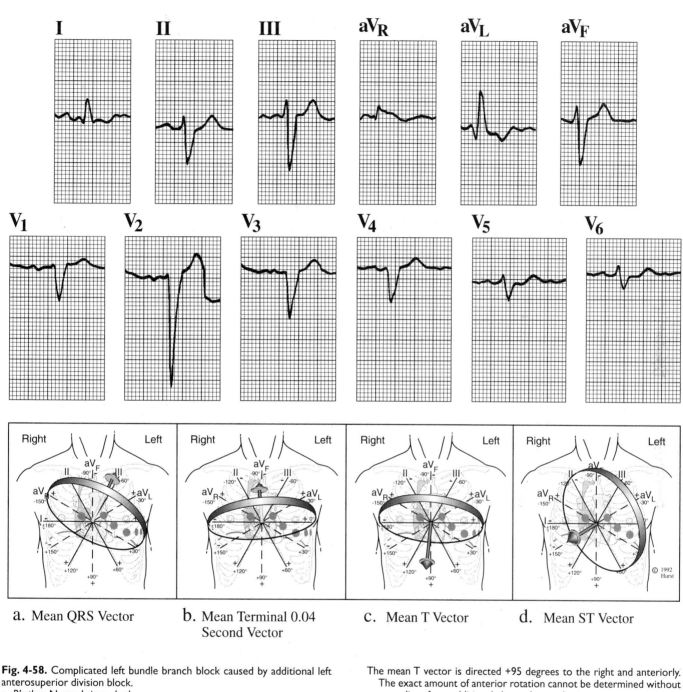

a. Mean QRS Vector

b. Mean Terminal 0.04 Second Vector

c. Mean T Vector

d. Mean ST Vector

Fig. 4-58. Complicated left bundle branch block caused by additional left anterosuperior division block.

- *Rhythm:* Normal sinus rhythm

  Rate: Undetermined in short strip. There were 73 depolarizations per minute in a longer strip.

  PR interval: 0.18 second

  QRS duration: 0.14 second

  QT interval: 0.42 second

- *Vector diagrams of electrical forces:* See *a, b, c,* and *d* below the ECG.

- *Electrophysiologic considerations:*

  The P waves are abnormal. There is an LA abnormality; note that the last half of the P wave is negative in leads V_1 and V_2.

  The mean QRS vector is directed -65 degrees to the left and posteriorly; the exact amount of posterior rotation cannot be determined without recordings from additional electrode sample sites.

  The mean terminal 0.04-second QRS vector is directed -95 degrees to the left. It is posteriorly directed; the exact amount of posterior rotation cannot be determined without recordings from additional electrode sample sites. This vector is directed abnormally in that it is directed much farther to the left than normal.

The mean T vector is directed +95 degrees to the right and anteriorly. The exact amount of anterior rotation cannot be determined without recordings from additional electrode sample sites.

The mean ST vector is directed about +150 degrees to the right and about 70 degrees anteriorly. It is probably about 60 degrees from the mean T vector.

The abnormal vectors indicate complicated left bundle branch, since there is additional left anterosuperior division block and the QRS duration is 0.14 second.

- *Clinical differential diagnosis:* Left bundle branch block plus left anterosuperior division block may occur in patients with dilated cardiomyopathy, severe coronary disease, primary disease of the conduction system (Lenegre disease), Lev disease, or severe aortic valve disease.

- *Discussion:* This ECG was recorded from a 58-year-old man with severe obstructive triple-vessel coronary atherosclerosis. The left anterior descending coronary artery was totally obstructed. The ejection fraction was 20% of normal, and the large LV contracted poorly. Severe heart failure was present.

Reproduced with permission from Hurst JW: *Cardiovascular diagnosis: the initial examination,* St Louis, 1993, Mosby, pp 335, 336.

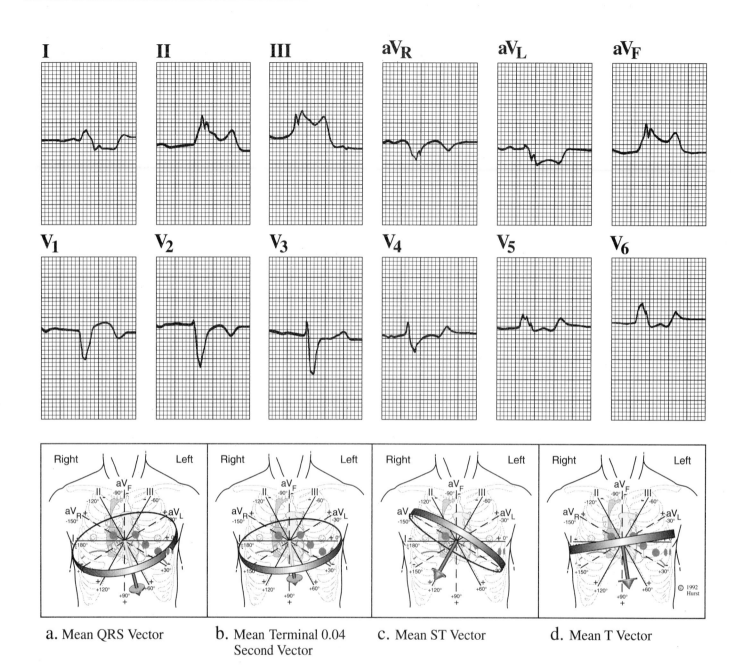

I II III aV_R aV_L aV_F

V₁ V₂ V₃ V₄ V₅ V₆

Right — Left (×4 torso diagrams)

aV_F, II, III, aV_R, aV_L with degree markings

© 1992 Hurst

a. Mean QRS Vector

b. Mean Terminal 0.04 Second Vector

c. Mean ST Vector

d. Mean T Vector

Fig. 4-59. Complicated left bundle branch block plus inferior and RV infarction.

- *Rhythm:* Atrial fibrillation

  Rate: Undetermined in short strip. There were 41 depolarizations per minute in a longer strip.

  PR interval: None

  QRS duration: 0.18 to 0.20 second

  QT interval: 0.48 second

- *Vector diagrams of electrical forces:* See *a, b, c,* and *d* below the ECG.

- *Electrophysiologic considerations:*

  Atrial fibrillation is present. The ventricular rate is quite slow.

  The duration of the QRS complex is 0.18 to 0.20 second. The mean QRS vector is directed about +75 degrees inferiorly and about 60 degrees posteriorly. The extremely wide duration of the QRS complex suggests an abnormality at the Purkinje-myocyte junction.

  The mean terminal 0.04-second QRS vector is directed about +80 degrees inferiorly and about 60 degrees posteriorly. The posterior direction of the vector indicates that depolarization of the LV is delayed.

The mean ST vector is directed about +120 degrees to the right and about 20 degrees anteriorly. The direction of this arrow suggests epicardial injury caused by inferior infarction plus an RV infarction.

The mean T vector is directed about +78 degrees inferiorly and parallel with the frontal plane. It is directed toward an inferior area of subendocardial ischemia.

The ECG shows atrial fibrillation, complicated left bundle branch block, and acute inferior RV infarction.

- *Clinical differential diagnosis:* The ST segment vector is diagnostic of inferior epicardial injury of the LV plus RV epicardial injury. Myocardial infarction is clearly present. The cause is most likely coronary atherosclerosis, but other causes of obstructive coronary artery disease may be considered.

- *Discussion:* This ECG was recorded from a 69-year-old man who had an RV infarction. Coronary arteriography revealed high-grade obstruction of the right coronary artery that was proximal to the RV branch of the right coronary artery.

Reproduced with permission from Hurst JW: *Cardiovascular diagnosis: the initial examination,* St Louis, 1993, Mosby, pp 386, 387.

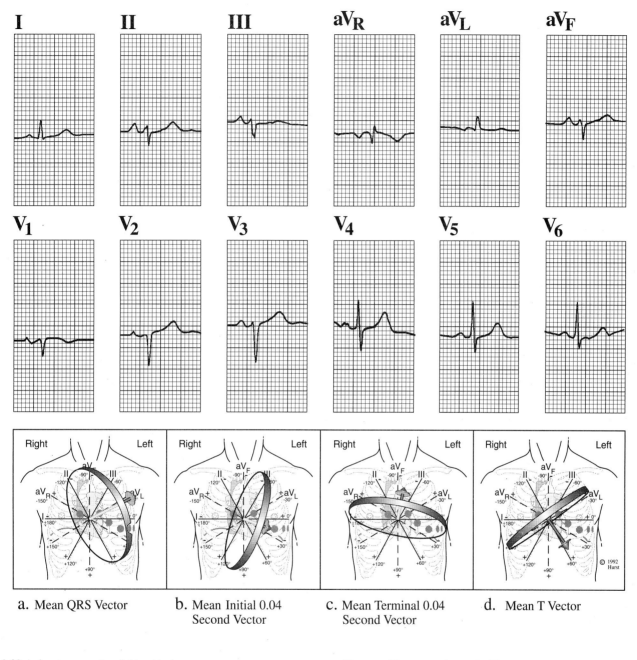

a. Mean QRS Vector

b. Mean Initial 0.04 Second Vector

c. Mean Terminal 0.04 Second Vector

d. Mean T Vector

Fig. 4-60. Left anterosuperior division block.
- *Rhythm:* Normal sinus rhythm
  Rate: Undetermined in short strip. There were 67 depolarizations per minute in a longer strip.
  PR interval: 0.14 second
  QRS duration: 0.08 second
  QT interval: 0.36 second
- *Vector diagrams of electrical forces:* See a, b, c, and d below the ECG.
- *Electrophysiologic considerations:*
  The mean QRS vector is directed -28 degrees to the left and about 40 degrees posteriorly. It is directed farther to the left than usual.
  The mean initial 0.04-second QRS vector is directed about +20 degrees inferiorly and about 25 degrees posteriorly. This vector is directed more posteriorly than usual and may represent an alteration of the conduction of the first portion of the septum; it could be misinterpreted as being caused by a septal infarction.
  The terminal 0.04-second QRS vector is directed -80 degrees to the left and more than 40 degrees posteriorly. This vector is directed farther to the left than normal and represents left anterosuperior division block.

The mean T vector is directed +55 degrees to the right and 5 degrees anteriorly.
The mean initial 0.04-second QRS vector suggest some type of initial conduction defect. The terminal 0.04-second QRS vector and the mean QRS vector are directed an abnormal degree to the left, suggesting left anterosuperior division block.
- *Clinical differential diagnosis:* Left anterosuperior division block can be associated with LV hypertrophy. It may occur in elderly individuals who have no other clinical evidence of heart disease. It may be caused by cardiomyopathy, atherosclerotic heart disease, or primary disease of the conduction system. Finally, it may occur for unexplained reasons.
- *Discussion:* This ECG was recorded from a 59-year-old woman who was asymptomatic and had no other evidence of heart disease. The ECG had not changed in nearly 2 decades. The cause of the abnormalities is unknown in this case but may be a congenital alteration of the conduction system.

Reproduced with permission from Hurst JW: *Cardiovascular diagnosis: the initial examination,* St Louis, 1993, Mosby, pp 316, 317.

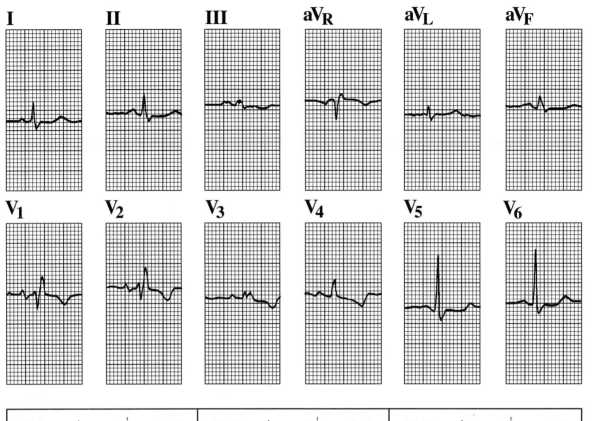

I **II** **III** **aV_R** **aV_L** **aV_F**

V_1 **V_2** **V_3** **V_4** **V_5** **V_6**

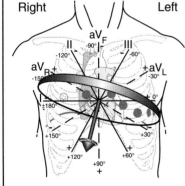

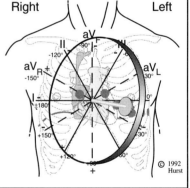

a. Mean QRS Vector   b. Mean Terminal 0.04 Second Vector   c. Mean T Vector

Fig. 4-61. Uncomplicated right bundle branch block (RBBB).

- *Rhythm:* Normal sinus rhythm
  Rate: Undetermined in short strip. There were 80 depolarizations per minute in a longer strip.
  PR interval: 0.14 second
  QRS duration: 0.12 second
  QT interval: 0.42 second
- *Vector diagrams of electrical forces:* See *a, b, c,* and *d* below the ECG.
- *Electrophysiologic considerations:*
  The duration of the QRS complex is 0.12 second. The mean QRS vector is directed about +105 degrees to the right and 15 to 20 degrees anteriorly.
  The mean terminal 0.04 second QRS vector is directed about -135 degrees superiorly and 60 degrees anteriorly. It points toward the RV, signifying RBBB.
  The mean T vector is directed +10 degrees inferiorly and about 70 degrees posteriorly. The ventricular gradient is normal.

The abnormalities in this ECG are characteristic of uncomplicated RBBB.

- *Clinical differential diagnosis:* RBBB may occur when no other evidence of heart disease exists. It may be caused by atherosclerotic coronary heart disease, cardiomyopathy, primary disease of the conduction system, or pulmonary embolism. The abnormal QRS vector associated with RV hypertrophy and dilatation from any cause may progress to RBBB. For example, the RV delay associated with RV hypertrophy and dilatation associated with a secundum atrial septal defect may gradually change to RBBB.
- *Discussion:* This ECG was recorded from a 65-year-old woman with an ostium secundum atrial septal defect. The abnormalities are caused by uncomplicated RBBB. A secondary T wave change occurs, and the ventricular gradient is normal.

Reproduction with permission from Hurst JW: *Cardiovascular diagnosis: the initial examination,* St Louis, 1993, Mosby, pp 324, 325.

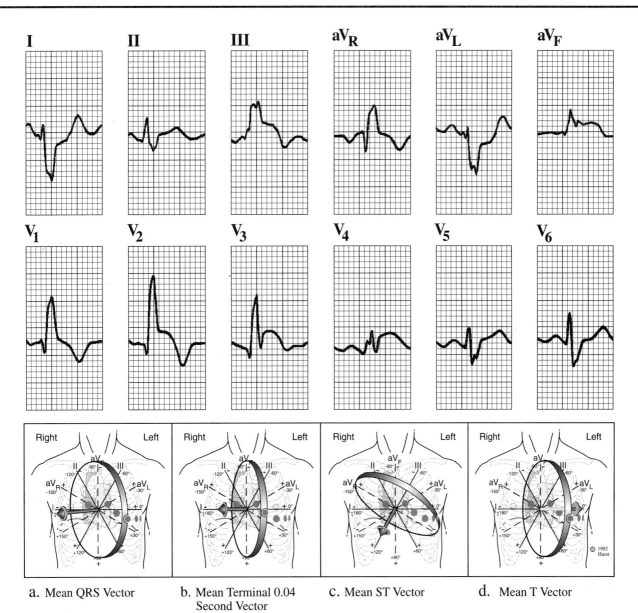

a. Mean QRS Vector

b. Mean Terminal 0.04 Second Vector

c. Mean ST Vector

d. Mean T Vector

Fig. 4-62. Complicated right bundle branch block (RBBB) plus postero-inferior division block, primary T wave abnormality, and primary ST segment abnormality. The ST segment abnormality could be caused by an inferoanterior infarction or a right ventricular infarction.

- *Rhythm:* Sinus tachycardia
  Rate: Undetermined in short strip. There were 104 depolarizations per minute in a longer strip.
  PR interval: 0.15 second
  QRS duration: 0.12 second
  QT interval: 0.36 second
- *Vector diagrams of electrical forces:* See *a, b, c,* and *d* below the ECG.
- *Electrophysiologic considerations:*
  The P waves are normal.
  The duration of the QRS complex is 0.12 second. The mean QRS vector is directed about +175 degrees to the right and about 50 degrees anteriorly. This degree of rightward deviation of the mean QRS vector is much more than it should be when there is uncomplicated RBBB.
  The mean terminal 0.04-second QRS vector is directed +180 degrees to the right and about 25 to 30 degrees anteriorly, signifying the presence of RBBB. The mean terminal 0.04-second QRS vector is directed farther to the right and more anteriorly than it is when uncomplicated RBBB is present.
  The extreme rightward deviation of the mean QRS vector and mean terminal 0.04-second QRS vector is probably caused by additional posteroinferior division block.

The mean ST vector points toward an area of epicardial injury. It is directed about +120 degrees inferiorly and about 30 degrees anteriorly and it could be caused by an inferoanterior myocardial infarction or a right ventricular infarction. Note that this is a primary ST segment abnormality because the mean ST vector is not parallel with the mean T vector, as it is when a secondary ST segment displacement occurs.

The mean T vector is directed at ±0 degrees in the frontal plane and about 35 degrees posteriorly. The ventricular gradient is abnormal, suggesting myocardial ischemia.

- *Clinical differential diagnosis:* This cluster of ECG abnormalities is caused by an acute myocardial infarction. The infarction could be located in the inferoanterior region or be located in the inferoseptal and right ventricular region. No other diagnostic option should be considered.
- *Discussion:* This ECG was recorded from a 56-year-old man with an acute myocardial infarction. Coronary arteriography revealed 80% obstruction of the left anterior descending coronary artery, which wrapped around the cardiac apex; 70% obstruction of the first diagonal; and 60% obstruction of the right coronary artery. There were no clinical signs of right ventricular infarction and the culprit artery was the left anterior descending coronary artery.

Reproduced with permission from Hurst JW: *Cardiovascular diagnosis: the initial examination,* St Louis, 1993, Mosby, pp 344, 345.

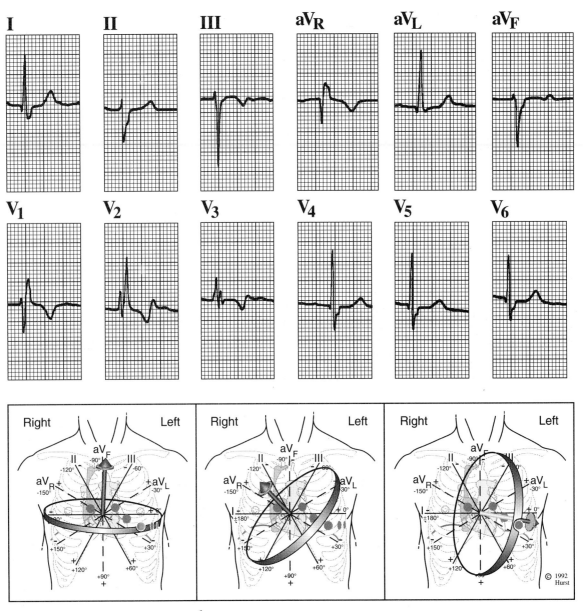

a. Mean QRS Vector   b. Mean Terminal 0.04 Second Vector   c. Mean T Vector

Fig. 4-63. Complicated right bundle branch block (RBBB) plus left antero-superior division block.

- *Rhythm:* Normal sinus rhythm
  Rate: Undetermined in short strip. There were 70 depolarizations per minute in a longer strip.
  PR interval: 0.21 second
  QRS duration: 0.12 second
  QT interval: 0.40 second
- *Vector diagrams of electrical forces:* See *a, b,* and *c* below the ECG.
- *Electrophysiologic considerations:*
  The P waves are normal. First-degree A-V block is present.
  The mean QRS vector is directed about -85 degrees to the left and about 30 degrees anteriorly. This vector is directed farther to the left than is usual for left bundle branch block (LBBB). In addition, the vector is directed anteriorly rather than posteriorly, as it is when LBBB exists.

The mean terminal 0.04-second QRS vector is directed about -135 degrees to the left and about 40 degrees anteriorly. The anterior direction of this vector indicates that the last portion of the myocardium to be depolarized is the RV.

The mean T vector is directed about +10 degrees inferiorly and about 40 degrees posteriorly. The ventricular gradient is abnormal.

This ECG is abnormal because of RBBB and left anterosuperior division block. First-degree A-V block is also present.

- *Clinical differential diagnosis:* This type of ECG can be caused by atherosclerotic coronary heart disease, cardiomyopathy, ostium primum septal defect, primary disease of the conduction system (Lenegre disease), Lev disease, or cardiac surgery for valvular or congenital heart disease.
- *Discussion:* This ECG was recorded from a 17-year-old woman with an ostium primum septal defect.

Reproduced with permission from Hurst JW: *Cardiovascular diagnosis: the initial examination,* St Louis, 1993, Mosby, pp 338, 339.

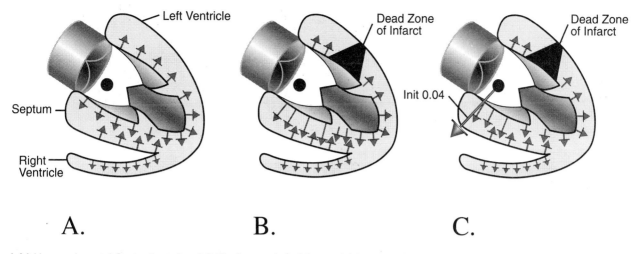

A. B. C.

Fig. 4-64. How an abnormal Q wave is produced. **A,** The first portion of the ventricles to undergo depolarization is the left upper portion of the interventricular septum. This occurs because the electrical impulse transmitted by an early twig of the left bundle branch stimulates this area of the heart. The left and right bundles transmit electrical impulses with rapid speed to the endocardial surfaces of the LV and RV. Electrical forces are produced as shown by the arrows. Those events occur during the initial 0.04 second of the depolariation of the LV and RV. **B,** Suppose a dead zone develops in the superolateral portion of the LV. This removes the electrical forces that are normally produced by this area of the endocardium during the initial 0.03 to

0.04 second of the QRS complex. The electrical forces (vectors) produced by the ventricular muscle that is located opposite the dead zone now dominate the electrical field. **C,** An arrow representing the electrical forces (vectors) responsible for a dead zone is directed away from the dead area. This produces an abnormal Q wave in the ECG. The location of the abnormal Q wave in the 12-lead ECG depends on the location and size of the infarct in the LV (and occasionally in the RV).

Reproduced with permission from Hurst JW: *Cardiovascular diagnosis: the initial examination,* St. Louis, 1993, Mosby, p358.

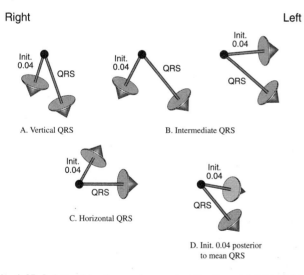

A. Vertical QRS

B. Intermediate QRS

C. Horizontal QRS

D. Init. 0.04 posterior to mean QRS

Fig. 4-65. Relationship of an arrow representing the mean initial 0.04-second QRS vector to an arrow representing the mean QRS vector in patients with myocardial infarction. The relationship of an arrow representing the normal mean initial 0.04-second QRS vector to an arrow representing the normal mean QRS vector is shown in Fig. 4-21. **A,** When an arrow representing the mean initial 0.04-second QRS vector is directed to the right of an arrow representing a vertically directed mean QRS vector, it is usually abnormal and often indicates the initial QRS abnormality of an anterolateral myocardial endocardial dead zone. **B,** When an arrow representing the mean initial 0.04-second QRS vector is directed 60 to 90 degrees to the right or left of an arrow representing an intermediately directed mean QRS vector, it often indicates, respectively, a lateral or inferior myocardial dead zone. **C,** When an arrow representing the mean initial 0.04-second QRS vector is directed superior to a horizontally directed arrow representing the mean QRS vector, it usually indicates an inferior myocardial dead zone. **D,** When an arrow representing the mean initial 0.04-second QRS vector is directed posterior to an arrow representing the mean QRS vector, it usually indicates an anterior myocardial dead zone.

Slightly modified with permission from Hurst JW: *Ventricular electrocardiography,* St. Louis, 1991, Mosby, fig 6.6.

Preexcitation of Ventricles

When the electrical activity spreads from the atria to the ventricles but circumvents the A-V node, it arrives at the ventricular myocytes earlier than usual. This is referred to as preexcitation of the ventricles. The path the electrical activity takes is called a bypass tract, and several such tracts have been identified.

The classic example of this condition is seen in the Wolff-Parkinson-White syndrome, in which the PR interval is short (0.12 second), the initial portion of the QRS complex is slurred, the QRS complex may be from 0.10 to 0.18 second in duration, and the patient is subject to episodes of supraventricular tachycardia or atrial fibrillation. When atrial fibrillations occur, the ventricular rate may be 220 depolarizations per minute.

An example of preexcitation of the ventricles is shown in Fig. 4-78. At times, an erroneous diagnosis of myocardial infarction is made because of the abnormal "Q waves."

Patients with idiopathic hypertrophic subaortic stenosis, Ebstein anomaly, or atrial septal defect may occasionally exhibit preexcitation, but as a common rule, the condition occurs in the absence of other cardiac conditions.

Low Amplitude of the QRS Complexes and T Waves

The normal range of total 12-lead QRS complex amplitude is 80 to 185 mm.[8] Because there are many causes for low amplitude of the T waves, it is customary to identify only low QRS complex amplitude. The QRS complex amplitude may be lower than normal because of: obesity; anasarca; pericardial effusion from many causes, including myxedema; constrictive pericarditis; pulmonary emphysema; and myocardial disease, such as amyloid infiltration, or myocarditis.

Pulmonary Emphysema

The ECG shows a RA abnormality, low QRS voltage, RV conduction delay, and a mean T vector directed away from the RV (Fig. 4-79).

Acute Pulmonary Embolism

The ECG does not usually change when a small pulmonary embolism is present. It may show sinus tachycardia, atrial fibrillation, RA abnormality, RV conduction delay, right bundle branch block, and a mean T vector directed to the left and posteriorly away from the RV (Fig. 4-80).

Effect of Digitalis on Electrocardiogram

- Digitalis does not alter the amplitude or contour of the QRS complex or the direction of a mean vector representing it.
- Digitalis more often shortens the QT interval than it prolongs the PR interval. The QT interval may become as short as 0.28 to 0.32 second when the heart rate is normal. This occurs because digitalis hastens the onset of the repolarization to the point that myocytes that are depolarized during the early part of depolarization begin to be repolarized before the remaining myocytes are depolarized.

- The mean T vector does not change direction as a result of digitalis medication. It does become shorter. A new ST vector develops as the T wave becomes smaller.
- A new ST vector develops; it is directed opposite to the mean T vector. As the T vector becomes shorter, the ST vector becomes larger. The ST vector is caused by early repolarization. Digitalis seems to eliminate the transmyocardial pressure gradient and permits repolarization to begin in the endocardium and travel to the epicardium. This reverses the direction of the repolarization vector. In other words, the ST segment vector caused by digitalis is, in reality, caused by the early part of the repolarization process (or T wave).

The effect of digitalis on the ECG is illustrated in Fig. 4-81. An ECG illustrating the effect of digitalis is shown in Fig. 4-82.

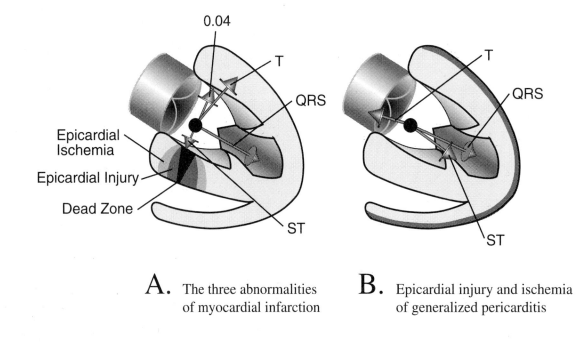

A. The three abnormalities of myocardial infarction

B. Epicardial injury and ischemia of generalized pericarditis

Fig. 4-66. Location of the dead zone, area of injury, and area of ischemia of myocardial infarction as compared with that of epicardial injury and ischemia of acute pericarditis. **A,** The dead zone is located inferiorly. It is largest in the endocardial area and smallest in the epicardial area. The zone of injury surrounds the dead zone and is largest in the epicardial area. The area of ischemia surrounds the area of injury and is largest in the epicardial area. The arrow representing the mean initial 0.03- to 0.04-second QRS vector is directed away from the dead zone. The arrow representing the mean ST vector points toward an area of epicardial injury. The arrow representing the mean T vector points away from the area of epicardial ischemia. **B,** Directions of arrows representing the mean ST and T vectors in a patient with pericarditis. Pericarditis is usually generalized, and the mean ST segment vector points toward the anatomic apex of the LV, whereas the mean T vector points away from the anatomic apex. An apical infarct can produce an ST segment vector that simulates the ST segment vector of pericarditis. No abnormal Q wave of infarction may be produced, since no ventricular myocardium is located opposite the apex. Pericarditis is usually generalized, as shown in this figure, but it can occasionally be localized. When this occurs, the arrow representing the mean ST vector may simulate the ST segment vector of myocardial infarction. This type of ST segment vector may be associated with pericarditis that follows cardiac surgery, trauma, or myocardial infarction.

Reproduced with permission form Hurst JW: *Cardiovascular diagnosis: the initial examination*, St. Louis, Mosby, 1993, p 362.

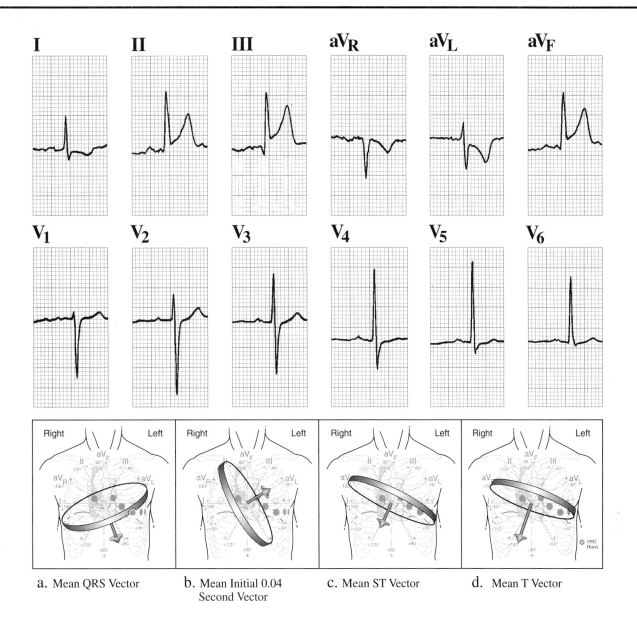

a. Mean QRS Vector   b. Mean Initial 0.04 Second Vector   c. Mean ST Vector   d. Mean T Vector

Fig. 4-67. Hyperacute T waves caused by inferior endocardial ischemia, inferior epicardial injury, and inferior dead zone.

- *Rhythm:* Normal sinus rhythm
  Rate: Undetermined in short strip. There were 75 depolarizations per minute in a longer strip.
  PR interval: 0.16 second
  QRS duration: 0.08 second
  QT interval: 0.36 second
- *Vector diagrams of electrical forces:* See *a, b, c,* and *d* below the ECG.
  Electrophysiologic considerations:
  The P waves are normal.
  The mean QRS vector is normally directed about +68 degrees inferiorly and about 35 to 40 degrees posteriorly.
  The mean initial 0.04-second QRS vector is directed about -30 degrees to the left and an undetermined number of degrees anteriorly (recordings from additional electrode sites would be needed to determine exactly how far anteriorly the mean initial 0.04-second QRS vector is directed). As drawn, however, the mean initial 0.04-second QRS vector is directed abnormally to the left of the mean QRS vector, which suggests an inferior myocardial dead zone.
  The mean ST vector is directed about +118 degrees to the right and about 15 degrees anteriorly. Note how the transitional pathway of the mean ST vector "interdigitates" with the precordial electrode position sites; all the precordial leads are very near the transitional pathway of the mean ST vector. This is why the ST segment shift is so small in the

lateral precordial leads. The mean ST vector represents inferior epicardial injury.
  The mean T vector is large and directed about +110 degrees to the right and about 25 degrees anteriorly. It is caused by inferior endocardial ischemia. These large, peaked T waves are referred to as *hyperacute T waves.*
  These abnormalities indicate the presence of a fresh myocardial infarction. There is an inferior endocardial dead zone and the expected inferior epicardial injury. The mean T vector ordinarily would point away from the epicardial area of ischemia that surrounds the epicardial injury. In this case, during the early phase of myocardial infarction, the endocardial ischemia is larger than the epicardial ischemia. This produces hyperacute T waves, and the mean T vector points toward the area of inferior endocardial ischemia.
- *Clinical differential diagnosis:* This tracing is diagnostic of a fresh myocardial infarction. There is likely to be an obstruction of the right coronary artery at its midpoint or just distal to the midpoint. The cause of such an obstruction is usually an atherosclerotic plaque and its complications.
- *Discussion:* This ECG was recorded from a 44-year-old man with an acute inferior myocardial infarction caused by atherosclerotic coronary heart disease. Coronary arteriography revealed total obstruction of the midportion of the right coronary artery.

Reproduced with permission from Hurst JW: *Cardiovascular diagnosis: the initial examination,* St. Louis, 1993, Mosby, pp 368, 369.

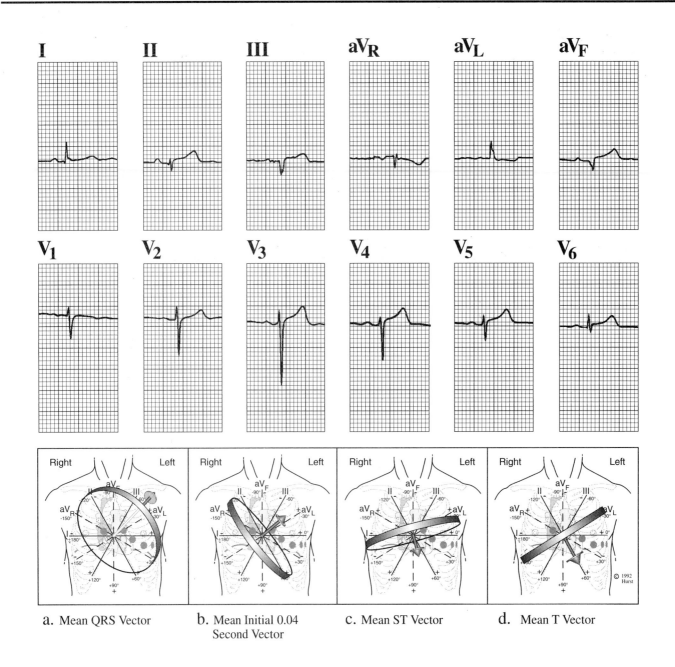

a. Mean QRS Vector

b. Mean Initial 0.04
Second Vector

c. Mean ST Vector

d. Mean T Vector

Fig. 4-68. Inferior myocardial infarction from thrombotic obstruction of a wraparound left anterior descending coronary artery.

- *Rhythm:* Normal sinus rhythm
  Rate: Undetermined in short strip. There were 71 depolarizations per minute on a longer strip.
  PR interval: 0.14 second
  QRS duration: 0.07 second
  QT interval: 0.32 second
- *Vector diagrams of electrical forces:* See *a, b, c,* and *d* below the ECG.
  Electrophysiologic considerations:
  The P waves are normal.
  The mean QRS vector is directed about -45 degrees to the left and about 60 degrees or more posteriorly. This abnormal degree of leftward deviation of the mean QRS vector is produced by the removal of the electrical forces ordinarily produced by the myocytes that are stimulated by the left anterosuperior division of the left bundle branch. The abnormal direction of the mean QRS vector could also be caused by a large inferior dead zone.
  The mean initial 0.04-second QRS vector is directed about -35 degrees to the left and about 10 degrees anteriorly. Careful scrutiny of leads I and II reveals small 0.01-second Q waves.

There is a large Q wave in leads III and aV$_F$, indicating the presence of an inferior dead zone.

The mean ST segment vector is directed about +75 degrees to the right and about 10 degrees anteriorly. This represents inferoanterior epicardial injury.

The mean T vector is directed +60 degrees inferiorly and is parallel with the frontal plane. This is due to endocardial ischemia.

- *Clinical differential diagnosis:* These ECG abnormalities indicate an inferolateral myocardial infarction. The direction of the ST segment vector indicates that the obstructed coronary artery is either the distal right coronary artery, the circumflex coronary artery, or a wraparound left anterior descending artery.
- *Discussion:* The ECG was recorded from a 24-year-old man who was a heavy smoker. He had severe, prolonged chest pain that was characteristic of myocardial ischemia. Coronary arteriography revealed a clot in the left anterior descending artery (LAD) with very little atherosclerosis. The left anterior descending artery wrapped around the apex of the heart. Isoembolism from a clot in the proximal LAD to the distal part of the LAD caused the infarction.

Reproduced with permission from Hurst JW: *Cardiovascular diagnosis: the initial examination,* St. Louis, 1993, Mosby, pp 372, 373.

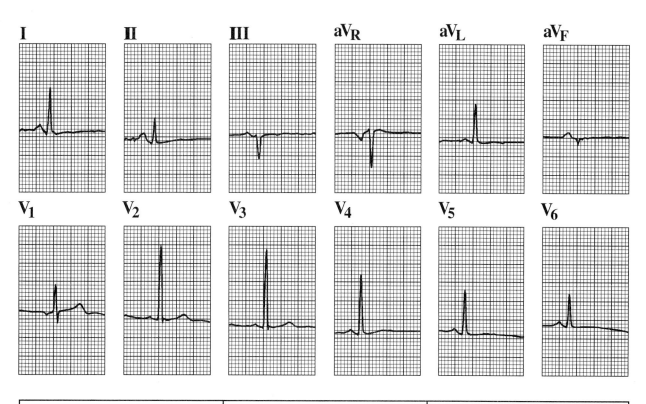

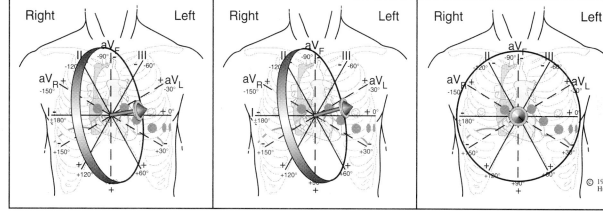

a. Mean QRS Vector

b. Mean Initial 0.04 Second Vector

c. Mean T Vector

Fig. 4-69. True posterior infarction

- *Rhythm:* Normal sinus rhythm

  Rate: Undetermined in short strip. There were 62 depolarizations per minute in a longer strip.

  PR interval: 0.16 second

  QRS duration: 0.08 second

  QT interval: 0.39 second

- *Vector diagrams of electrical forces:* See *a, b,* and *c* below the ECG.

  Electrophysiologic considerations:

  The P waves are normal.

  The mean QRS vector is directed about -10 degrees to the left and about 45 degrees anteriorly (note that the QRS amplitude is approximately the same in leads V_1 and V_6). The direction of the mean QRS vector is abnormal; it is directed too far anteriorly. This could be caused by RV hypertrophy or true posterior infarction. RV hypertrophy is very unlikely because the mean QRS vector is directed to the left.

  The mean initial 0.04-second QRS vector is directed about -10 degrees to the left and approximately 45 degrees anteriorly. This abnormality could be caused by RV hypertrophy or a true posterior infarction.

The mean T vector is directed 90 degrees anteriorly. Note that the T waves are not visible in the extremity leads and that there is a tall T wave in lead V_1 and a flat T wave in lead V_6. It indicates a repolarization abnormality in the posterior epicardial portion of the LV.

- *Clinical differential diagnosis:* The mean QRS vector and the mean initial 0.04-second vector are directed abnormally anteriorly. They are both directed leftward, which makes RV hypertrophy unlikely. The most likely cause of these abnormalities is true posterior infarction from coronary artery disease. The mean T vector points away from an area of true posterior epicardial ischemia surrounding the dead zone.

- *Discussion:* This ECG shows a true posterior infarction. It was recorded from a man who had coronary bypass surgery 9 years before this tracing was recorded. A coronary arteriogram revealed 40% obstruction of the left main coronary artery, 60% to 70% obstruction of a ramus artery, 70% to 80% obstruction of an obtuse marginal artery, 50% obstruction of the ostium of the right coronary artery, and 90% obstruction of the proximal portion of the right coronary artery.

Reproduced with permission from Hurst JW: *Cardiovascular diagnosis: the initial examination,* St. Louis, 1993, Mosby, pp 374, 375.

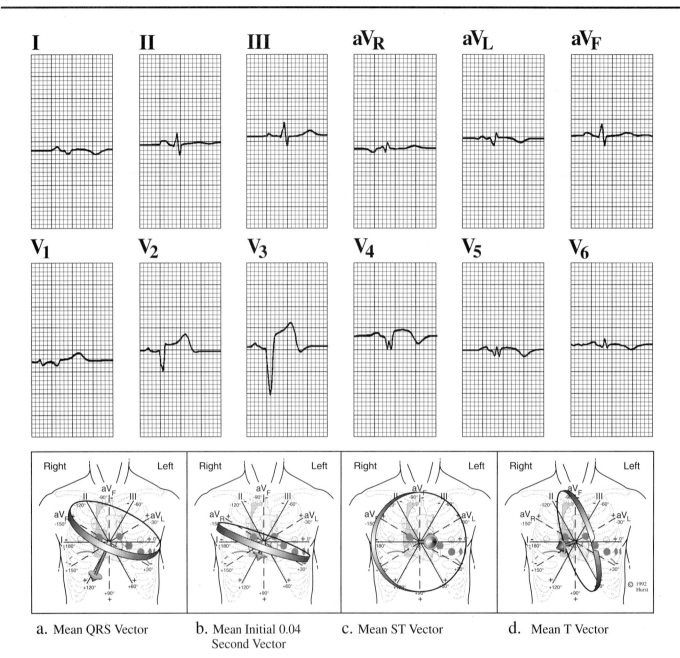

I II III aV_R aV_L aV_F

V_1 V_2 V_3 V_4 V_5 V_6

a. Mean QRS Vector

b. Mean Initial 0.04 Second Vector

c. Mean ST Vector

d. Mean T Vector

Fig. 4-70. Anterolateral myocardial infarction.
- *Rhythm:* Normal sinus rhythm
- *Rate:* Undetermined in short strip. There were 77 depolarizations per minute in a longer strip.
  PR interval: 0.16 second
  QRS duration: 0.08 second
  QT interval: 0.35 second
- *Vector diagrams of electrical forces:* See *a, b, c,* and *d* below the ECG.
- *Electrophysiologic considerations:*
  The P waves are normal.
  The mean QRS vector is directed about +125 degrees to the right and about 20 degrees posteriorly. The abnormal direction of the mean QRS vector may be caused by an endocardial dead zone of the lateral portion of the LV, left posteroinferior division block, or both.
  The mean initial 0.04 second QRS vector is directed about +125 degrees to the right and 5 to 10 degrees posteriorly. The direction of this vector is caused by a dead zone in the endocardial region of the anterolateral portion of the LV.

The mean ST vector is directed at 0 degrees in the frontal plane and 85 to 90 degrees anteriorly. It is produced by extensive anterolateral LV epicardial injury.

The mean T vector is directed about +170 degrees to the right and about 20 degrees anteriorly. It is produced by lateral epicardial ischemia.

These abnormalities are caused by an anterolateral myocardial infarction.

- *Clinical differential diagnosis:* These ECG abnormalities are diagnostic of anterolateral myocardial infarction, which is usually caused by obstruction of the proximal portion of the left anterior descending artery or the first diagonal. The obstruction in the artery is usually related to coronary atherosclerosis, but other causes such as coronary embolism may be responsible.

- *Discussion:* The ECG was recorded from a 59-year-old man with prolonged chest pain that was characteristic of myocardial ischemia. A coronary arteriogram revealed a high-grade obstruction of a long segment of the proximal portion of the left anterior descending coronary artery.

Reproduced with permission from Hurst JW: *Cardiovascular diagnosis: the initial examination,* St. Louis, 1993, Mosby, pp 380, 381.

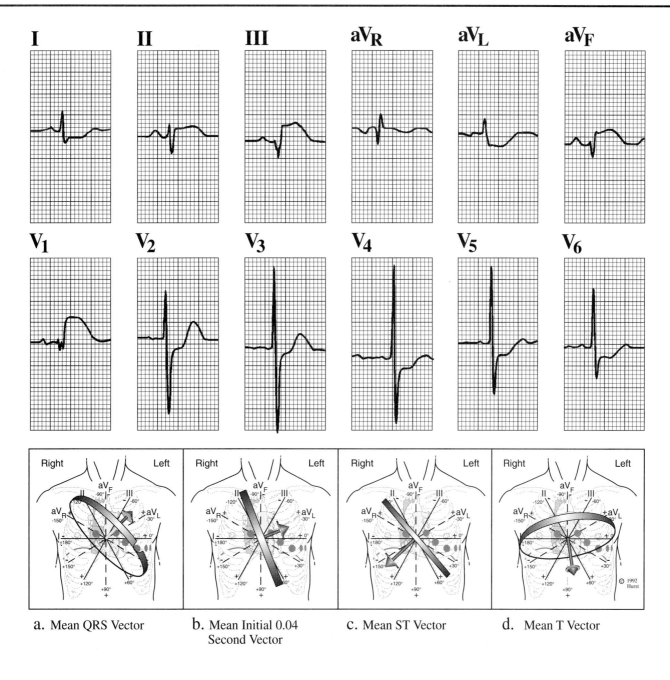

a. Mean QRS Vector

b. Mean Initial 0.04 Second Vector

c. Mean ST Vector

d. Mean T Vector

Fig. 4-71. Acute inferior infarction plus RV myocardial infarction

- *Rhythm:* Normal sinus rhythm

  Rate: Undetermined in short strip. There were 85 depolarizations per minute in a longer strip.

  PR interval: 0.16 second

  QRS duration: 0.08 second

  QT interval: 0.40 second

- *Vector diagrams of electrical forces:* See *a, b, c,* and *d* below the ECG.

- *Electrophysiologic considerations:*

  The P waves are normal.

  The mean QRS vector is directed about -50 degrees to the left and about 20 degrees posteriorly. This abnormal direction could be caused by myocardial damage (dead zone) inferiorly or left anterosuperior division block.

  The mean initial 0.04-second QRS vector is directed about -20 degrees to the left and is parallel with the frontal plane. Note the small R wave that is 0.02 second in duration in lead aV$_F$. The direction of the mean initial 0.04-second QRS vector could be, but is not definitely, caused by an inferior myocardial dead zone.

The mean ST vector is large. It is directed about +120 degrees to the right and is parallel with the frontal plane. It is produced by epicardial injury in the inferior portion of the septum and lower portion of the RV.

The mean T vector is directed about +80 degrees to the right and about 30 to 40 degrees anteriorly. This is probably a hyperacute ischemic T wave abnormality. As such, it is directed toward an area of inferior endocardial ischemia.

The most easily explained abnormality is the large ST segment vector. It is directed toward epicardial injury of the inferior portion of the LV (probably the lowest portion of the septum) and the lowest portion of the RV.

- *Clinical differential diagnosis:* The mean ST segment of this ECG suggests an inferior LV infarction that also involves the RV.

- *Discussion:* This ECG was recorded from a 46-year-old man with an acute inferior-RV myocardial infarction. A coronary arteriogram revealed a 90% obstruction of the right artery proximal to the RV branch of the right coronary artery.

Reproduced with permission from Hurst JW: *Cardiovascular diagnosis: the initial examination,* St. Louis, Mosby, 1993, pp 376, 377.

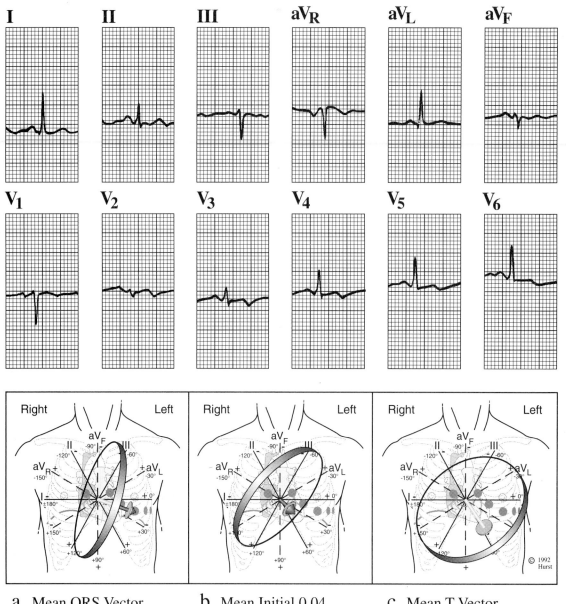

a. Mean QRS Vector

b. Mean Initial 0.04 Second Vector

c. Mean T Vector

Fig. 4-72 Non–Q wave myocardial infarction

- *Rhythm:* Sinus tachycardia

  Rate: Undetermined in short strip. There were 93 depolarizations per minute in a longer strip.

  PR interval: 0.12 second

  QRS duration: 0.08 second

  QT interval: 0.32 second

- Vector diagrams of electrical forces: See *a, b,* and *c* below the ECG.

  Electrophysiologic considerations:

  The P waves are normal.

  The mean QRS vector is normally directed at about +20 degrees inferiorly and 20 degrees posteriorly.

  The mean initial 0.04-second QRS vector is directed normally at +40 degrees inferiorly and about 45 degrees anteriorly. It is directed inferior to and anterior to the mean QRS vector.

  The mean T vector is directed about +58 degrees inferiorly and about 80

degrees posteriorly. It is directed away from the anterolateral surface of the LV and represents a primary repolarization abnormality.

- *Clinical differential diagnosis:* The abnormal mean T vector is most likely caused by anterolateral epicardial myocardial ischemia from obstructive coronary artery disease. The usual cause is coronary arteriosclerosis, but other causes of coronary disease must be remembered and sought. Pericarditis is unlikely because the mean T vector is usually directed away from the centroid of generalized epicardial ischemia, whereas in this ECG the mean T vector is directed away from the anterolateral portion of the LV.

- *Discussion:* This ECG was recorded from a 67-year-old man with unstable angina pectoris and episodes of prolonged chest discomfort that were characteristic of myocardial ischemia. This ECG illustrates the ECG signs of a non–Q wave myocardial infarction.

Reproduced with permission from Hurst JW: *Cardiovascular diagnosis: the initial examination,* St. Louis, Mosby, 1993, pp 382, 383.

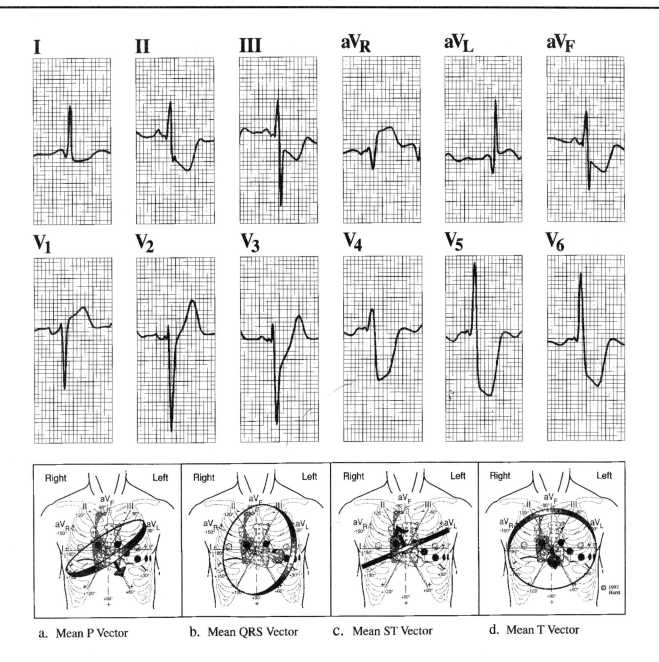

I II III aV$_R$ aV$_L$ aV$_F$

V$_1$ V$_2$ V$_3$ V$_4$ V$_5$ V$_6$

a. Mean P Vector   b. Mean QRS Vector   c. Mean ST Vector   d. Mean T Vector

Figure 4-73. Prolonged subendocardial injury and infarction.

- *Rhythm:* Sinus tachycardia

  Rate: Undetermined in short strip. There were 115 depolarizations per minute in a longer strip.

  PR interval: 0.13 second

  QRS duration: 0.09 second

  QT interval: 0.40 second

- *Vector diagrams of electrical forces:* See *a, b, c,* and *d* below the ECG.

- *Electrophysiologic considerations:*

  The P waves are abnormal.

  The mean P vector is a little more posteriorly directed than usual. The second half of the P wave is negative in leads V$_1$ and V$_2$ and measures -0.04 mm·sec in lead V$_1$. This indicates an LA abnormality, which is usually caused by an abnormality of the LV or mitral valve.

  The mean QRS vector is directed at +15 degrees in the frontal plane and about 70 degrees posteriorly. The initial 0.04-second vector is normal.

  The mean ST vector is quite large. It is directed -115 degrees to the left

and is parallel with the frontal plane. It is directed away from the centroid of generalized subendocardial injury.

The mean T vector is directed at +85 degrees in the frontal plane and is directed more than 45 to 60 degrees anteriorly. The QRS-T angle is abnormally large.

- *Clinical differential diagnosis:* The ST segment displacement is characteristic of subendocardial injury caused by myocardial ischemia. When the ST segment displacement lasts for hours, it indicates subendocardial infarction. This often occurs in patients with LV hypertrophy and obstructive coronary atherosclerosis.

- *Discussion:* This ECG was recorded from a 54-year-old man who experienced severe retrosternal pain and later developed ventricular fibrillation. Defibrillation and cardiac resuscitation were successful. He gave a history of hypertension and had LV hypertrophy. Subendocardial infarction was diagnosed because of the persistence of the ST vector that is directed away from the centroid of the generalized subendocardial injury.

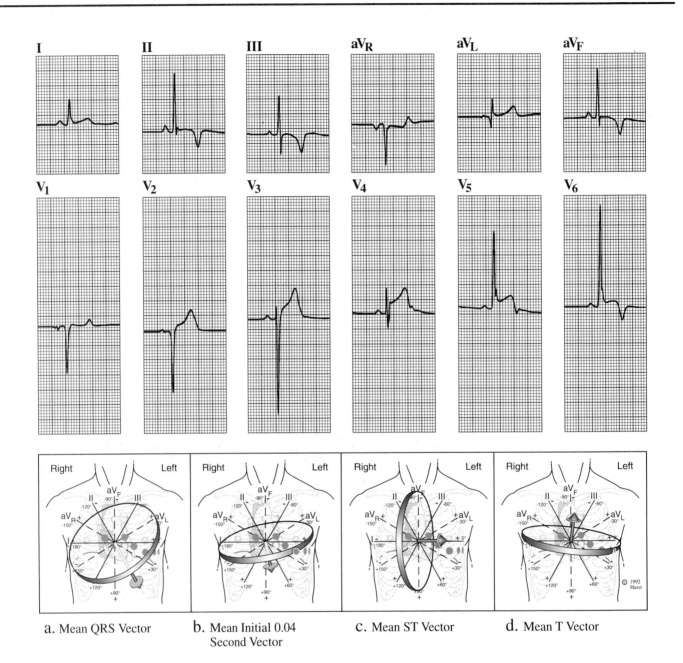

a. Mean QRS Vector b. Mean Initial 0.04
Second Vector c. Mean ST Vector d. Mean T Vector

Fig. 4-74. Pseudomyocardial infarction caused by hypertrophic cardiomy-opathy.

- *Rhythm:* Sinus bradycardia
  Rate: Undetermined in short strip. There were 53 depolarizations per minute in a longer strip.
  PR interval: 0.16 second
  QRS duration: 0.09 second
  QT interval: 0.14 second
- *Vector diagrams of electrical forces:* See *a, b, c,* and *d* below ECG.
- *Electrophysiologic considerations:*
  The P waves are normal.
  The mean QRS vector is directed about +60 degrees inferiorly and about 50 degrees posteriorly. The total amplitude of the QRS complex is about 243 mm, indicating LV hypertrophy.
  The mean initial 0.04-second QRS vector is directed about +80 degrees inferiorly and about 35 degrees posteriorly. This direction is more posterior than usual and could be caused by LV hypertrophy or a dead zone anteriorly.
  The mean ST vector is directed at +0 degree and 30 degrees anteriorly. It is not parallel with the mean T vector. This abnormal ST vector could

be caused by acute lateral epicardial injury secondary to myocardial infarction, or, as will become apparent, it may be associated with hypertrophic cardiomyopathy.
  The mean T vector is directed -85 degrees to the left and about 30 degrees anteriorly. The vector in this tracing may result from LV hypertrophy plus a primary T wave abnormality. The ventricular gradient is obviously abnormal.
- *Clinical differential diagnosis:* The LV hypertrophy, abnormal 0.04-second QRS vector, epicardial injury, and primary T wave abnormality may be caused by myocardial infarction from coronary atherosclerosis plus some other cause of LV hypertrophy, such as hypertension or aortic valve disease, or it may be caused by hypertrophic cardiomyopathy alone. Finally, on rare occasions, patients may have both hypertrophic cardiomyopathy and myocardial infarction resulting from coronary atherosclerosis.
- *Discussion:* This ECG was recorded from a 37-year-old man with nonobstructive hypertrophic cardiomyopathy. He gave a history of cardiac arrhythmia and syncope.

Reproduced with permission from Hurst JW: *Cardiovascular diagnosis: the initial examination,* St. Louis, 1993, Mosby, pp 390, 391.

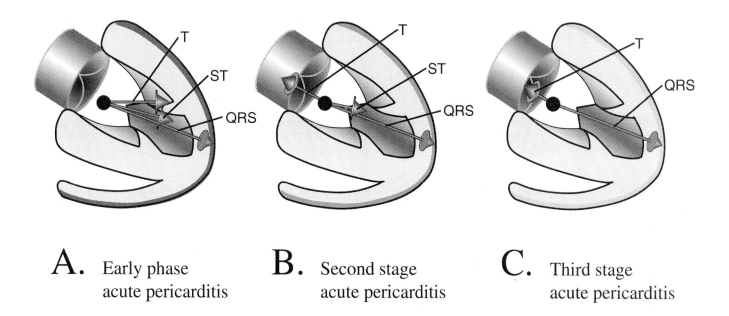

A. Early phase acute pericarditis

B. Second stage acute pericarditis

C. Third stage acute pericarditis

Fig. 4-75. ECG abnormalities produced by acute pericarditis. **A,** Pericarditis usually produces generalized epicardial myocardial injury *(dark area)*. Initially, during the early stage of pericarditis, an arrow representing the mean of the electrical forces (vectors) responsible for the ST segment is directed toward the anatomic apex of the LV. It is produced by generalized epicardial injury. The PQ segment may become displaced downward in leads where the P waves are upright. It cannot be represented by an arrow, since it is rarely seen in all leads. **B,** During the second stage of acute pericarditis, the arrow representing the ST segment vector becomes smaller than it was in **A,** and an arrow representing the mean of the electrical forces (vectors) responsible for the T wave is directed somewhat opposite to the anatomic apex of the LV; it results from generalized epicardial ischemia. **C,** During the third stage of acute pericarditis, an arrow representing the mean of the electrical forces (vectors) responsible for the ST segment decreases greatly, and the arrow representing the mean of the electrical forces (vectors) responsible for the T wave may become larger than it was in **B.** The T waves may then decrease in size, as shown here. When pericardial fluid develops, the amplitude of the QRS complexes and T waves decreases, and electrical alternans of the QRS complexes and T waves my appear.

Reproduced with permission from Hurst JW: *Cardiovascular diagnosis: the initial examination.* St Louis, 1992, Mosby, p 392.

Effect of Quinidine and Other Drugs on the Electrocardiogram

- *Quinidine* medication may increase the duration of the QRS complex and prolong the QT interval. Premature ventricular depolarizations may develop and may cause ventricular tachycardia and fibrillation with or without the classic findings of torsades de pointes. The drug can also cause sinus arrest, A-V conduction prolongation, wider than normal QRS complexes, and primary T wave abnormalities.
- *Procainamide* may produce the same abnormalities as those discussed for quinidine.
- *Disopyramide* may cause the same abnormalities as those discussed for quinidine.

Electrolyte Abnormalities and Electrocardiogram

- Hypokalemia causes the U waves to become prominent and join the T waves. This causes the T waves to appear longer than normal and the QT interval to appear longer than normal. Atrial tachycardia or atrial fibrillation may be present (Fig. 4-83).
- Hyperkalemia can produce any type of QRS conduction abnormality as well as sinus node arrest. The T waves become large and peaked; the ascending limb of the T wave becomes as acutely slanted as the descending limb of the T wave, and thus the name "tent-like" T waves (Fig. 4-84).
- Hypocalcemia produces a long QT interval because of prolongation of the ST segment (Fig. 4-83).
- Hypercalcemia produces a short QT interval and may appear similar to the abnormalities produced by digitalis. Occasionally an ST vector is created that is directed anteriorly, suggesting epicardial injury, but its cause is unknown.

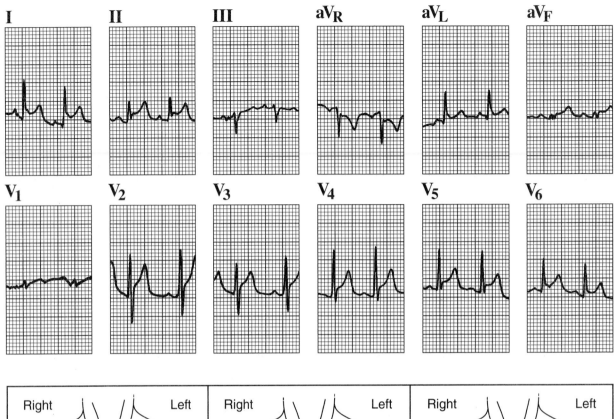

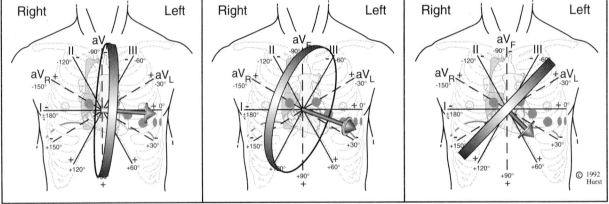

a. Mean QRS Vector   b. Mean ST Vector   c. Mean T Vector

Fig. 4-76. Acute pericarditis.
- *Rhythm:* Sinus tachycardia
  Rate: 130 depolarizations per minute
  PR interval: 0.14 second
  QRS duration: 0.08 second
  QT interval: 0.28 second
- *Vector diagrams of electrical forces:* See *a, b,* and *c* below the ECG.
- *Electrophysiologic considerations:*
  The P waves are normal. The PQ segment in lead II may be displaced
    downward, but one cannot be certain of this observation.
  The mean QRS vector is directed about +5 degrees inferiorly and about
    5 to 10 degrees posteriorly.
  The mean ST vector is directed about +20 degrees inferiorly and about
    20 to 30 degrees anteriorly. The ST segment vector indicates the pres-
    ence of generalized epicardial injury.
  The mean T vector is directed about +45 degrees inferiorly and is parallel
    with the frontal plane.
- *Clinical differential diagnosis: Generalized epicardial injury* is a clue to generalized
  pericarditis. This ECG abnormality occurs early; it precedes the T wave

abnormality, which tends to occur as the ST segment vector decreases in
size. When the abnormal T wave vector appears, it can be represented by
a vector that is directed opposite to the mean ST vector. An *apical myocardial infarction* can produce such an ST segment vector, but such an
infarct is unusual. An abnormal Q wave may not appear with apical
infarction, since there is no myocardium opposite the apex; the aortic
and mitral valves are opposite the cardiac apex. *Segmental pericarditis*
may cause the ST segment vector to be directed toward the epicardium
of a segment of myocardium, as it does with infarction. For example,
postoperative pericarditis, traumatic pericarditis, and the pericarditis of
infarction may be segmental rather than generalized, as it is with viral
pericarditis.
- *Discussion:* This ECG was recorded from a 68-year-old man with acute
  pericarditis. He had rheumatoid arthritis and clinical clues suggesting lupus
  erythematosus.

Reproduced with permission from Hurst JW: *Cardiovascular diagnosis: the initial
examination,* St. Louis, 1993, Mosby, pp 394, 395.

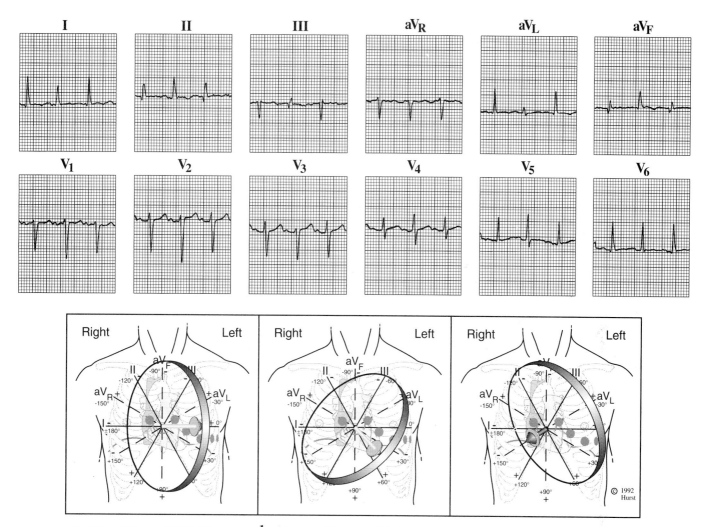

a. First Mean QRS Vector   b. Second Mean QRS Vector   c. Mean T Vector

Fig. 4-77. Pericardial effusion.

- *Rhythm:* Sinus bradycardia
  Rate: 140 depolarizations per minute
  PR interval: 0.13 second
  QRS duration: 0.08 second
  QT interval: 0.28 second
- *Vector diagrams of electrical forces:* See *a, b,* and *c* below the ECG.
- *Electrophysiologic considerations:*
  Sinus tachycardia is present.
  The direction and amplitude of the mean QRS vector alternates with every other depolarization. This is called *electrical alternans.* The total QRS amplitude (97 mm) is on the low side of the normal range.

The T waves are small. The mean T vector is directed +150 degrees to the right and about 85 to 90 degrees anteriorly. This is a primary T wave abnormality.

- *Clinical differential diagnosis:* Electrical alternans, QRS voltage on the low side of normal, low-amplitude T waves, and a primary T wave abnormality indicate the presence of pericardial effusion. Electrical alternans may also be associated with supraventricular tachycardia.
- *Discussion:* This ECG was recorded from a 40-year-old man with a pericardial effusion caused by what was presumed to be a sarcoma of the thymus gland with involvement of the pericardium.

Reproduced with permission form Hurst JW: *Cardiovascular diagnosis: the initial examination,* St. Louis, 1993, Mosby, pp 396, 397.

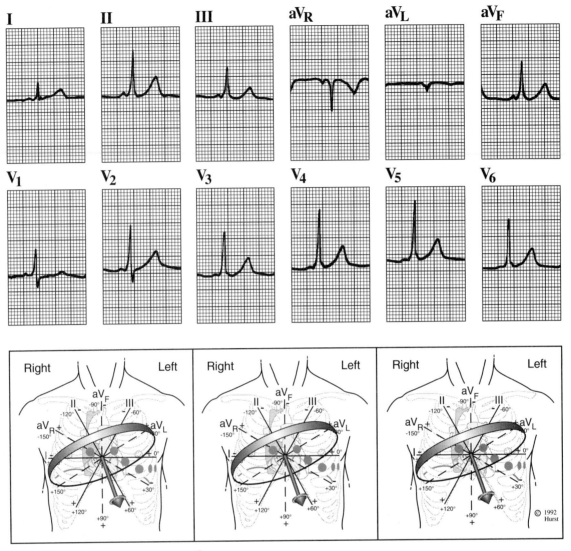

a. Mean QRS Vector

b. Mean Initial 0.04 Second Vector

c. Mean T Vector

Fig. 4-78. Preexcitation of the ventricle responsible for the Wolff-Parkinson-White syndrome.

- *Rhythm:* Normal sinus rhythm
  Rate: Undetermined in a short strip. There were 74 depolarizations per minute in a longer strip.
  PR interval: 0.08 to 0.09 second
  QRS duration: 0.09 second
  QT interval: 0.42 second
- *Vector diagrams of electrical forces:* See a, b, and c below the ECG.
- *Electrophysiologic considerations:*
  The PR interval is abnormally short. This finding alone should lead one to consider the possibility of a bypass tract that circumvents the A-V node, causing early electrical activation of the ventricles.
  The mean QRS vector is directed about +70 degrees inferiorly and anteriorly (the exact number of degrees cannot be determined without recording from additional electrode sample sites). There are two unusual features of the QRS complex:
  1. The slur of the first portion of the QRS complex, called a delta wave.
  2. The mean initial 0.04-second QRS vector is directed +70 degrees inferiorly and anteriorly, producing a tall R wave in leads V_1 and V_2. This is abnormal and could be produced by a true posterior myocardial infarction.

The mean T vector is directed +70 degrees inferiorly and anteriorly.
  It is probably directed about 20 degrees anteriorly, because the T wave in lead V_1 is much smaller than the T wave in lead V_6.
- *Clinical differential diagnosis:* The short PR interval and delta wave are diagnostic of preexcitation of the ventricles caused by a bypass tract that circumvents the A-V node. This type of ECG is usually seen in patients who have episodes of supraventricular tachycardia (including atrial fibrillation) and who have no other evidence of heart disease. The clinician should, however, search for idiopathic hypertrophic cardiomyopathy, an ostium secundum atrial septal defect, or Ebstein's anomaly, since the abnormality is more common in patients with these conditions compared with a population without such diseases.
- *Discussion:* This ECG was recorded from a 22-year-old woman who had experienced episodes of rapid heartbeat since age 6. The ECG abnormalities plus the episodes of rapid heartbeat qualify her as having Wolff-Parkinson-White syndrome. Abnormal Q waves are typically seen in the ECGs of patients who have preexcitation of the ventricles. Because of this, clinicians must be alert to the characteristics of preexcitation so that an erroneous diagnosis of myocardial infarction is not made. Once this is learned, the clinician must then be alert to the fact that patients whose ECGs show preexcitation of the ventricles may also have myocardial infarction. Preexcitiation does not prevent coronary atherosclerosis.

Reproduced with permission from Hurst JW: *Cardiovascular diagnosis: the initial examination,* St. Louis, 1993, Mosby, pp 406, 407.

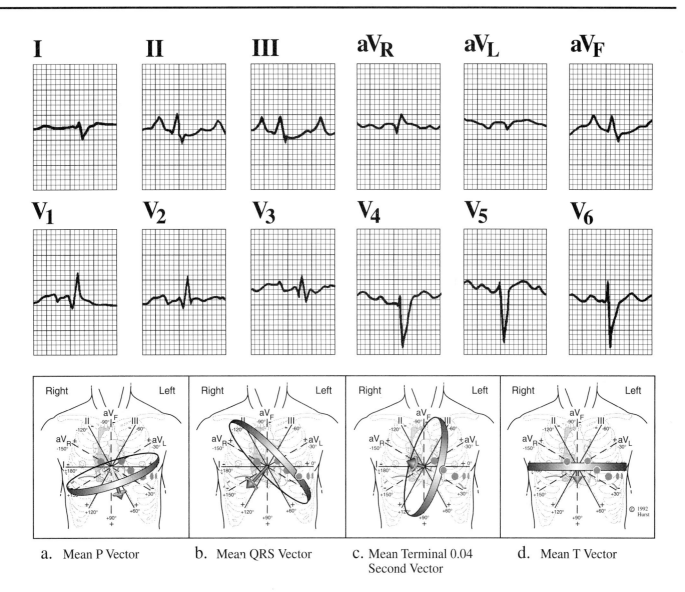

a. Mean P Vector

b. Mean QRS Vector

c. Mean Terminal 0.04 Second Vector

d. Mean T Vector

Fig. 4-79. Pulmonary emphysema.

- *Rhythm:* Normal sinus rhythm
  Rate: Undetermined in short strip
  PR interval: 0.14 second
  QRS duration: 0.09 second
  QT interval: 0.48 second
- *Vector diagrams of electrical forces:* See *a, b, c,* and *d* below the *ECG.*
- *Electrophysiologic considerations:*
  The amplitude of the P wave in lead II is 2.5 mm. Note the peaked shape of the P waves in leads II, III, and aV_F. The mean P vector is directed +73 degrees inferiorly and 30 degrees posteriorly. There is a right atrial abnormality.
  The mean QRS vector is directed about +135 degrees to the right and about 20 degrees anteriorly. This abnormality is due to right ventricular conduction delay or right ventricular hypertrophy (or both). The 12-lead QRS amplitude is about 84 mm, which is on the low side of the normal range.

The mean terminal 0.04-second QRS vector is directed at -170 degrees and 20 degrees anteriorly as a result of right ventricular conduction delay.
The mean T vector is small and difficult to plot. It seems to be directed +90 degrees inferiorly and parallel with the frontal plane.
There is a right atrial abnormality, right ventricular conduction delay, and low amplitude of the QRS complexes.

- *Clinical differential diagnosis:* The most common cause of this type of ECG is extensive pulmonary emphysema due to obstructive lung disease. Other conditions could be responsible for these abnormalities. For example, a patient with secundum atrial septal defect who also had a pericardial effusion might exhibit such an ECG.
- *Discussion:* This patient had severe pulmonary emphysema and cor pulmonale. The right atrial abnormality, low QRS amplitude, and right ventricular conduction delay should strongly suggest emphysema and cor pulmonale.

Electrocardiogram reproduced with permission from Fowler NO, Daniels C, Scott RC et al: The electrocardiogram in cor pulmonale with and without emphysema, *Am F Cardiol* 16:501, 1965.

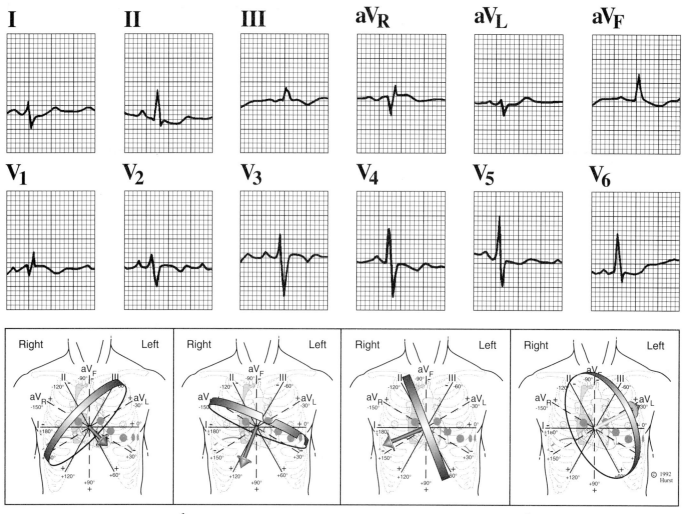

a. Mean P Vector

b. Mean QRS Vector

c. Mean Terminal 0.04 Second Vector

d. Mean T Vector

Fig. 4-80. Acute pulmonary embolism.
- *Rhythm:* Normal sinus rhythm
  Rate: Undetermined in short strip
  PR interval: 0.16 second
  QRS duration: 0.08 second
  QT interval: 0.32 second
- *Vector diagrams of electrical forces:* See *a, b, c,* and *d* below the ECG.
- *Electrophysiologic considerations:*
  The mean P vector is directed +45 degrees inferiorly and about 20 degrees anteriorly. The anterior rotation suggests an RA abnormality, but this is not definite.
  The mean QRS vector is directed +110 degrees to the right and about 10 degrees anteriorly. Note that the QRS complexes in leads V_5 and V_6 are resultantly positive, whereas the transitional pathway of the mean QRS shown in *b* would cause QRS complexes in leads V_5 and V_6 to be resultantly zero. This discrepancy occurs because the electrode positions for leads V_5 and V_6 are near the transitional pathway of the mean QRS vector. Accordingly, a small electrode placement error could cause such a variance.

The mean terminal 0.04-second QRS vector is directed +160 degrees to the right and is parallel with the frontal plane. This is characteristic of RV conduction delay.

The mean T vector is directed almost -30 degrees to the left and 70 degrees posteriorly. The mean T vector points away from a repolarization abnormality of the RV.

The possible RA abnormality, RV conduction defect, and anterior repolarization abnormality strongly indicate an acute pulmonary embolism. Such patients may have right bundle branch block. Also, the mean initial 0.04-second QRS vector may shift to the left, producing a Q wave in leads III and aV_F, suggesting an inferior myocardial infarction.
- *Clinical differential diagnosis:* When these ECG abnormalities appear in a patient with syncope, acute dyspnea, or acute pleuritic pain and when a previous ECG is normal (or does not show the same abnormalities), the clinician should diagnose acute pulmonary embolism.
- *Discussion:* This ECG was recorded from a 54-year-old patient with an acute pulmonary embolism.

ECG from Hurst JW, Woodson GC Jr: *Atlas of spatial vector electrocardiography,* New York, 1952, Blakiston, p203. Reprinted with permission from the author.

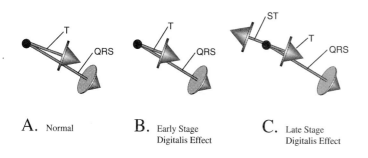

A. Normal

B. Early Stage Digitalis Effect

C. Late Stage Digitalis Effect

Fig. 4-81. ECG effects of digitalis. **A,** The direction and magnitude of arrows representing the mean of the electrical forces (vectors) responsible for the normal QRS complex and normal T wave before digitalis medication are illustrated. The QT interval is 0.36 second. **B,** Early signs of digitalis medication may be recognized as a decrease in the amplitude of the T wave.

Note in this illustration that the arrow representing the T wave becomes shorter than in **A** but that the direction of the arrow has not changed. The QT interval is now 0.30 second. The direction and magnitude of the arrow representing the mean of the electrical forces (vectors) responsible for the QRS complex show no change from the direction and magnitude of the arrow shown in **A. C,** More advanced ECG changes of digitalis medication are shown here. An arrow representing the mean of the electrical forces (vectors) responsible for the T waves is shorter, but its direction has not changed from that shown in **A** and **B.** An arrow representing the mean of the electrical forces (vectors) responsible for the ST segment displacement is shown; it is actually caused by the early forces of repolarization and is directed opposite to the arrow representing the mean T vector. The QT interval is 0.28 second. The direction and magnitude of the arrow representing the QRS vector show no change from the direction and magnitude of the arrows shown in **A** and **B.**

Reproduced with permission from Hurst JW: *Cardiovascular diagnosis: the initial examination,* St. Louis, 1993, Mosby, p 414.

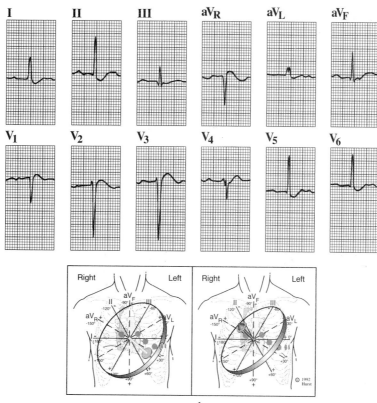

a. Mean QRS Vector   b. Mean ST Vector

Fig. 4-82. ECG effects of digitalis and a high serum calcium level.
- *Rhythm:* Sinus tachycardia
  Rate: Undetermined in short strip. There were 96 depolarizations per minute in a longer strip.
  PR interval: 0.28 second
  QRS duration: 0.08 second
  QT interval: 0.29 second
- *Vector diagrams of electrical forces:* See *a* and *b* below the ECG.
- *Electrophysiologic considerations:*
  The PR interval is prolonged, indicating first-degree A-V block.
  The QT interval is shorter than normal.
  The mean QRS vector is directed +40 degrees inferiorly and 70 degrees posteriorly. It is more posteriorly directed than usual.
  The mean ST segment vector is large. It is directed at -140 degrees and 30 to 40 degrees anteriorly.
  The T waves are not seen in all leads. Therefore, a mean vector for the T waves cannot be drawn. The T waves are small and upright in leads aV$_L$, V$_5$, and V$_6$.

The longer than normal PR interval, the shorter than normal QT interval, and an ST segment vector that is opposite in direction to the mean QRS vector are characteristic of the effect of digitalis on the ECG. The same effect occurs with hypercalcemia.
- *Clinical differential diagnosis:* There are two causes of these abnormalities: the digitalis effect and hypercalcemia. Subendocardial injury can produce an ST segment displacement of this magnitude, but the QT interval is usually prolonged and the T waves are usually more obvious than those shown here.
- *Discussion:* This ECG was recorded from a 66-year-old woman with *Staphylococcus aureus* and *Streptococcus viridans* endocarditis of the aortic valve, a history of hypertension, severe heart failure, a digoxin blood level of 3.2 ng/ml, and a serum calcium level of 12.2 mg%. The patient also had hyperparathyroidism.

The ST segment and T wave abnormalities in this ECG are undoubtedly caused by digitalis plus hypercalcemia.

Reproduced with permission from Hurst JW: *Cardiovascular diagnosis: the initial examination,* St. Louis, 1993, Mosby, pp 416, 417.

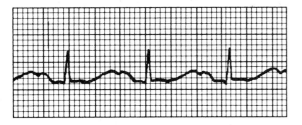

Fig. 4-83. ECG signs of hypokalemia and hypocalcemia.
- *Rhythm:* Sinus tachycardia
  Rate: Undetermined in short strip. There were about 100 depolarizations per minute in a longer strip.

PR interval: Approximatley 0.20 second
QRS duration: 0.06 second
QT interval: 0.44 second
- *Electrophysiologic considerations:* The long QT interval is abnormal, and the amplitude of the T waves is low. In this tracing the T waves abut the P waves, and it is not possible to identify U waves.
- *Clinical differential diagnosis:* The long QT interval and low-amplitude T waves suggest the possibility of hypokalemia. The ST segment seems a little long, suggesting hypocalcemia.
- *Discussion:* This ECG was recorded from a 57-year-old woman with cirrhosis of the liver. The serum potassium level was 2.7mEq/L, and the serum calcium level was 4.4 mg%.

Reproduced with permission from Hurst JW: *Cardiovascular diagnosis: the initial examination,* St. Louis, 1993, Mosby, p 410.

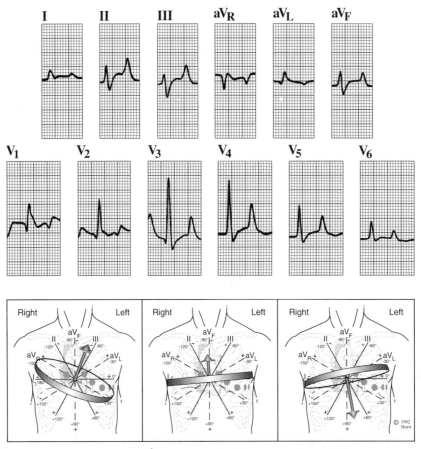

a. Mean QRS Vector   b. Mean Terminal 0.04 Second Vector   c. Mean T Vector

Fig. 4-84. ECG signs of hyperkalemia.
- *Rhythm:* Junctional rhythm
  Rate: Undetermined in short strip. There were 90 depolarizations per minute in a longer strip.
  PR interval: None
  QRS duration: 0.12 second
  QT interval: 0.44 second
- *Vector diagrams of electrical forces:* See *a ,b,* and *c* below the ECG.
- *Electrophysiologic considerations:*
  P waves cannot be identified.
  The mean QRS vector is directed about -70 degrees to the left and about 20 degrees anteriorly. The direction of the mean QRS vector is characteristic of right bundle branch block (RBBB) plus left anterosuperior division block.

The mean terminal 0.04-second QRS vector is directed -95 degrees to the left and is parallel with the frontal plane. This, too is typical of RBBB plus left anterosuperior division block.
The mean T vector is directed about +80 degrees to the right and 5 to 10 degrees anteriorly. Note the shape of the T waves. They are tall and narrow, and the ascending and descending limbs are sloped to the same degree. Such T waves are referred to as being tent-shaped.
The long QT interval, abnormal rhythm, RBBB plus left anterosuperior division block, and tent-shaped T waves characteristic of hyperkalemia.
- *Clinical differential diagnosis:* This cluster of abnormalities is almost diagnostic of hyperkalemia.
- *Discussion:* This ECG was recorded from an 85-year-old man with diabetic ketoacidosis. His serum potassium level was 9.1 mEq/L.

Reproduced with permission from Hurst JW: *Cardiovascular diagnosis: the initial examination,* St. Louis, 1993, Mosby, pp 412, 413.

REFERENCES

1. Hurst JW: The ECG. In *Cardiovascular diagnosis: the initial examination*, St Louis, 1993, Mosby.
2. Grant RP, Estes EH: *Spatial vector electrocardiography*, Philadelphia, 1951, Blakiston.
3. Hurst JW: The hypothetical myocardial cell. In *Ventricular electrocardiography*, St. Louis, 1991, Mosby.
4. Bayley R: *Electrocardiographic analysis.* Vol 1, Biophysical principles, New York, 1958, Hoeber.
5. Wilson FN, Johnston FD, MacLeod AG, Barker PS: Electrocardiograms that represent potential variation of single electrode, *Am Heart J* 9:447, 1934.
6. Goldberger E: Simple indifferent, electrocardiographic electrode of zero potential and a technique of obtaining augmented, unipolar, extremity leads, *Am Heart J* 23:483, 1942.
7. Wilson FN. Foreword. In Barker JM: *The unipolar electrocardiogram: a clinical interpretation*, New York, 1952, Appleton-Century-Crofts.
8. Odom H II, Davis JL, Dinh HA, et al: QRS voltage measurements in autopsied men free of cardiopulmonary disease: a basis for evaluating total QRS voltage as an index of left ventricular hypertrophy, *Am J Cardiol* 58:801, 1986.
9. Morris JJ, Estes EH Jr, Whalen RE, et al: P wave analysis in valvular heart disease, *Circulation* 29:242, 1964.
10. Romhilt DW, Estes EH Jr: A point-score system for the ECG diagnosis of left ventricular hypertrophy, *Am Heart J* 75:752, 1968.

Table 4-1 Upper limits of the normal PR intervals

Rate	Below 70	71-90	91-110	111-130	Above 130
Large adults	0.21	0.20	0.19	0.18	0.17
Small adults	0.20	0.19	0.18	0.17	0.16
Children ages 14-17	0.19	0.18	0.17	0.16	0.15
Children ages 7-13	0.18	0.17	0.16	0.15	0.14
Children ages 1 1/2 to 6	0.17	0.165	0.155	0.145	0.135
Children ages 0 to 1 1/2	0.16	0.15	0.145	0.135	0.125

From Ashman R, Hull E: *Essentials of electrocardiography*, ed 2, New York, 1941, Macmillan, p 341. The copyright was transferred to the authors in 1956. The authors are deceased.

Table 4-2 Normal QT intervals and the upper limits of normal

Cycle lengths (sec)	Heart rate (per min)	Men and children (sec)	Women (sec)	Upper limits of normal Men and children (sec)	Women (sec)
1.50	40	0.449	0.461	0.491	0.503
1.40	43	0.438	0.450	0.479	0.491
1.30	46	0.426	0.438	0.466	0.478
1.25	48	0.420	0.432	0.460	0.471
1.20	50	0.414	0.425	0.453	0.464
1.15	52	0.407	0.418	0.445	0.456
1.10	54.5	0.400	0.411	0.438	0.449
1.05	57	0.393	0.404	0.430	0.441
1.00	60	0.386	0.396	0.422	0.432
0.95	63	0.378	0.388	0.413	0.423
0.90	66.5	0.370	0.380	0.404	0.414
0.85	70.5	0.361	0.371	0.395	0.405
0.80	75	0.352	0.362	0.384	0.394
0.75	80	0.342	0.352	0.374	0.384
0.70	86	0.332	0.341	0.363	0.372
0.65	92.5	0.321	0.330	0.351	0.360
0.60	100	0.310	0.318	0.338	0.347
0.55	109	0.297	0.305	0.325	0.333
0.50	120	0.283	0.291	0.310	0.317
0.45	133	0.268	0.276	0.294	0.301
0.40	150	0.252	0.258	0.275	0.282
0.35	172	0.234	0.240	0.255	0.262

From Ashman R, Hull E: *Essentials of electrocardiography*, ed 2, New York, 1941, Macmillan, p 344. The copyright was transferred to the authors in 1956. The authors are deceased.

PART II

PATIENT PUZZLES

INTRODUCTION

The clues required to solve, or at least begin to unravel, most cardiac mysteries were discussed in Part I. In Part II, you, the physician-detective, will have the opportunity to search for the clues that will solve 50 cardiac puzzles.

The data used to describe each of the 50 patients were derived from patients I have seen in the office, on teaching rounds at Emory University Hospital, and in teaching conferences. Accordingly, each patient is a composite of several patients. This method of presentation is used in order to teach some of the principles of clinical cardiology and to challenge the reader's analytical ability, correlative ability, and ability to synthesize data into a correct diagnosis. Except for patient 1, the sequence of presentations has been randomized. At times, a major diagnostic clue establishes the cardiac diagnosis. At other times, a cluster of minor clues, when added together, point toward the disease. Diagrams are used to illustrate abnormal physical signs and abnormalities noted in the chest x-ray film and the electrocardiogram (ECG). This method of presentation is used because clues can be highlighted in the diagrams just as facial features are emphasized in cartoons. It is hoped that this approach will assist the readers in their efforts to remember the clues. At times the reader is referred to actual chest x-ray films that are shown in Chapter 3 of Part I. Vectors are used to illustrate the ECGs because of the belief that basic electrophysiologic principles should be used to interpret each ECG. At times the reader is referred to actual ECGs that are presented in Chapter 4 of Part I of this set.

Wherever illustrations are used from other sources, they are identified by the statement, "see figure credits." The figure credit, in turn, is shown at the end of each patient presentation.

The diagnostic clues for each patient are listed on the right-hand page of the book, and the answer and discussion are presented on subsequent pages.

It is hoped that if readers master the diagnostic lessons of the 50 patients presented here, they will, with practice, improve their examination of the heart and will be able to come to diagnostic conclusions more easily.

Now, to the reader, please don't turn the page until you have answered the questions posed in the patient presentations. Who would destroy the joy and excitement of a detective story by reading the last few pages of a mystery novel before coming to a conclusion regarding "who did it?"

HISTORY

The patient is a 47-year-old asymptomatic man who needs a medical examination as part of his application for life insurance. The form supplied by the insurance company requires a statement indicating the presence or absence of heart disease. His father died in an automobile wreck at age 45, and his mother is living and well at age 72. He has no brothers or sisters. He does not smoke. He plays tennis three times each week and jogs two miles daily.

PHYSICAL EXAMINATION

He is 6 feet tall and weighs 185 pounds.

The systolic blood pressure is 130 mm Hg, and the diastolic blood pressure is 80 mm Hg.

The jugular venous pulsation, carotid artery pulsation, and precordial movements are normal.

Auscultation of the heart reveals the heart sounds shown on the right. No murmurs are heard.

The pulsations of the peripheral arteries are normal.

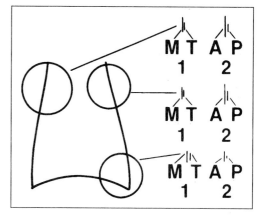

1, First heart sound; *2*, second heart sound; *M*, mitral valve closure sound; *T*, tricuspid valve closure sound; *A*, aortic valve closure sound; *P*, pulmonary valve closure sound. See figure credit.

CHEST X-RAY FILM

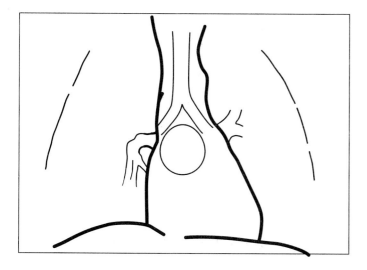

ELECTROCARDIOGRAM

The heart rate and rhythm are normal. The PR interval is 0.16 second. The QRS duration is 0.08 second. The QT interval is 0.34 second. The total 12-lead QRS amplitude is 160 mm.

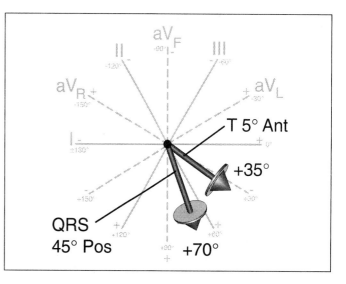

WHAT IS DIFFERENTIAL DIAGNOSIS?

WHAT WOULD YOU DO?

HISTORY

The patient is an active, nonsmoking, asymptomatic 47-year-old male. He is an avid tennis player and jogs daily. His father died at a young age as the result of an automobile accident. Accordingly, no judgment can be made regarding a history of coronary atherosclerotic heart disease. His mother is well at age 72.

PHYSICAL EXAMINATION

The blood pressure is normal. The patient is not obese. The heart sounds are normal. The second is louder than the first heart sound in the second right intercostal space near the sternum. The second heart sound is normally split. The intensity of the heart sounds at the cardiac apex is normal. The pulmonary valve closure sound is barely heard at the apex. There are no murmurs. Auscultation of the heart is normal.

CHEST X-RAY FILM

The heart size is normal. The size of each cardiac chamber is normal. The size of the aorta is normal. The pulmonary artery and its branches are normal. The pulmonary blood flow is normal. There are no signs of heart failure. The lungs and bony structures are normal.

See Fig. 3-1, which shows a cartoon of a normal chest x-ray film.

ELECTROCARDIOGRAM

The heart rhythm and rate are normal. The PR interval, QRS duration and QT interval are normal. The direction and size of the mean QRS vector are normal. The mean T vector has a normal relationship to the mean QRS vector. The QRS-T angle is 50 degrees. The ECG is normal.

See Fig. 4-24 which shows a normal electrocardiogram.

DIFFERENTIAL DIAGNOSIS; WHAT TO DO

There are only two possibilities.
1)   The heart is normal.
2)   Despite the negative history, normal physical examination, normal chest x-ray film, and normal ECG, the patient could have coronary atherosclerotic heart disease.

The normal physical examination rules out hypertension, cardiac valve disease, cardiomyopathy, and pericardial disease. Con-genital heart disease, with a few rare exceptions, is excluded because the heart sounds are normal and there are no murmurs. Despite the absence of known risk factors, it would be wise to pursue the possibility of asymptomatic coronary atherosclerotic heart disease. His father died in an accident at age 45, so the status of the patient's coronary arteries cannot be determined. The level of his blood lipids is not known.

Because the patient participates in vigorous exercise and the insurance form must be completed, it would be wise to have the patient undergo an exercise stress ECG test. If it is positive, a coronary arteriogram should be performed. His blood lipids should be measured.

DIAGNOSTIC PRINCIPLE

This presentation has been included to emphasize that the heart of an asymptomatic patient over age 40 who has a normal physical examination, normal chest x-ray film, and normal ECG at rest may be normal, but that such a patient could have asymptomatic coronary atherosclerotic heart disease. Coronary atherosclerotic heart disease can occur in men and women under age 40, but it occurs more frequently in men who are over age 40 and women who are over age 50.

This presentation can also serve as background information for the following 49 cardiac puzzles.

BIBLIOGRAPHY

Hurst JW, Morris DC: The history: symptoms and past events related to cardiovascular disease. In Schlant RC, Alexander RW, editors: *Hurst's the heart*, ed 8, New York, 1994, McGraw-Hill, pp 205-216.

Hurst JW: *Cardiovascular diagnosis: the initial examination*, St Louis, 1993, Mosby.

FIGURE CREDIT

Reproduced with permission from Hurst JW: The examination of the heart: the importance of initial screening, *Dis Mon* 36(5):294, 1990.

HISTORY

The patient is a 30-year-old asymptomatic woman who has been referred by her gynecologist.

PHYSICAL EXAMINATION

General inspection of the patient is normal.

The systolic blood pressure is 120 mm Hg, and the diastolic blood pressure is 70 mm Hg.

The abnormal physical findings are not given here. Diagrams of the abnormal physical findings should be drawn by the reader after studying the chest x-ray and electrocardiogram.

CHEST X-RAY FILM

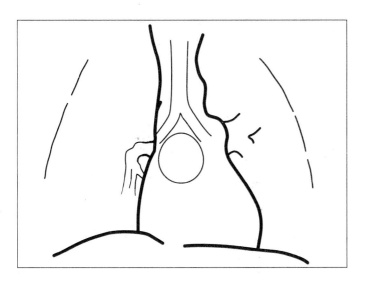

ELECTROCARDIOGRAM

The heart rhythm is normal. There are 68 depolarizations per minute. The P wave in lead II is 3 mm high, and its duration is 0.12 second. The PR interval is 0.14 second. The QRS duration is 0.08 second. The QT interval is 0.40 second. The 12-lead amplitude of the QRS is 175 mm.

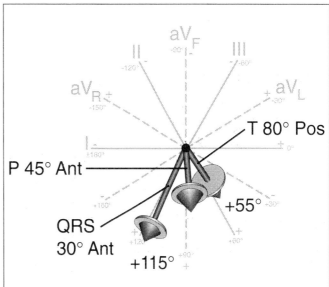

WHAT IS DIFFERENTIAL DIAGNOSIS?

DIAGRAM ABNORMAL PHYSICAL FINDINGS

WHAT IS FINAL DIAGNOSIS?

HISTORY

The gynecologist did not state why she referred the 30-year-old patient for consultation. A common reason for referral is that some type of heart murmur is heard or the patient gives a history of paroxysmal rapid heartbeat. The murmur is usually caused by mitral valve prolapse, but other causes may be present.

PHYSICAL EXAMINATION

The systemic blood pressure is normal. See figures under *Abnormal Physical Findings.*

CHEST X-RAY FILM

The main pulmonary artery and the left branch of the pulmonary artery are larger than normal. The right branch of the pulmonary artery appears to be normal in size and shape. The right lower border of the heart may be larger than normal. This could be caused by a large right atrium.

The large main pulmonary artery, large left pulmonary artery, normal right pulmonary artery, and possible right atrial (RA) enlargement suggest the presence of pulmonary valve stenosis.

See Patient 1 for a normal chest x-ray film.

ELECTROCARDIOGRAM

The mean P vector is larger than normal and is directed +85 degrees in the frontal plane and 45 degrees anteriorly indicating an RA abnormality. Such an abnormality may be caused by tricuspid valve disease or RV disease.

The duration of the QRS complexes is normal.

The mean QRS vector is directed +115 degrees in the frontal plane and 30 degrees anteriorly, indicating RV hypertrophy.

The mean T vector is directed +55 degrees in the frontal plane and 80 degrees posteriorly. The QRS-T angle is about 110 degrees.

The ECG is diagnostic of RV hypertrophy. It is not possible to indicate the cause of the RV hypertrophy from the ECG.

See Fig. 4-55 for an ECG showing RV hypertrophy.

See Patient 1 for a normal ECG.

DIFFERENTIAL DIAGNOSIS

RV hypertrophy, which is definitely present, could be caused by:
• Primary pulmonary hypertension. The normal right branch of the pulmonary artery conflicts with this diagnosis.
• A patient with Eisenmenger physiology related to patent ductus arteriosus, interventricular septal defect, or atrial septal defect has a large main pulmonary artery and large, but tapering, right pulmonary artery. The left pulmonary artery is also larger than normal and tapers quickly, but it is not as easily seen as the right pulmonary artery. The right branch of the pulmonary artery is normal in this patient and makes Eisenmenger physiology less likely.
• Pulmonary hypertension caused by longstanding, severe mitral stenosis could produce RV hypertrophy. However, there are no other signs of mitral stenosis in the chest x-ray film or in the ECG.

• Pulmonary valve stenosis is the likely diagnosis because of a dilated main pulmonary artery and large left pulmonary artery branch associated with a normal right pulmonary artery branch.

ABNORMAL PHYSICAL FINDINGS

The reader should create diagrams that resemble those shown below.
• Internal jugular vein pulsation

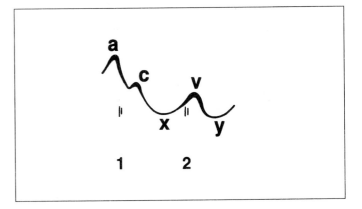

Note the large a wave. *1,* First heart sound; *2,* second heart sound. See figure credits.

• Precordial movement

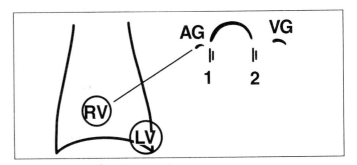

Note the sustained systolic movement of the anterior chest wall caused by RV hypertrophy and the palpable RA gallop and RV gallop. *RV,* right ventricle; *LV,* left ventricle; *AG,* atrial gallop; and *VG,* ventricular gallop. See figure credits.

• Auscultation of the heart

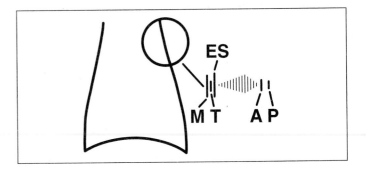

Note the systolic ejection sound (*ES*), diamond-shaped systolic murmur, and the delayed pulmonary valve closure (*P*) sound, which may be inaudible in some patients. *M,* mitral; *T,* tricuspid; and *A,* aortic valve closure sounds. *RA* and *RV* gallop sounds are shown. See figure credits.

FINAL DIAGNOSIS

Congenital heart disease due to pulmonary valve stenosis.

DIAGNOSTIC PRINCIPLE

It is important to study the size of the main pulmonary artery and the size of its right and left branches. It is often possible to determine if there is normal, increased, or decreased pulmonary blood flow. Pulmonary valve stenosis creates a large main pulmonary artery because of poststenotic dilatation. The left pulmonary artery may also be large, but the size of the right pulmonary artery is usually normal. Idiopathic dilatation of the pulmonary artery can be ruled out because of the evidence for RV hypertrophy in the ECG.

BIBLIOGRAPHY

Nugent EW, Plauth WH, Edwards JE, Williams WH: The pathology, pathophysiology, recognition, and treatment of congenital heart disease. In Schlant RC, Alexander RW, editors: *Hurst's the heart*, ed 8, New York, 1994, McGraw-Hill, pp 1796-1799.

FIGURE CREDITS

Diagram of abnormal venous pulsation, reproduced with permission. Diagrams of precordial movements and auscultation are slightly modified and reproduced with permission, from Hurst JW: The examination of the heart: the importance of initial screening, *Dis Mon* 36(5):262 (middle), 280 (upper), 285 (lower), 1990.

HISTORY

A 58-year-old man is being admitted to the intensive care unit because of a cerebrovascular accident (CVA, stroke) that produced aphasia and right hemiplegia. The past history cannot be obtained from the patient. A neighbor, who did not know him, saw him fall and called the ambulance. The neighbor, who followed the ambulance in his car, states that the man never lost consciousness.

PHYSICAL EXAMINATION

The systolic blood pressure is 150 mm Hg, and the diastolic blood pressure is 85 mm Hg.

The patient is aphasic, and there is evidence of right hemiplegia. The neck veins and the pulsations of the peripheral arteries are normal. Funduscopic examination of the eyes is normal. An ectopic systolic bulge is felt just above the cardiac apex impulse. The first heart sound is faint, and the second heart sound is normal. Atrial and ventricular gallop sounds are heard at the cardiac apex.

CHEST X-RAY FILM

ELECTROCARDIOGRAM

There is normal sinus rhythm. There are 88 depolarizations per minute. The PR interval is 0.22 second, the QRS duration is 0.10 second, and the QT interval is 0.44 second.

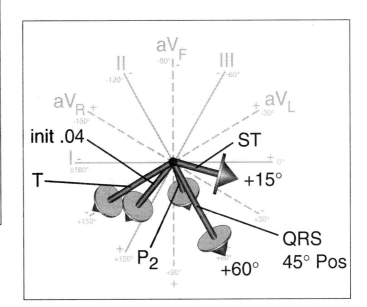

WHAT IS LIKELY CAUSE OF THE STROKE?

HISTORY

The patient obviously had a stroke, most likely caused by an embolus. The diagnostic task is to find the source of the embolus.

PHYSICAL EXAMINATION

The peripheral pulses are normal, which speaks against a dissection of the aorta as the cause for the stroke. The heart rhythm is normal, eliminating atrial fibrillation as the cause of an embolic stroke. The first heart sound is faint, suggesting a longer-than-normal PR interval. The precordial movement is not normal; the abnormal movement suggests a ventricular aneurysm secondary to myocardial infarction (MI). The ventricular gallop sound heard in diastole indicates left ventricular (LV) dysfunction, and the atrial gallop sound heard at the cardiac apex indicates poor LV compliance.

CHEST X-RAY FILM

There is a bulge noted just above the apex of the heart. It could represent a ventricular aneurysm.

See Patient 1 for a normal chest x-ray film.

ELECTROCARDIOGRAM

The PR interval is abnormally long, as is the QT interval.

A mean vector representing the last half of the P wave, designated as P_2, is directed abnormally posteriorly, indicating a left atrial (LA) abnormality. This is usually caused by LV disease or mitral valve disease.

The mean QRS vector is directed 60 degrees in the frontal plane and 45 degrees posteriorly. The mean initial 0.04-second vector is directed far to the right and posteriorly, as is the mean T vector. These abnormalities indicate an anterior dead zone and anterior epicardial ischemia, respectively.

The mean ST vector is directed +15 degrees in the frontal plane and is parallel with the frontal plane. It is caused by epicardial injury.

The ECG shows an extensive anterolateral MI. An ST segment shift of this type, when persistent, suggests a ventricular aneurysm.

See Patient 1 for a normal ECG.

LIKELY CAUSE OF THE STROKE

The stroke was most likely caused by an embolus that originated in a mural thrombus located in a ventricular aneurysm because of an anterolateral MI that occurred several weeks previously. The patient fell at the time of the recent stroke.

DIAGNOSTIC PRINCIPLE

Many strokes are caused by cerebral emboli, and the physician must search for a cardiovascular cause of the emboli.

A ventricular aneurysm can often be palpated. Ventricular aneurysms are almost always caused by an MI related to coronary atherosclerotic heart disease.

BIBLIOGRAPHY

Broderick JP: Heart disease and stroke. *Heart Disease and Stroke* 2:355-359, 1993.

Roberts R, Morris DC, Pratt CM, Alexander RW: Pathophysiology, recognition, and treatment of acute myocardial infarction and its complications. In Schlant RC, Alexander RW, editors: *Hurst's the heart*, ed 8, New York, 1994, McGraw-Hill, p 1153.

HISTORY

The patient is a 72-year-old man. He gives a history of retrosternal discomfort that is precipitated by walking up the slight incline from his mailbox to his home. This discomfort has occurred daily for 2 weeks. He has had one episode of syncope.

PHYSICAL EXAMINATION

The systolic blood pressure is 135 mm Hg, and the diastolic pressure is 75 mm Hg.

The abnormal physical findings are not given here. Diagrams of the abnormal physical findings should be drawn after studying the chest x-ray film and electrocardiogram.

CHEST X-RAY FILM

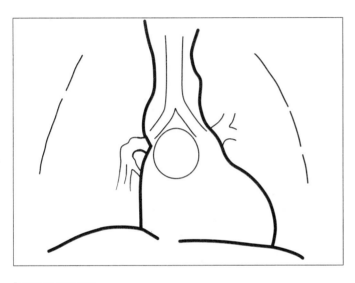

Posteroanterior view

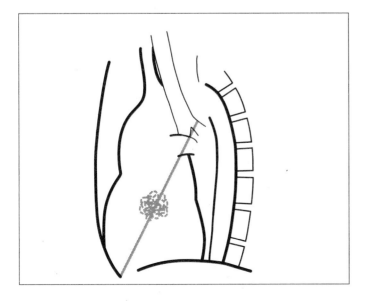

Left lateral view

ELECTROCARDIOGRAM

The rhythm is normal. There are 70 depolarizations per minute. The PR interval is 0.20 second. The QRS duration is 0.09 second. The QT interval is 0.40 second. The 12-lead QRS amplitude is 200 mm.

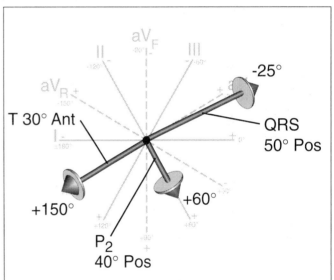

WHAT IS DIFFERENTIAL DIAGNOSIS?

WHAT ARE POSSIBLE CARDIOVASCULAR ABNORMALITIES?

WHAT IS FINAL DIAGNOSIS?

HISTORY

The possible diagnoses based on the history of chest discomfort and syncope precipitated by effort are aortic valve stenosis, hypertrophic cardiomyopathy, coronary atherosclerotic heart disease with a cardiac dysrhythmia, or aortic valve stenosis plus coronary atherosclerotic heart disease.

PHYSICAL EXAMINATION

The systemic blood pressure is normal. This makes hypertensive cardiovascular disease unlikely.

See figures under *Possible Cardiovascular Abnormalities*.

CHEST X-RAY FILM

The heart is enlarged. The left ventricle is large. The root of the aorta is dilated. These abnormalities could be caused by hypertension, but the blood pressure is normal. The abnormalities could be caused by aortic valve regurgitation, but the diastolic blood pressure and pulse pressure are normal. The abnormalities could be caused by aortic valve stenosis.

It is necessary to look for valve calcification in the left lateral x-ray film. Calcification of the aortic valve is located in the center of the heart. It straddles a line drawn from the carina to the anterior costophrenic angle. Note the aortic valve calcification in this diagram.

See Patient 1 for a normal chest x-ray film.

ELECTROCARDIOGRAM

The heart rhythm and rate are normal. The PR interval, QRS duration, and QT interval are normal.

The mean vector representing the last half of the P wave is directed at +60 degrees in the frontal plane and 40 degrees posteriorly. It indicates left atrial abnormality that can result from mitral valve disease or left ventricular (LV) disease.

The mean QRS vector is directed at -25 degrees in the frontal plane and 50 degrees posteriorly. It is abnormally large; the 12-lead amplitude of the QRS complexes is larger than normal. The mean T vector is directed to the right of the mean QRS vector. It is directed +150 degrees in the frontal plane and 30 degrees anteriorly.

All these abnormalities combined indicate LV hypertrophy. They favor a systolic pressure overload type of LV hypertrophy. Such abnormalities could be caused by hypertension, aortic valve stenosis, or primary hypertrophy of the heart.

See Patient 1 for a normal ECG.

See ECG shown in Fig. 4-53, Part 1.

DIFFERENTIAL DIAGNOSIS

The level of systolic and diastolic blood pressure rule out hypertension and aortic regurgitation as a cause of the LV hypertrophy and a dilated aortic root.

The patient could have hypertrophic cardiomyopathy, but the aortic root is not usually dilated in this condition. Mitral valve regurgitation is unlikely for the same reason.

The presence of calcium in the aortic valve is diagnostic of aortic valve disease. The episode of syncope was undoubtedly caused by aortic stenosis and indicates that the stenosis is severe. Other data are needed to determine if the retrosternal discomfort (unstable angina pectoris) produced by effort is caused by aortic valve stenosis alone or if there is additional obstructive coronary atherosclerosis.

POSSIBLE CARDIOVASCULAR ABNORMALITIES

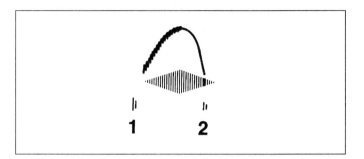

I, 2, First, second heart sounds. See figure credits.

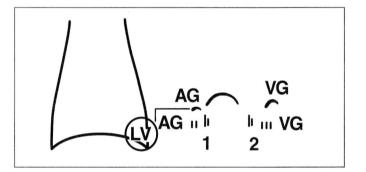

LV, left ventricle; *AG,* atrial gallop; *VG,* ventricular gallop. See figure credits.

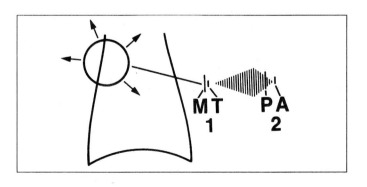

M, mitral; *T,* tricuspid; *P,* pulmonary; and *A,* aortic valve closure sounds. See figure credits.

The aortic upstroke is slow, and a shudder is felt during systole (upper figure). No pulsus bisferiens is felt in the carotid artery.

The apex impulse lasts longer than normal. Abnormal atrial and ventricular movements can be palpated (middle figure).

There is a coarse systolic murmur heard in the second right intercostal space near the sternum (lower figure). It radiates to the neck. A systolic thrill is also located in that area. The murmur is heard at the apex, but is a little higher pitched in this area. The murmur does not radiate laterally from the apex, which excludes mitral valve regurgitation. The aortic valve closure sound is diminished in intensity and may follow the pulmonary valve closure sound. The latter may be masked by the murmur. Atrial and ventricular gallop sounds are commonly heard at the apex (not shown in the illustration).

FINAL DIAGNOSIS

The diagnosis is calcific aortic stenosis of elderly persons. It is severe. The aortic-left ventricular gradient would be at least 100 mm Hg. The unstable angina and syncope also indicate the severe nature of the condition.

The patient should have cardiac catheterization, including a coronary arteriogram, before aortic valve surgery to determine the status of the coronary arteries, which may or may not be diseased with atherosclerosis. The patient *should not* have an exercise stress test of any type. An echocardiogram is not needed because all the information required can be obtained at the time of cardiac catheterization which must be done because echocardiography cannot, as yet, adequately assess the status of the coronary arteries.

DIAGNOSTIC PRINCIPLE

Syncope plus stable or unstable angina should always lead one to consider the possibility of aortic valve stenosis or idiopathic hypertrophic subaortic stenosis (IHSS). In such cases the angina may or may not be caused by associated coronary atherosclerosis. Calcific aortic stenosis can usually be diagnosed because the early portion of the aorta is dilated and calcium can be seen in the aortic valve in the lateral x-ray view. In addition, the murmur and diminished aortic valve closure sounds are characteristic of aortic valve stenosis, whereas the murmur of IHSS is associated with an audible aortic valve closure sound and the murmur decreases with isometric exercise (handgrip).

Remember, patients who have angina pectoris alone rarely have electrocardiographic signs of LV hypertrophy. When LV hypertrophy is evident in the ECG, one must search for a cause other than coronary disease or in addition to coronary disease.

BIBLIOGRAPHY

Rapaport E, Rackley CE, Cohn LH. Aortic valvular disease. In Schlant RC, Alexander RW, editors: *Hurst's the heart*, ed 8, New York, 1994, McGraw-Hill, pp 1457-1466.

FIGURE CREDITS

Left, reproduced with permission, *middle*, modified and reproduced with permission, and *right*, reproduced with permission from Hurst JW: The examination of the heart: the importance of initial screening, *Dis Mon* 36(5):278 (middle), 262 (upper), 285 (lower), 1990.

HISTORY

The patient is an asymptomatic 43-year-old woman. She is referred by her primary care physician because of an abnormal chest x-ray film.

PHYSICAL EXAMINATION

The systolic blood pressure is 120 mm Hg, and the diastolic blood pressure is 80 mm Hg.

Remainder of examination withheld for now.

CHEST X-RAY FILM

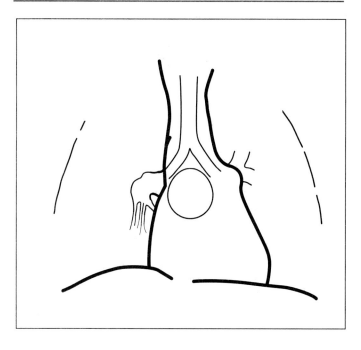

ELECTROCARDIOGRAM

The rhythm is regular. There are 70 depolarizations per minute. The PR interval is 0.16 second. The QRS duration is 0.10 second. The QT interval is 0.40 second. The 12-lead QRS amplitude is 170 mm.

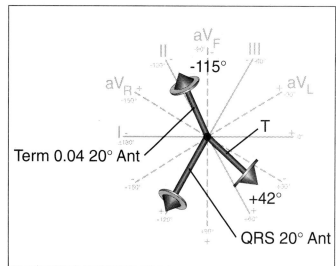

WHAT IS DIFFERENTIAL DIAGNOSIS?

DIAGRAM HEART SOUNDS AND MURMURS HEARD IN SECOND LEFT INTERCOSTAL SPACE NEAR STERNUM

HISTORY

The patient is an asymptomatic 43-year-old-female with an abnormal chest x-ray film. The cause of the abnormal chest x-ray film cannot be determined from the history.

PHYSICAL EXAMINATION

The blood pressure is normal.

See figure in *Heart Sounds and Murmurs Heard in Second Left Intercostal Space Near Sternum.*

CHEST X-RAY FILM

The aortic knob is not seen. The main pulmonary artery is large. The right pulmonary artery is large, and its branches extend deep into the lung. The left pulmonary artery is barely visible in the posteroanterior view, but it appears to be large. These abnormalities suggest the presence of an increased pulmonary artery blood flow.

The abnormalities are characteristic of a left-to-right shunt at the atrial level. The diagnosis is most likely an ostium secundum atrial septal defect. The left atrium and left ventricle are not large, which tends to exclude the presence of an ostium primum type of defect.

See x-ray film in Fig. 3-10.

See Patient 1 for a normal chest x-ray film.

ELECTROCARDIOGRAM

The ECG is abnormal because of right ventricular (RV) conduction delay. This abnormality is consistent with a diagnosis of ostium secundum atrial septal defect. It is not characteristic of the abnormalities associated with an ostium primum atrial septal defect.

See ECG in Fig. 4-56.

See Patient 1 for a normal ECG.

DIFFERENTIAL DIAGNOSIS

Very few conditions could produce the abnormalities found in the chest x-ray film and ECG other than an ostium secundum atrial septal defect. The large main pulmonary artery and large right and left branches suggest an increase in pulmonary arterial blood flow. We are accustomed to seeing large superior pulmonary veins when there is an elevated left atrial pressure, as occurs with mitral stenosis. Superior pulmonary veins may also become larger than normal when there is an increase in pulmonary arterial blood flow.

The ECG indicates RV conduction delay, which is almost always seen in patients with an ostium secundum atrial septal defect. It may occasionally be seen in patients with no other evidence of heart disease. The combination of the abnormalities seen in the chest x-ray film *plus* those seen in the ECG indicate the presence of an ostium secundum atrial septal defect.

HEART SOUNDS AND MURMURS HEARD IN SECOND LEFT INTERCOSTAL SPACE NEAR STERNUM

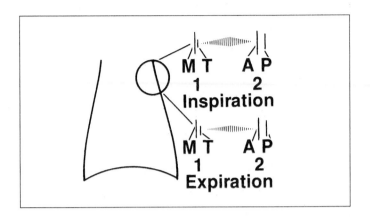

Fixed, wide splitting of the second heart sound (2) during inspiration and expiration, characteristic of a secundum atrial septal defect. The abnormally large lapse of time between the aortic (A) and pulmonary (P) valve closure sounds remains constant during inspiration and expiration. Note the systolic diamond-shaped pulmonary artery murmur that is caused by a large RV stroke volume. Also note that the pulmonary valve closure sound is louder than normal in the second left intercostal space and at the apex, because the pulmonary artery pressure may be slightly or moderately elevated. M, Mitral; T, tricuspid valve closure; I, first heart sound. See figure credits.

Fixed splitting of the second heart sound occurs during inspiration and expiration. The grade 2 midsystolic murmur heard in the same area may increase in intensity during inspiration.

DIAGNOSTIC PRINCIPLE

Fixed splitting of the second heart sound is virtually diagnostic of an ostium secundum type of septal defect.

RV conduction delay in the ECG usually indicates the presence of an ostium secundum type of atrial septal defect. It can occur, however, in the absence of any additional recognizable heart disease.

BIBLIOGRAPHY

Nugent EW, Plauth WH, Edwards JE, Williams WH: The pathology, pathophysiology, recognition, and treatment of congenital heart disease. In Schlant RC, Alexander RW, editors: *Hurst's the heart*, ed 8, New York, 1994, McGraw-Hill, pp 1773-1777.

FIGURE CREDIT

Reproduced with permission from Hurst JW: The examination of the heart: the importance of initial screening, *Dis Mon* 36(5):284, 1990.

HISTORY

The patient is a 45-year-old man who is complaining of chest pain.

PHYSICAL EXAMINATION

The systolic blood pressure, neck veins, and carotid pulsation are normal.

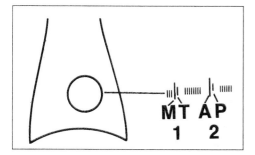

M, mitral; T, tricuspid; A, aortic; and P, pulmonary valve closure sounds; 1, 2, first, second heart sounds. See figure credits.

CHEST X-RAY FILM

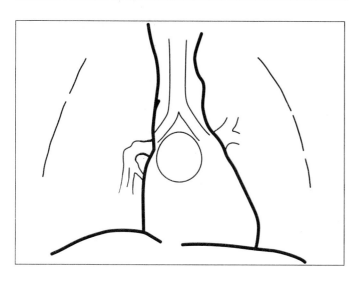

ELECTROCARDIOGRAM

Sinus tachycardia is present. There are 130 depolarizations per minute. The PR interval is 0.14 second. The QRS duration is 0.08 second. The QT interval is 0.28 second. The 12-lead QRS complex amplitude is 155 mm.

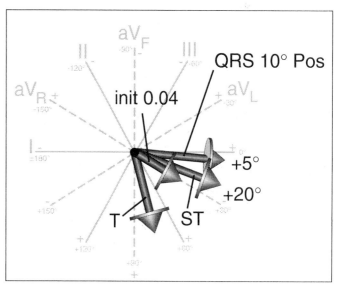

WHAT IS DIFFERENTIAL DIAGNOSIS?

WAS HISTORY ADEQUATE? WHAT QUESTIONS WOULD YOU ASK?

WHAT IS FINAL DIAGNOSIS?

HISTORY

The history is inadequate. The patient could have a myocardial infarction (MI), pericarditis, dissection of the aorta, pulmonary infarction, or any one of a number of noncardiac causes of chest pain.

PHYSICAL EXAMINATION

There is a scratchy sounding, three-component "murmur" or rub heard over the precordium. To be diagnostic of pericarditis, a rub should have three components, each occurring when the heart moves. Accordingly, there is a presystolic rub when the atria contract, a systolic rub that results from ventricular systole, and a diastolic rub related to ventricular diastole. This patient has a three-component rub, which is diagnostic 'of acute pericarditis. On the other hand, pericarditis can be present when there is no precordial rub, a one-component rub, or a two-component rub.

CHEST X-RAY FILM

The chest x-ray film of this patient is normal. The patient with chest pain caused by MI, pericarditis, dissection of the aorta, or pulmonary infarction may have a normal chest x-ray film.

See Patient 1 for a normal chest x-ray film.

ELECTROCARDIOGRAM

The ECG is characteristic of pericarditis. The mean QRS vector is directed +5 degrees in the frontal plane and 10 degrees posteriorly. This is normal, as is the mean initial 0.04-second vector.

The mean ST vector is large. It is directed toward the cardiac apex and is parallel with the frontal plane. It indicates generalized epicardial "injury."

The mean T vector is directed at +75 degrees and is parallel with the frontal plane. Later, the ST vector will become smaller, and the mean T vector will be directed away from the cardiac apex.

There is only one condition other than pericarditis that can, on rare occasion, produce an ECG such as this. An apical MI can produce the ECG abnormalities found in this patient.

See ECG shown in Fig. 4-76.

See Patient 1 for a normal ECG.

DIFFERENTIAL DIAGNOSIS

Two conditions should be considered. The patient either has acute pericarditis or the rare apical MI caused by atherosclerotic coronary heart disease.

HISTORY AND QUESTIONS

The history, as given in *History*, is inadequate. The history of chest pain should always include the answer to the following questions. When did it begin? Is it continuous? What precipitates the discomfort? Where is it located? Where does the pain radiate? Does taking a deep breath cause the pain to increase?

The chest pain of dissection of the aorta begins abruptly and reaches its maximum intensity instantly, whereas the pain of MI builds to its maximum intensity more gradually. The chest pain of pericarditis varies with inspiration, expiration, swallowing, and turning the trunk.

The pain of dissection of the aorta is typically felt more severely in the back, whereas the pain of MI is usually felt in the retrosternal area with radiation into the neck, jaw, arms, and elbows. The pain of pericarditis usually radiates to the top of the shoulders and is aggravated by inspiration.

In this patient the pain is aggravated by a deep breath, with swallowing, and by turning the trunk side to side. The pain is characteristic of pericarditis.

FINAL DIAGNOSIS

Acute pericarditis (etiology to be determined).

DIAGNOSTIC PRINCIPLE

This patient serves to emphasize the importance of the history. The initial evaluation of chest pain, based on an evaluation of symptoms, is one of the most important acts performed by the physician because such an evaluation determines if other diagnostic procedures are needed. Then, too, the chest discomfort must be correlated with the abnormalities found as the result of other procedures because, unfair as it is to the patient and physician, there may be more than one cause of chest pain in the patient.

In this patient the history (when questioned properly) assists in the exclusion of the rare apical MI that can occasionally produce ECG abnormalities that are more often caused by pericarditis.

BIBLIOGRAPHY

Shabetai R: Diseases of the pericardium. In Schlant RC, Alexander RW, editors: *Hurst's the heart*, ed 8, New York, 1994, McGraw-Hill, pp 1649-1651.

FIGURE CREDIT

Reproduced with permission from Hurst JW: The examination of the heart: the importance of initial screening, *Dis Mon* 36(5):284, 1990.

HISTORY

The patient is a 64-year-old man. He is complaining of constant retrosternal chest discomfort that has been present for 2 hours. He feels weak and is slightly confused.

PHYSICAL EXAMINATION

The patient appears pale and is sweating profusely.

The systolic blood pressure is 90 mm Hg, and the diastolic blood pressure is 50 mm Hg.

The pulse rate is 60 beats per minute. The external jugular veins are noted to be distended several centimeters above the clavicle when the patient's trunk is elevated 30 degrees. The *a* wave is easily seen in the internal jugular veins.

The first heart sound is faint. No murmurs are heard.

The lungs are clear on auscultation.

The peripheral arteries pulsate normally.

CHEST X-RAY FILM

There is no evidence of pulmonary congestion.

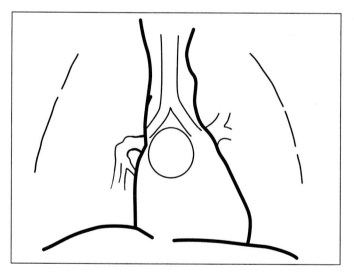

ELECTROCARDIOGRAM

There is sinus bradycardia. There are 58 depolarizations per minute. The PR interval is 0.24 second. The QRS duration is 0.09 second. The QT interval is 0.38 second. The 12-lead QRS amplitude is 170 mm.

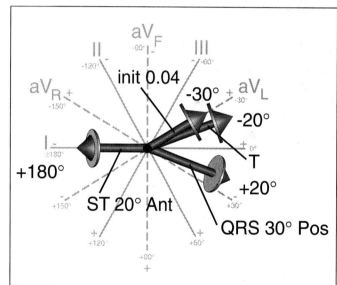

WHAT IS DIFFERENTIAL DIAGNOSIS?

WHAT IS FINAL DIAGNOSIS?

HISTORY

The history of retrosternal discomfort suggests that the patient is having a myocardial infarction (MI). Dissection of the aorta is also possible.

PHYSICAL EXAMINATION

The patient is pale, sweaty, and hypotensive, with a heart rate of 60 beats per minute. This, along with the chest pain, suggests inferior MI. The neck veins are abnormally distended, suggesting a high venous pressure. The *a* wave is easily seen, suggesting a long PR interval in the ECG. The faint first heart sound also suggests that the PR interval is long. Abnormal neck veins are present, whereas the lungs are clear, suggesting right ventricular (RV) MI as part of inferior MI.

The peripheral arteries pulsate normally.

CHEST X-RAY FILM

The posteroanterior view shows that the heart size is normal.

The lungs show no evidence of pulmonary congestion. This, along with abnormal distension of the neck veins, suggests RV MI as part of inferior MI.

The size of the aorta is normal.

See Patient 1 for a normal chest x-ray film.

ELECTROCARDIOGRAM

There is first-degree atrioventricular block and sinus bradycardia. This is why the *a* wave is seen easily and the first heart sound is faint.

The mean QRS vector is directed +20 degrees in the frontal plane and 30 degrees posteriorly.

The directions of the mean initial 0.04-second vector and the mean T vector are abnormal; they are directed abnormally to the left of the mean horizontally directed QRS vector and indicate an inferior dead zone and inferior epicardial ischemia.

The mean ST vector is directed +180 degrees in the frontal plane and 20 degrees anteriorly. The right ventricle is usually infarcted when the mean ST vector is directed to the right and anteriorly to this degree.

As the mean ST vector shifts more to the right of +120 degrees and anteriorly, the more likely the body of the right ventricle is to be infarcted.

See ECG in Fig. 4-71. The ECG of Patient 7 also shows RV MI.

See Patient 1 for a normal ECG.

DIFFERENTIAL DIAGNOSIS

The clues indicate an inferior MI plus RV MI caused by atherosclerotic coronary heart disease. No other reasonable possibility exists.

FINAL DIAGNOSIS

RV MI associated with inferior MI resulting from atherosclerotic coronary heart disease.

DIAGNOSTIC PRINCIPLE

The ST vector related to MI typically points toward the area of epicardial injury related to the MI. When the ST segment vector is directed +130 degrees to +150 degrees or more to the right in the frontal plane and is directed anteriorly or parallel with the frontal plane, it often signifies an RV MI associated with an inferior MI. The farther the ST segment vector is directed to the right, the more likely the body of the right ventricle is to be infarcted.

When a patient with anterior chest pain exhibits hypotension, bradycardia, distended neck veins, and clear lungs, it is highly likely that the patient is experiencing an inferior MI with RV MI.

BIBLIOGRAPHY

Dell'Italia LJ: Right ventricular infarction. In Hurst JW, editor: *Current therapy in cardiovascular disease*, ed 4, St Louis, 1994, Mosby, pp 167-170.

Hurst JW: Detection of right ventricular myocardial infarction associated with inferior myocardial infarction from the standard 12-lead electrocardiogram, *Heart Dis Stroke* 2(6):464-467, 1993.

HISTORY

The patient is a 32-year-old woman who has noted retrosternal discomfort while sitting in a chair watching television. The discomfort was first noted 2 days previously. She has noticed the discomfort on five occasions. The discomfort appeared to be related to walking rapidly on two occasions. Each of the previous episodes lasted several minutes, but the last episode lasted more than an hour. The pain was not aggravated by inspiration.

The patient has lupus erythematosus and mild renal failure but continues to work. She had pericarditis a year ago that responded to corticosteroid treatment.

PHYSICAL EXAMINATION

The systolic blood pressure is 148 mm Hg, and the diastolic blood pressure is 88 mm Hg.

The typical "butterfly" rash of lupus is noted on her face.

There is a left atrial (LA) gallop sound. No murmurs are heard.

CHEST X-RAY FILM

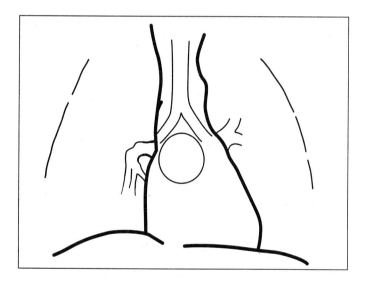

ELECTROCARDIOGRAM

The rhythm is normal. There are 86 depolarizations per minute. The PR interval is 0.18 second. The QRS duration is 0.09 second. The QT interval is 0.38 second. The 12-lead QRS amplitude is 180 mm.

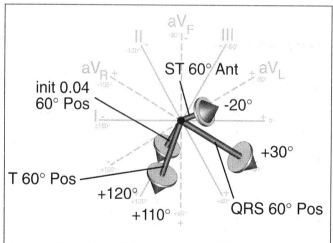

WHAT IS DIFFERENTIAL DIAGNOSIS?

WHAT IS FINAL DIAGNOSIS?

HISTORY

Although the patient has a past history of pericarditis, the chest discomfort she is now experiencing is not related to inspiration. The patient's chest discomfort has the features of myocardial ischemia. The first four episodes lasted several minutes, and two of the episodes were related to effort. These episodes could represent unstable angina pectoris. The last episode lasted an hour and was not aggravated with deep inspiration. It could be caused by myocardial infarction.

Although obstructive coronary atherosclerosis can develop in a 32-year-old woman, it is wise to consider a nonatherosclerotic cause in a young patient with lupus erythematosus.

PHYSICAL EXAMINATION

The blood pressure is borderline high. The skin lesions of lupus should lead one to consider the cardiovascular complications of this disease. The patient's chest pain could be pericarditis, which is common in patients with lupus. However, there is no pericardial friction rub. The LA gallop suggests poor compliance of the left ventricle.

CHEST X-RAY FILM

The chest x-ray film is normal. This does not exclude pericarditis or MI.

See Patient 1 for a normal chest x-ray film.

ELECTROCARDIOGRAM

The QRS amplitude is 180 mm. This suggests left ventricular hypertrophy that may be related to hypertension.

The initial 0.04-second vector is directed to the right and posteriorly away from an anterolateral myocardial dead zone.

The mean ST vector points toward an area of anterolateral epicardial injury.

The mean T vector is directed away from an area of anterolateral epicardial ischemia.

The ECG abnormalities are typical of acute anterolateral MI. See ECG in Fig. 4-70.

See Patient 1 for a normal ECG.

DIFFERENTIAL DIAGNOSIS

Only two reasonable possibilities exist: pericarditis or MI. All data support the diagnosis of MI. The episodes of chest pain before the last episode are typical of myocardial ischemia. The pain is not made worse by inspiration, and no pericardial friction rub is present. The ECG is diagnostic of acute anterolateral MI.

FINAL DIAGNOSIS

Acute MI related to lupus erythematosus. Occlusion of the coronary artery may be part of the antiphospholipid syndrome or may result from coronary arteritis.

DIAGNOSTIC PRINCIPLE

First, the patient had unstable angina pectoris for several days before the final episode of prolonged chest discomfort. *Unstable angina* is defined as angina occurring for the first time, angina occurring with less effort than formerly, angina occurring at rest, and angina that has developed during the last 60 days. Unstable angina must be viewed as being different from stable angina (see Patient 45). The vascular biology, pathophysiology, clinical manifestations, and treatment of unstable angina are different from those of stable angina. As a rule, the myocardial ischemia associated with unstable angina pectoris is caused by a change in the coronary artery rather than resulting from an increase in myocardial oxygen demand, as it is with stable angina. Chest pain that lasts more than an hour should not be labeled as angina pectoris. When chest pain caused by myocardial ischemia lasts 20 minutes or longer, it must be referred to as *prolonged myocardial ischemia*. It is labeled as an MI when there are QRS complex, ST segment or T wave changes in the ECG or a rise in the blood level of creatine phosphokinase.

Second, this patient is presented to emphasize that coronary atherosclerosis is not the only cause of MI. This patient probably had the antiphospholipid syndrome or coronary arteritis as a cause of her MI. MI is a common cause of death in patients with lupus erythematosus. An antiphospholipid antibody test should be ordered.

BIBLIOGRAPHY

Galve E, Ordi-Ros J: Primary antiphospholipid syndrome and the heart. In Hurst JW, editor: *New types of cardiovascular diseases*, New York, 1994, Igaku Shoin, pp 77-88.

HISTORY

The patient is a 24-year-old man who is complaining of chills, fever, fatigue, and dyspnea. He has been ill for several weeks.

The history as stated is inadequate. The omissions will be discussed under the heading *Other Questions*. In the meantime, think of the questions you would like to ask the patient.

PHYSICAL EXAMINATION

The patient appears acutely ill.

The temperature is 102 degrees F (38.8 degrees C).

The systolic blood pressure is 118 mm Hg, and the diastolic blood pressure is 68 mm Hg.

The pulse is 110 beats per minute.

The external jugular veins are extremely distended with the patient sitting. The pulsations of the internal jugular vein with the patient sitting are shown in the diagram on the right.

The apex impulse is located a little to the left of its normal position.

There is a loud systolic murmur heard at the lower end of the sternum.

The liver edge is palpated 4 cm below the lower ribs on the right. It seems to move with each cardiac systole.

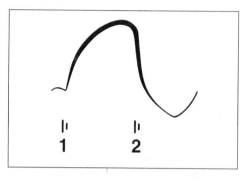

1, 2, First, second heart sounds. See figure credits.

CHEST X-RAY FILM

There is moderate pulmonary congestion.

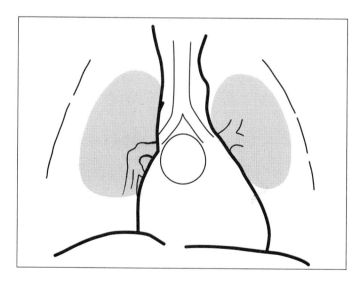

ELECTROCARDIOGRAM

The heart rhythm is normal. There are 105 depolarizations per minute. The PR interval is 0.17 second. The QRS duration is 0.09 second. The QT interval is 0.34 second. The 12-lead QRS amplitude is 150 mm.

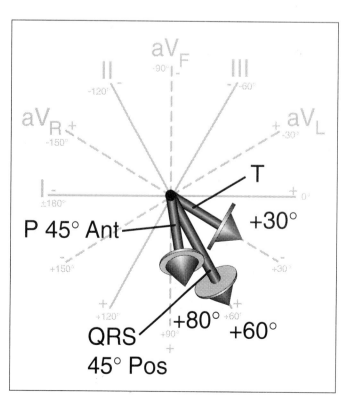

WHAT OTHER QUESTIONS WOULD YOU ASK PATIENT?

WHAT IS DIFFERENTIAL DIAGNOSIS?

WHAT IS FINAL DIAGNOSIS?

HISTORY

The data presented suggest that the patient has an acute infection. The type cannot be determined from the history as given. (See discussion under *Other Questions*.)

PHYSICAL EXAMINATION

The temperature is elevated.

The external jugular veins are abnormally distended, and the abnormal pulsation of the internal jugular veins is caused by severe tricuspid valve regurgitation. This type of pulsation is often misinterpreted as being an arterial pulsation. One can separate the two and identify it as being venous in origin when the pulsation increases with inspiration, when the pulsation can be eliminated by external pressure on the jugular veins that is not sufficient to eliminate the carotid artery pulse, and when the pulsation increases with pressure on the abdomen.

The location of the apex impulse suggests that the heart is slightly enlarged.

There is a loud systolic murmur heard at the lower end of the sternum indicating tricuspid valve regurgitation. It should be pointed out that most patients with tricuspid regurgitation have no murmur; tricuspid regurgitation is more often recognized by identifying the abnormal pulsation of the internal jugular veins.

The patient's liver is enlarged and moves downward with each cardiac systole. The enlargement and movement indicates tricuspid regurgitation.

CHEST X-RAY FILM

The heart is slightly enlarged. The right atrium appears to be larger than normal. There is pulmonary congestion, indicating the presence of heart failure.

See Patient 1 for a normal chest x-ray film.

ELECTROCARDIOGRAM

There may be a right atrial (RA) abnormality because the mean P vector is directed more vertically and farther anteriorly than usual.

See Patient 1 for a normal ECG.

OTHER QUESTIONS

The physician should ask the patient if he has "mainlined" cocaine or narcotics such as heroin. Patients who give themselves intravenous (IV) injections are likely to develop: hepatitis; acquired immunodeficiency syndrome (AIDS); endocarditis; and cocaine coronary spasm, myocardial infarction, systemic hypertension, and dysrhythmia. The patient replied "yes" to the question.

Because the patient has "right-sided" heart disease and little evidence of "left-sided" disease, the patient should be asked if he ever has a flushed sensation, diarrhea, or wheezing because carcinoid heart disease may be responsible for the condition.

DIFFERENTIAL DIAGNOSIS

Chills occur infrequently in patients with hepatitis. Also, there is ample evidence of heart disease.

AIDS cannot be completely excluded. However, the nature of the illness would force one to consider a superimposed infection of the heart.

There is no evidence for cocaine-induced infarction or hypertension.

The history of chills and fever eliminates the possibility of carcinoid heart disease.

The development of a febrile illness with severe tricuspid valve regurgitation indicates bacterial endocarditis of the tricuspid valve. This is especially likely to occur in patients who use IV drugs.

FINAL DIAGNOSIS

Endocarditis of the tricuspid valve leading to heart failure. The patient admitted "mainlining" drugs. Blood cultures should be obtained and treatment started immediately.

DIAGNOSTIC PRINCIPLE

Any patient with a heart murmur and unexplained fever must be viewed as having infective endocarditis until proved otherwise. Today, because of the common use of self-administered IV narcotics, tricuspid valve involvement occurs frequently.

BIBLIOGRAPHY

Durack DT: Infective and noninfective endocarditis. In Schlant RC, Alexander RW, editors: *Hurst's the heart*, ed 8, New York, 1994, McGraw-Hill, pp 1681-1709.

FIGURE CREDIT

Modified and reproduced with permission from Hurst JW: The examination of the heart: the importance of initial screening, *Dis Mon* 36(5):280, 1990.

HISTORY

The patient is a 43-year-old female who is complaining of acute episodes of dyspnea and occasional syncope. She has no history of palpitation or chest discomfort. She gives a history of migraine headaches and uses one to two tablets of an ergot preparation each month for relief.

PHYSICAL EXAMINATION

The systolic blood pressure is 120 mm Hg, and the diastolic blood pressure is 80 mm Hg.

The pulsations of the neck veins are normal, as are the pulsations of the peripheral arteries.

The precordial movements are normal.

Auscultation at the apex reveals the abnormalities shown in the diagram on the right.

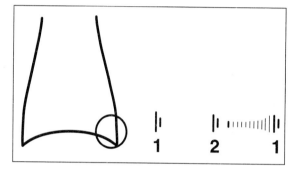

1, 2, First, second heart sounds.

CHEST X-RAY FILM

Pulmonary edema is noted just after an attack of acute dyspnea.

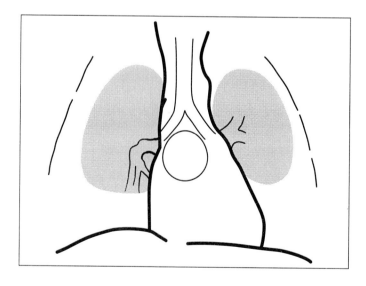

ELECTROCARDIOGRAM

There is normal heart rhythm and 82 depolarizations per minute. The PR interval is 0.14 second. The QRS duration is 0.09 second. The QT interval is 0.36 second. The 12-lead QRS amplitude is 140 mm.

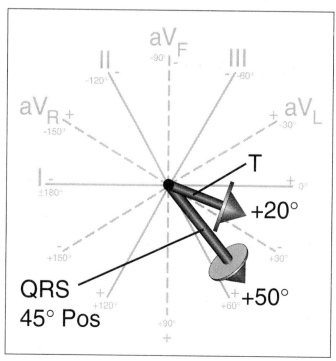

WHAT IS DIFFERENTIAL DIAGNOSIS?

WHAT IS FINAL DIAGNOSIS?

HISTORY

The history of acute episodes of dyspnea and occasional syncope could be caused by pulmonary emboli, mitral stenosis with episodes of atrial fibrillation, aortic stenosis with episodes of atrial fibrillation, idiopathic hypertrophic subaortic stenosis, or left atrial (LA) myxoma.

PHYSICAL EXAMINATION

A diastolic rumble is heard at the cardiac apex. The rumble is introduced by a loud sound. The intensity of the first heart sound is thought to be normal.

The diastolic rumble could be caused by any abnormality that reduces the size of the mitral valve orifice, including mitral stenosis or LA myxoma. The loud sound in early diastole could be the opening snap of mitral stenosis or could be caused by a tumor "plop."

CHEST X-RAY FILM

Pulmonary edema is present in the film made shortly after an episode of dyspnea. The heart size and shape are normal.

See Patient 1 for a normal chest x-ray film.

ELECTROCARDIOGRAM

The ECG is normal. This does not exclude coronary disease, mild valve disease, LA myxoma, hypertrophic cardiomyopathy, restrictive cardiomyopathy, dysrhythmias, and previous pericarditis.

See Patient 1 for a normal ECG.

DIFFERENTIAL DIAGNOSIS

This patient has the triad of dyspnea, syncope and a diastolic rumble at the apex.

The patient could have mitral stenosis. The most likely cause is rheumatic heart disease. Congenital mitral stenosis is not likely, and she ingested too little ergot to suspect an ergot etiology of mitral valve disease. There are no signs of mitral stenosis noted in the chest x-ray film. That is, the LA size is normal, and the LA appendage is not seen.

The patient could have a mobile LA myxoma that is attached to the atrial septum by a stalk. It could swing back and forth in the LA and occlude the mitral valve and orifice during ventricular diastole.

FINAL DIAGNOSIS

Although calcification of the tumor may occasionally be identified in the left lateral chest x-ray film, one cannot consistently separate the mitral valve blockade caused by an LA myxoma from rheumatic mitral stenosis without additional studies (e.g., echocardiogram).

The excessive use of an ergot preparation for migraine headache may cause mitral and aortic valve disease. However, the patient did not use excessive amounts of the drug. Accordingly, she does not have ergot-induced mitral stenosis.

Finally, because the LA myxoma continues to beat against the mitral valve leaflets, it may produce mitral valve regurgitation. This is known as the "wrecking ball" effect.

The echocardiogram made on this patient showed an LA myxoma.

DIAGNOSTIC PRINCIPLE

All that rumbles is not mitral stenosis. Apical diastolic rumbles can be heard in patients with aortic regurgitation (Austin Flint murmur, or rumble), mitral valve regurgitation, patent ductus arteriosus, ventricular septal defect, LA tumor, idiopathic hypertrophy of the heart (including hypertrophy of the papillary muscles), severe anemia, as well as mitral stenosis caused by rheumatic heart disease, congenital disease, or ergot heart disease.

A tricuspid diastolic rumble may be heard in patients with an atrial septal defect, tricuspid valve regurgitation, or tricuspid stenosis caused by rheumatic heart disease or carcinoid heart disease.

BIBLIOGRAPHY

Gaasch WH, O'Rourke RA, Cohn LH, Rackley CE: Mitral valve disease. In Schlant RC, Alexander RW, editors: *Hurst's the heart*, ed 8, New York, 1994, McGraw-Hill, pp 1483-1491.

Hall RJ, Cooley DA, McAllister HA, Frazier OH: Neoplastic heart disease. In Schlant RC, Alexander RW, editors: *Hurst's the heart*, ed 8, New York, 1994, McGraw-Hill, pp 2010-2012.

HISTORY

The patient, a 70-year-old man, is complaining of dyspnea on effort. He first noted the dyspnea 3 months earlier. He had coronary bypass surgery 1 1/2 years ago but denies angina pectoris, palpitation, or syncope. He has noted slight edema of the feet and "fullness" in his abdomen.

PHYSICAL EXAMINATION

The systolic blood pressure is 130 mm Hg and the diastolic blood pressure is 80 mm Hg.

The external jugular veins are distended as high as the ears when the patient is in the sitting position. The pulsation of the internal jugular veins is shown in the upper diagram on the right.

The apex impulse could not be felt.
Auscultation reveals the following:
(See figure at right)

The liver edge is felt 3 cm below the rib cage on the right.
There is slight edema of the feet.

CHEST X-RAY FILM

Slight pulmonary congestion is noted.

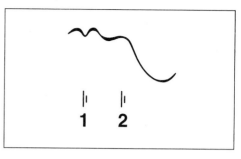

1, 2, First, second heart sounds. See figure credit.

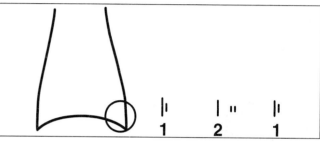

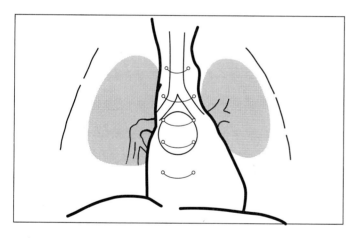

Left

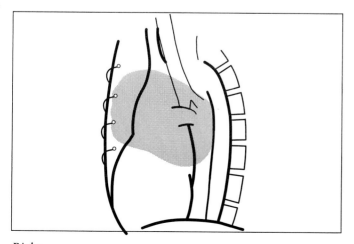

Right

ELECTROCARDIOGRAM

There is normal sinus rhythm. There are 82 depolarizations per minute. The PR interval is 0.16 second. The QRS duration is 0.10 second. The QT interval is 0.36 second. The total QRS amplitude is 100 mm.

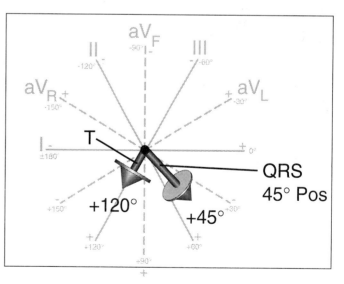

WHAT IS DIFFERENTIAL DIAGNOSIS?

WHAT LOW-TECHNOLOGY PROCEDURE WOULD YOU PERFORM?

WHAT IS FINAL DIAGNOSIS?

HISTORY

The patient had coronary bypass surgery 18 months ago. He now denies angina pectoris, palpitation, and syncope.

His symptoms could be related to chronic lung disease of some type or recurrent pulmonary emboli, or the patient has pulmonary congestion and edema related to heart failure. The latter could be related to coronary atherosclerotic heart disease or a complication of coronary bypass surgery. Finally, the patient could have developed a new type of heart disease such as dilated cardiomyopathy.

PHYSICAL EXAMINATION

The neck veins are abnormal. The external jugular veins are distended up to the patient's ears, and the internal jugular venous pulsation shows a rapid *y* descent. These abnormalities suggest the presence of constrictive pericarditis.

The apex impulse could not be felt.

The first and second heart sounds are normal. An extra sound is heard in early diastole at the apex. It is slightly higher pitched than a ventricular gallop sound. Such a sound is referred to as a *pericardial knock*.

The liver is enlarged, and there is slight edema of the feet.

This cluster of abnormalities suggests the possibility of constrictive pericarditis.

CHEST X-RAY FILM

There is slight congestion of the lungs. No pericardial calcification is seen. The heart is not enlarged. Sternal wires and vascular clips are seen.

Lung disease can be excluded. Heart failure with a normal heart size must be considered. Although no pericardial calcification is seen, constrictive pericarditis must be considered a good diagnostic possibility.

See Patient 1 for a normal chest x-ray film.

ELECTROCARDIOGRAM

The ECG shows low QRS amplitude and a primary T-wave abnormality. The low QRS amplitude could be caused by constrictive pericarditis, pericardial effusion, dilated or restrictive cardiomyopathy, anasarca, myxedema, or improper standardization of the electrocardiogram.

See Patient 1 for a normal electrocardiogram.

DIFFERENTIAL DIAGNOSIS

The abnormal neck veins, pericardial knock heard at the apex, normal-size heart, enlarged liver, and low total QRS amplitude indicate constrictive pericarditis. This is especially likely in a patient who has had coronary bypass surgery because this is one of the complications of this procedure.

There are no data to support a diagnosis of heart failure caused by a new infarction of the myocardium.

LOW-TECHNOLOGY PROCEDURE

You should determine if a pulsus paradoxus is present. When tested, this patient had 20 mm Hg pulsus paradoxus. This confirms the diagnosis of constrictive pericarditis, although pulsus paradoxus is less common with constrictive pericarditis than with cardiac tamponade from pericardial fluid.

FINAL DIAGNOSIS

Constrictive pericarditis following coronary bypass surgery.

DIAGNOSTIC PRINCIPLE

Whenever a patient has surgery for any problem and later becomes sick, it is wise to consider three diagnostic possibilities:
- The original condition was not cured.
- The patient's new medical problem is caused by the surgery.
- A new condition has developed.

Constrictive pericarditis is a well-known complication of coronary bypass surgery. Calcification of the pericardium does not appear on the x-ray film because too little time has passed since surgery.

BIBLIOGRAPHY

Shabetai R: Diseases of the pericardium. In Schlant RC, Alexander RW, editors: *Hurst's the heart*, ed 8, New York, 1994, McGraw-Hill, pp 1662-1665.

FIGURE CREDIT

Modified and reproduced with permission from Hurst JW: The examination of the heart: the importance of initial screening, *Dis Mon* 36(5):280, 1990.

HISTORY

The patient is a 36-year-old woman. She gives a history of episodes of rapid heart-beat that start abruptly, last 2 to 4 hours, and stop suddenly.

PHYSICAL EXAMINATION

Her systolic blood pressure is 118 mm Hg, and the diastolic blood pressure is 76 mm Hg.

The pulsations of the neck veins are normal, and the arterial pulse is slightly hyperdynamic.

The first (1) and second (2) heart sounds are normal. Auscultation at the cardiac apex revealed the abnormalities shown in the diagram to the right.

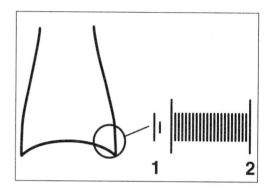

1, 2, First, second heart sounds.

CHEST X-RAY FILM

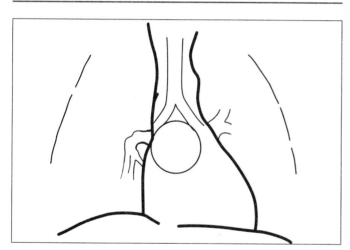

Left

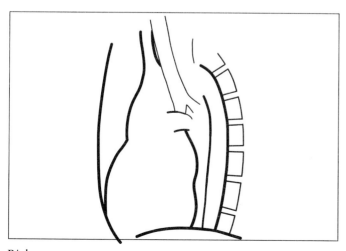

Right

ELECTROCARDIOGRAM

There is normal rhythm. The heart rate is 88 depolarizations per minute. The PR interval is 0.17 second. The QRS duration is 0.09 second. The QT interval is 0.34 second. There is no delta wave. The total QRS amplitude is 180 mm.

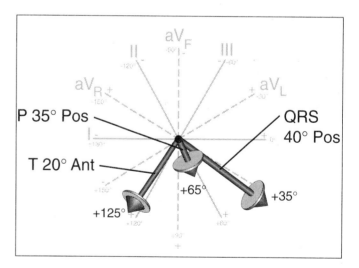

WHAT ADDITIONAL LOW-TECHNOLOGY PROCEDURE WOULD YOU PERFORM?

WHAT IS DIFFERENTIAL DIAGNOSIS?

WHAT IS FINAL DIAGNOSIS?

HISTORY

The history of paroxysmal rapid heart action in a young woman should lead one to consider the presence of mitral stenosis with episodes of atrial fibrillation, Wolff-Parkinson-White syndrome with paroxysmal atrial tachycardia or atrial fibrillation, mitral valve prolapse with atrial or ventricular tachycardia, or supraventricular tachycardia in an otherwise normal heart.

PHYSICAL EXAMINATION

The circulation is slightly hyperdynamic. This can occur as a result of aortic regurgitation, peripheral arteriovenous fistula, mitral valve regurgitation, thyrotoxicosis, excess catecholamines, and fever.

The neck veins are normal.

There is a grade 3 holosystolic murmur at the apex. An early systolic click introduces the murmur. The murmur radiates laterally. The murmur and systolic click are characteristic of mitral valve prolapse.

CHEST X-RAY FILM

Posteroanterior and lateral views show that the left ventricle is slightly enlarged. The left atrium is a little enlarged, suggesting mitral valve disease.

See Patient 1 for a normal chest x-ray film.

ELECTROCARDIOGRAM

There is a left atrial abnormality. The PR interval is longer than 0.12 second, and there is no delta wave; this rules out Wolff-Parkinson-White syndrome.

The total QRS voltage is 180 mm.

The QRS-T angle is 90 degrees, indicating a repolarization abnormality.

The ECG abnormalities suggest slight left ventricular hypertrophy.

See Patient 1 for a normal electrocardiogram.

LOW-TECHNOLOGY PROCEDURE

Auscultation at the cardiac apex should be performed as the patient moves from the squatting position to the standing position. The systolic click should become louder and occur later in systole as a result of this maneuver. This is characteristic of mitral valve prolapse.

DIFFERENTIAL DIAGNOSIS

No evidence indicates preexcitation in the ECG, and the systolic click and murmur are diagnostic of mitral valve regurgitation resulting from mitral valve prolapse.

FINAL DIAGNOSIS

Mitral valve prolapse with moderate mitral valve regurgitation. There is a history of paroxysmal rapid heart action. The rhythm disturbance is most likely supraventricular tachycardia, but other studies are needed to be certain of this diagnosis.

DIAGNOSTIC PRINCIPLE

The most common cause of isolated mitral valve regurgitation is mitral valve prolapse. The systolic click should be sought in every patient with mitral regurgitation because it is diagnostic of the condition.

Mitral valve prolapse may be mild or severe and serious or inconsequential. The severe examples are usually caused by myxomatous degeneration of the mitral valve.

Patients with severe mitral valve prolapse may develop heart failure or paroxysmal dysrhythmias or may experience rupture of a mitral valve chordae tendineae or endocarditis.

BIBLIOGRAPHY

Gaasch WH, O'Rourke RA, Cohn LH, Rackley CE: Mitral valve disease. In Schlant RC, Alexander RW, editors: *Hurst's the heart*, ed 8, New York, 1994, McGraw-Hill, pp 1502-1518.

HISTORY

The patient is a 5-month-old boy. The parents have noted persistent cyanosis, an increase in respiratory rate, and failure to gain weight.

PHYSICAL EXAMINATION

Cyanosis is obvious.

The heart rate is 120 beats per minute.

Peripheral arterial pulsations are normal, and neck vein pulsations cannot be examined because of crying and an increase in respiratory rate.

There is a prominent anterior systolic movement of the precordium. The apex impulse is larger than normal and is located to the left of its normal position.

There are two components of the second heart sound. In fact, both components are easily heard.

There is a grade 3 systolic murmur located in the third intercostal space near the sternum.

CHEST X-RAY FILM

ELECTROCARDIOGRAM

Sinus tachycardia is present. The heart rate is 120 depolarizations per minute. The PR interval is 0.13 second. The QRS duration is 0.07 second. The QT interval is 0.30 second.

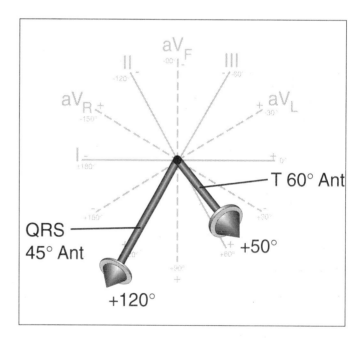

WHAT IS DIFFERENTIAL DIAGNOSIS?

WHAT IS FINAL DIAGNOSIS?

HISTORY

The persistent cyanosis indicates that a right-to-left intracardiac shunt is present in this infant boy. The rapid breathing suggests the presence of heart failure.

Conditions such as tricuspid atresia, truncus arteriosus, tetralogy of Fallot, and complete transposition of the great arteries should be considered.

PHYSICAL EXAMINATION

Cyanosis is present, indicating a right-to-left intracardiac shunt.

The heart is large; note the abnormal anterior systolic movement and the abnormal apical impulse. The former suggests right ventricular (RV) enlargement, and the latter suggests left ventricular (LV) enlargement. The presence of LV hypertrophy excludes tetralogy of Fallot.

Two components of the second heart sound are heard. This excludes truncus arteriosus because the second sound is always single in this condition. (This is because there is no separate aortic or pulmonary valves present with this anomaly.) Tetralogy of Fallot and tricuspid atresia are not likely to be present because the two components of the second sound are easily heard.

The systolic murmur suggests the presence of an interventricular septal defect, but this alone would not cause cyanosis. It is part of a more complex anomaly.

CHEST X-RAY FILM

The heart is larger than normal. The main pulmonary artery is not seen and the shadow created by the aorta is narrow. Blood flow to the lungs is increased.

The large heart with an increase in pulmonary arterial blood flow excludes tetralogy of Fallot and tricuspid atresia. The narrow aortopulmonary shadow helps to exclude truncus arteriosus. The abnormalities are typical of transposition of the great arteries with increase in pulmonary arterial blood flow to the lungs. There must be an associated interventricular septal defect, patent ductus, or atrial septal defect for a patient with transposition of the great arteries to survive.

See Patient 1 for a normal chest x-ray film.

ELECTROCARDIOGRAM

The ECG excludes tricuspid atresia because, with this condition, it always shows LV dominance.

The mean QRS vector is large and directed to the right +120 degrees and 45 degrees anteriorly. The direction could be normal for the patient's age but the amplitude indicates right ventricular dominance.

The mean T vector is directed at +50 degrees in the frontal plane and 60 degrees anteriorly. The anterior direction of the T vector is abnormal in an infant and suggests RV hypertrophy. This excludes truncus arteriosus, but it could be caused by tetralogy of Fallot or transposition of the great arteries.

See Patient 1 for a normal electrocardiogram.

DIFFERENTIAL DIAGNOSIS

The persistent cyanosis indicates a right-to-left intracardiac shunt.

Tricuspid atresia is excluded because the chest x-ray film shows an increase in blood flow to the lungs and the ECG does not show LV hypertrophy.

Truncus arteriosus is excluded because two components of the second heart sound are heard.

Tetralogy of Fallot is excluded because: (1) the heart is large with evidence of RV and LV hypertrophy on physical examination; (2) the two components of the second heart sound are easily heard; and, (3) an increase in pulmonary arterial blood flow is detected on the x-ray film.

Transposition of the great arteries with an interventricular septal defect is the best choice because of persistent cyanosis, a large heart, two components to the second sound, narrow aortopulmonary shadow, and an increase in pulmonary arterial blood flow. The typical x-ray findings are produced because the aorta and pulmonary artery are transposed, which creates a narrow aortopulmonary shadow in the posteroanterior (PA) view and a wider shadow than normal in the left lateral view.

FINAL DIAGNOSIS

Transposition of the great arteries plus an interventricular septal defect.

DIAGNOSTIC PRINCIPLE

- Persistent cyanosis indicates lung disease or a right-to-left intracardiac shunt.
- Truncus arteriosus can be excluded when two components of the second sound are heard.
- A loud pulmonary closure sound excludes tetralogy of Fallot.
- Evidence of an increase in pulmonary arterial blood flow on the chest x-ray film excludes tetralogy of Fallot, tricuspid atresia, and type 4 truncus arteriosus.
- Tricuspid atresia can be diagnosed by the triad of cyanosis, decrease in pulmonary arterial blood flow, and LV hypertrophy in the ECG.
- Transposition of the great arteries is recognized when there is cyanosis, evidence of RV and LV hypertrophy, an increase in pulmonary arterial blood flow, and a narrow aortopulmonary shadow on the PA chest film.

BIBLIOGRAPHY

Nugent EW, Plauth WH, Edwards JE, Williams WH: The pathology, pathophysiology, recognition, and treatment of congenital heart disease. In Schlant RC, Alexander RW, editors: *Hurst's the heart*, ed 8, New York, 1994, McGraw-Hill, pp 1808-1811.

HISTORY

The patient is a 74-year-old man. He has had symptoms of a peptic ulcer intermittently for years. He has noticed black stools for several days and has just vomited blood. He felt weak and collapsed to the floor but did not lose consciousness. He began to notice retrosternal tightness, which was still present when he arrived at the emergency clinic.

PHYSICAL EXAMINATION

The patient is pale and sweaty. His pulse rate is 110 beats per minute. The systolic blood pressure is 90 mm Hg. The diastolic blood pressure is 65 mm Hg.

Neck veins are normal.

Auscultation reveals the clues shown in the diagram to the right.

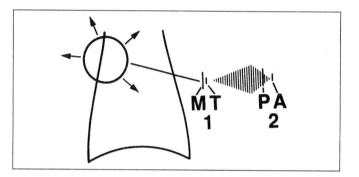

1, 2, First, second heart sounds; *M,* mitral; *T,* tricuspid; *P,* pulmonary; and *A,* aortic valve closure sounds. See figure credit.

PORTABLE CHEST X-RAY FILM

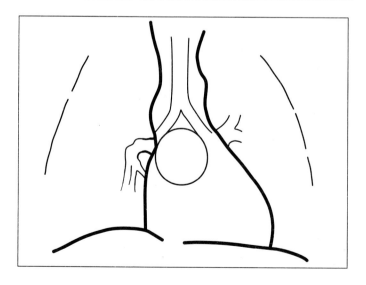

ELECTROCARDIOGRAM

Sinus tachycardia is present. The heart rate is 105 depolarizations per minute. The PR interval is 0.18 second. The QRS duration is 0.10 second. The QT interval is 0.36 second. The total QRS amplitude is 190 mm Hg.

A tracing made 6 hours later showed no change.

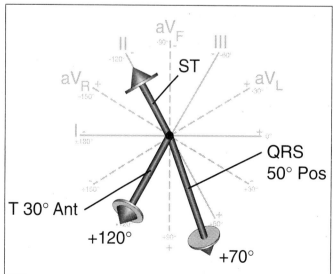

WHAT IS DIFFERENTIAL DIAGNOSIS?

WHAT IS FINAL DIAGNOSIS?

121

HISTORY

The signs of gastrointestinal bleeding are obvious. The patient apparently had been bleeding from his peptic ulcer for several days and now has bled profusely. The collapse and retrosternal tightness could represent myocardial ischemia precipitated by hypotension caused by bleeding.

PHYSICAL EXAMINATION

The patient has many early signs of cardiovascular shock. The murmur is typical of aortic valve stenosis. It peaks in late systole, and the aortic valve closure sound is decreased in intensity. In some patients the pulmonary valve closure sound may appear before the delayed aortic valve closure sound and may be masked by the murmur.

CHEST X-RAY FILM

The proximal portions of the aorta and left ventricle appear to be larger than normal. It is difficult to evaluate the size of the heart and aorta in a portable x-ray film of the chest. From the x-ray film alone, one could suspect that the patient either has aortic valve stenosis, aortic valve regurgitation, or hypertension.

See Patient 1 for a normal chest x-ray film.

ELECTROCARDIOGRAM

Sinus tachycardia is present. There are 105 depolarizations per minute.

The mean QRS vector is directed +70 degrees in the frontal plane and 50 degrees posteriorly. The QRS amplitude is sufficiently large to state that left ventricular (LV) hypertrophy is highly likely to be present.

The mean T vector is directed at +120 degrees in the frontal plane and 30 degrees anteriorly, which also supports the diagnosis of LV hypertrophy.

The large mean ST vector is directed away from the cardiac apex and is not parallel with the mean T vector as it should be when it is caused by LV hypertrophy; rather, this results from subendocardial injury. Its persistence for many hours suggests subendocardial infarction.

See the ECG in Fig. 4-53. It is characteristic of the ECG that is caused by aortic valve stenosis. Subendocardial injury is not shown in Fig. 4-53.

Also, see Fig. 4-73 for an example of subendocardial infarction. See Patient 1 for a normal ECG.

DIFFERENTIAL DIAGNOSIS

The patient has aortic valve stenosis of elderly persons and subendocardial myocardial infarction caused by associated coronary atherosclerosis. No other diagnostic possibilities are reasonable.

FINAL DIAGNOSIS

Severe aortic valve stenosis of elderly persons and subendocardial infarction related to coronary atherosclerosis.

DIAGNOSTIC PRINCIPLE

There are three types of infarction:
- *Q wave infarction.* The abnormal Q waves, which are produced by an abnormally directed mean initial 0.03- or 0.04-second QRS vector, plus a mean ST vector from epicardial injury and a mean T vector from epicardial ischemia. This type of tracing was formerly labeled as a "transmural" infarction.
- *Non–Q wave infarction.* The mean ST vector and mean T wave vector are abnormally directed, indicating epicardial injury and ischemia, respectively. The vector representing initial 0.04 second of the QRS complex is directed normally and is related properly to the mean QRS vector. These abnormalities were formerly labeled as resulting from subendocardial infarction or a "nontransmural" infarction.
- *Subendocardial infarction.* The mean ST vector is directed away from the centroid of the entire endocardial area and represents generalized endocardial injury. Infarction of the entire subendocardial area is thought to occur when the mean ST vector persists for hours and the proper clinical setting exists.

The pathophysiology responsible for the subendocardial infarction in this patient is worth reviewing. The patient has LV hypertrophy caused by aortic valve stenosis. The LV diastolic pressure was probably elevated above normal. When the systemic diastolic pressure falls to 50 mm Hg as the result of gastrointestinal bleeding, the entire subendocardial area of the left ventricle was not perfused properly. When diffuse obstructive coronary atherosclerosis is also present, the entire subendocardial area may become infarcted.

BIBLIOGRAPHY

Rapaport E, Rackley CE, Cohn LH: Aortic valve disease. In Schlant RC, Alexander RW, editors: *Hurst's the heart*, ed 8, New York, 1994, McGraw-Hill, pp 1457-1466.

FIGURE CREDIT

Reproduced with permission from Hurst JW. The examination of the heart: the importance of initial screening, *Dis Mon* 36(5):285, 1990.

HISTORY

The patient is a 20-year-old man with a history of paroxysmal rapid heart action.

PHYSICAL EXAMINATION

A malar flush is noted.

The systolic blood pressure is 118 mm Hg and the diastolic blood pressure is 68 mm Hg.

A large *a* wave is seen in the internal jugular vein when the patient's trunk is elevated 45 degrees. There is also a prominent wave noted in the internal jugular vein during ventricular systole.

Auscultation in the second left intercostal space near the sternum reveals that the second sound is more widely split than normal and is a little more widely split during inspiration than during expiration. No murmurs are heard at the cardiac apex.

CHEST X-RAY FILM

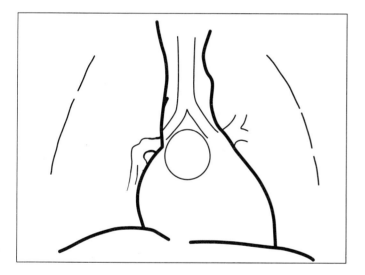

ELECTROCARDIOGRAM

The heart rhythm is normal. The heart rate is 84 depolarizations per minute; the P wave duration is 0.11 second, and its amplitude is 4 mm in lead II. The PR interval is 0.24 second. The QRS duration is 0.12 second. The QT interval is 0.36 second.

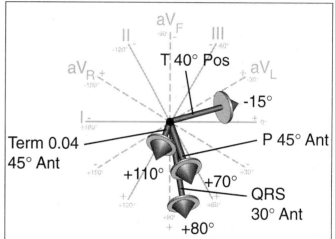

WHAT IS DIAGNOSIS?

HISTORY

The history of paroxysmal rapid heart beat in a young man should lead the physician to consider the possibility of Wolff-Parkinson-White syndrome, mitral valve prolapse, ostium secundum, atrial septal defect, and Ebstein anomaly. The condition can also occur when there is no other evidence of heart disease.

PHYSICAL EXAMINATION

A malar flush may occur in a patient with mitral stenosis or Ebstein anomaly.

The large *a* wave in the internal jugular vein indicates poor compliance of the right ventricle. The large prominent wave during systole indicates tricuspid valve regurgitation.

Wide splitting of the second heart sound that becomes more widely split on inspiration than during expiration suggests right bundle branch block.

These abnormalities suggest the presence of right-sided heart disease that causes tricuspid valve regurgitation and RBBB. There is no evidence of left-sided heart disease. Mitral stenosis as a cause of malar flush is excluded because no diastolic murmur is heard at the apex.

Ebstein anomaly is a good diagnostic choice.

CHEST X-RAY FILM

The chest x-ray film is abnormal; the cardiac silhouette suggests the presence of pericardial effusion. Careful scrutiny of the shape of the silhouette reveals that its right lower portion is probably produced by a large right atrium (note how it curves in toward the center of the chest rather than extending farther to the right and inferiorly as it would be when caused by pericardial effusion). The abnormalities suggest Ebstein anomaly.

See Patient 1 for a normal chest x-ray film.

See Fig. 3-7.

ELECTROCARDIOGRAM

The duration of the P wave is 0.11 second, and its amplitude is 4 mm. The large mean P vector is directed +70 degrees in the frontal plane and 45 degrees anteriorly, indicating a right atrial abnormality.

The mean QRS vector is directed +80 degrees in the frontal plane and 30 degrees anteriorly. The QRS duration is 0.12 second. The terminal 0.04-second QRS vector is directed +110 degrees in the frontal plane and 45 degrees anteriorly, indicating RBBB. The terminal 0.04-second vector is not very large.

The mean T vector is directed -15 degrees to the left and 40 degrees posteriorly.

The extremely tall P waves suggest the diagnosis of Ebstein anomaly. There is a right ventricular conduction defect that is not typical of RBBB (see following discussion).

See Patient 1 for a normal electrocardiogram.

DIAGNOSIS

The diagnosis is Ebstein anomaly. In this condition the tricuspid valve is displaced downward into the right ventricle. Tricuspid regurgitation may be evident, and, rarely, tricuspid stenosis may be present. An ostium secundum atrial septal defect or Wolff-Parkinson-White syndrome may be associated with Ebstein anomaly. Paroxysmal atrial tachycardia or atrial fibrillation often occurs.

DIAGNOSTIC PRINCIPLE

Ebstein anomaly is not rare and may be seen in elderly persons. Whenever there are signs of a malar flush, right-sided heart disease with large *a* waves, and tricuspid valve regurgitation, what appears at first to be a pericardial effusion on the chest x-ray film (but is in reality a large right atrium) and right conduction delay that is often called RBBB, one should consider the diagnosis of Ebstein anomaly. The typical abnormalities of RBBB may not be present because the right ventricle is quite small.

The mean P vector may be directed posteriorly, suggesting a left atrial abnormality when there is actually a large right atrium. This probably occurs because the depolarization process of the huge right atrium is initially directed anteriorly, but then is directed posteriorly but remains in the right atrium on its way to the left atrium.

BIBLIOGRAPHY

Nugent EW, Plauth WH, Edwards JE, Williams WH: The pathology, pathophysiology, recognition, and treatment of congenital heart disease. In Schlant RC, Alexander RW, editors: *Hurst's the heart*, ed 8, New York, 1994, McGraw-Hill, pp 1802-1806.

HISTORY

The patient is a 43-year-old woman. She was well until 2 days before admission to the hospital. She developed a "flulike" syndrome consisting of fever, myalgia, and weakness. This was followed by increasing shortness of breath.

PHYSICAL EXAMINATION

The temperature is 101 degrees F (38.3 degrees C).

The systolic blood pressure is 96 mm Hg, and the diastolic blood pressure is 68 mm Hg. The heart rate is 120 beats per minute.

The arterial pulse wave is illustrated in the diagram below.

The external neck veins are abnormally distended, and the internal jugular pulsations are noted higher in the neck than normal when the patient is sitting.

The apex impulse cannot be felt.

A left ventricular (LV) gallop sound and a grade 1 systolic murmur are heard at the apex.

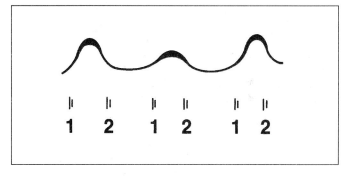

1, 2, First, second heart sounds. See figure credit.

CHEST X-RAY FILM

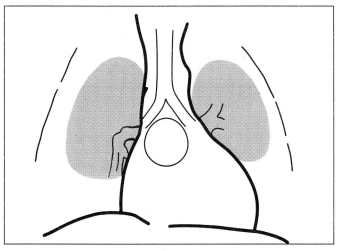

WHAT LOW-TECHNOLOGY PROCEDURE WOULD YOU PERFORM?

WHAT IS DIFFERENTIAL DIAGNOSIS?

WHAT IS FINAL DIAGNOSIS?

ELECTROCARDIOGRAM

Sinus tachycardia is present. The heart rate is 120 depolarizations per minute. The PR interval is 0.14 second. The QRS duration is 0.09 second. The QT interval is 0.36 second. The total 12-lead QRS amplitude is 75 mm.

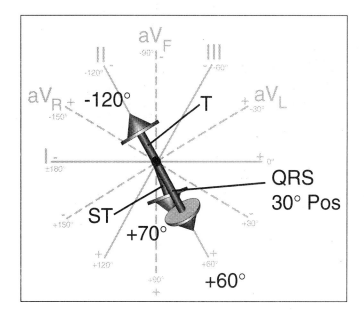

HISTORY

The symptoms should lead one to consider pneumonia or some other acute lung disease, pericarditis, myocarditis, or a combination of myocarditis and pericarditis.

PHYSICAL EXAMINATION

In this clinical setting, the temperature elevation should lead one to consider an infectious process.

The abnormalities of the neck veins suggest heart failure. The heart rate is rapid, and thus perfect observations are difficult. Therefore, the neck vein abnormalities of cardiac tamponade could be missed. Accordingly, cardiac tamponade cannot be excluded.

The diagram of the arterial pulse shows pulsus alternans. This indicates severe LV dysfunction.

The apex impulse could not be felt; this suggests the possibility of pericardial effusion.

The LV gallop indicates LV dysfunction.

CHEST X-RAY FILM

Heart failure with pulmonary edema is evident. The cardiac silhouette is larger than normal, and there is no evidence of primary lung disease.

The cardiac silhouette could be larger than normal because of acute myocarditis, pericardial effusion, or both. Pulmonary edema favors myocardial disease, but pericardial effusion could also be present.

See Fig. 3-2A for an x-ray film showing pericardial effusion.

See Patient 1 for a normal chest x-ray film.

ELECTROCARDIOGRAM

The total QRS amplitude of 75 mm is abnormally low.

The mean ST vector is directed toward the cardiac apex, and the mean T vector is directed 150 degrees from the mean QRS vector.

These abnormalities can be caused by pericarditis with effusion, myocarditis, or both. Actually, there may be myopericarditis.

See Fig. 4-77 for an ECG showing the effect of pericarditis with effusion.

See Patient 1 for a normal ECG.

LOW-TECH PROCEDURE

The patient should be tested for pulsus paradoxus. When tested, no pulsus paradoxus was detected in this patient.

DIFFERENTIAL DIAGNOSIS

There is abundant evidence of myocardial dysfunction and heart failure. The acute onset of the condition and the associated "flulike" symptoms and elevated body temperature indicate that the patient had acute myocarditis. Pericardial effusion may be present because the apex impulse could not be felt. However, no additional sign of cardiac tamponade was found.

FINAL DIAGNOSIS

Myopericarditis with possible pericardial effusion, most likely caused by a viral infection.

DIAGNOSTIC PRINCIPLE

Pulsus alternans is a useful sign of LV dysfunction. The ejection fraction is usually under 30% when there is a pulsus alternans.

The development of heart failure, pulsus alternans, an LV gallop, and low QRS amplitude in the ECG following a "flulike" syndrome indicates the development of myocarditis. Pericarditis with effusion may also be present, but pericarditis alone does not produce pulsus alternans or an LV gallop.

BIBLIOGRAPHY

O'Connell JB, Renlund DG: Myocarditis and specific myocardial diseases. In Schlant RC, Alexander RW, editors: *Hurst's the heart*, ed 8, New York, 1994, McGraw-Hill, pp 1591-1598.

FIGURE CREDIT

Reproduced with permission from Hurst JW: The examination of the heart: the importance of initial screening, *Dis Mon* 36(5):278, 1990.

HISTORY

The patient is a 32-year-old woman who has suddenly developed severe dyspnea. She indicates that she can hear a noise in her chest. She states a physician told her previously that she has a heart murmur, but she has not seen a physician in many years.

PHYSICAL EXAMINATION

She is extremely dyspneic.

Her systolic blood pressure is 144 mm Hg, and the diastolic blood pressure is 82 mm Hg. The heart rate is 115 beats per minute.

Coarse rales are heard in both lungs. The arterial pulse is normal except for tachycardia. Neck veins cannot be evaluated because of tachycardia and the tensing of neck muscles as she struggles to breathe. The apex impulse is located in the fifth intercostal space 1 to 2 cm to the left of the left midclavicular line.

Auscultation of the heart reveals the following (note figure on the right):

The grade 4 systolic murmur radiates laterally and can be heard over the cervical and thoracic vertebrae. The murmur is easily heard over the sacrum and is heard faintly on top of the head.

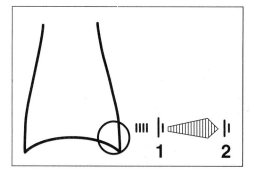

I, 2, First, second heart sounds.

CHEST X-RAY FILM

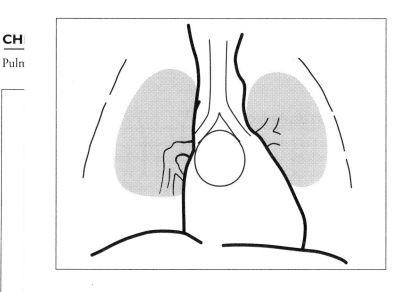

ELECTROCARDIOGRAM

There is sinus rhythm. The heart rate is 120 depolarizations per minute. The PR interval is 0.14 second. The QRS duration is 0.08 second. The QT interval is 0.34 second. The total 12-lead QRS amplitude is 170 mm.

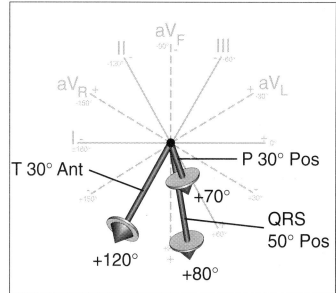

WHAT IS DIFFERENTIAL DIAGNOSIS?

WHAT IS FINAL DIAGNOSIS?

HISTORY

Increasing dyspnea on effort for a year could be caused by pulmonary disease, such as interstitial fibrosis; heart disease such as mitral or aortic valve disease, cardiomyopathy, or certain types of congenital heart disease, such as ostium secundum atrial septal defect; or primary pulmonary artery hypertension. Within this context the syncope leads one to consider mitral stenosis, aortic valve stenosis, hypertrophic subaortic stenosis, a cardiac dysrhythmia, left atrial tumor, pulmonary hypertension, or vasovagal syncope.

PHYSICAL EXAMINATION

The presence of cyanosis indicates that the patient may have severe chronic lung disease or a right-to-left cardiac shunt.

There is an abnormal prominent *a* wave in the jugular venous pulsation (see upper figure). This indicates poor compliance of the right ventricle.

A prominent prolonged systolic pulsation is felt in the second left intercostal space near the sternum (see middle figure). This indicates dilatation of the main pulmonary artery. Furthermore, the movement is typical of an increase in pressure rather than an increase in volume.

There is an abnormally prolonged anterior movement of the precordium, indicating right ventricular (RV) hypertrophy (see middle figure). The movement is typical of that caused by an increase in pressure rather than an increase in volume.

Auscultation in the second left intercostal area reveals that the pulmonary valve closure sound is abnormally loud (see lower figure). The pulmonary valve closure sound is easily heard at the apex and this is abnormal.

A grade 1 or 2 systolic murmur may be heard in the second left intercostal space adjacent to the sternum. This murmur is usually associated with a dilated pulmonary artery.

These abnormalities indicate the presence of RV hypertrophy and severe pulmonary arterial hypertension.

CHEST X-RAY FILM

On posteroanterior and lateral views, the lungs appear normal.

The right atrium is large, as is the main pulmonary artery. The right pulmonary artery is large and tapers promptly. There is evidence of RV hypertrophy in the lateral view.

The abnormalities indicate the presence of right ventricular hypertrophy and pulmonary artery hypertension. There is no evidence of lung disease. It follows that the heart disease is either caused by Eisenmenger physiology, primary pulmonary hypertension, or repeated pulmonary emboli.

See Patient 1 for a normal chest x-ray film.

ELECTROCARDIOGRAM

The amplitude of the P wave is abnormally large. The mean P vector is directed +70 degrees in the frontal plane and 60 degrees anteriorly. The abnormalities indicate a right atrial abnormality.

The mean QRS vector is directed +100 degrees to the right in the frontal plane and 60 degrees anteriorly. The QRS duration is 0.10 second. This indicates right ventricular hypertrophy.

The mean T vector is directed 0 degrees in the frontal plane and 45 degrees posteriorly. This abnormality is caused by RV hypertrophy and is related to systolic pressure overload of the right ventricle.

The abnormalities should lead one to consider all the causes of RV hypertrophy.

The ECG shown in Fig. 4-55 shows RV hypertrophy caused by subpulmonic stenosis. The RV hypertrophy shown in Fig. 4-55 is similar to that caused by primary pulmonary hypertension.

See Patient 1 for a normal ECG.

DIFFERENTIAL DIAGNOSIS

The patient could have Eisenmenger physiology, primary pulmonary hypertension, or repeated pulmonary emboli.

Eisenmenger physiology is excluded because there is no history of heart disease before a year ago and no evidence of left ventricular disease such as might be present when Eisenmenger physiology is caused by patent ductus or interventricular septal defect. The toes were not more cyanotic than the fingers, as they are with a patent ductus arteriosus with reversed shunt resulting from Eisenmenger physiology. The second heart sound is not characteristic of Eisenmenger physiology associated with an atrial septal defect.

There is no evidence for discrete episodes of pulmonary emboli.

It must be emphasized that these three diagnostic possibilities cannot always be separated using only low technology, because when the pulmonary artery pressure, RV pressure, and right atrial pressure reach certain levels, the shunts associated with them diminish. Accordingly, the heart murmurs become altered to the point they may not have diagnostic value. It also must be pointed out that patients can have small pulmonary emboli without experiencing discrete episodes of dyspnea.

FINAL DIAGNOSIS

Pulmonary hypertension. The most likely diagnosis is *primary pulmonary hypertension*, but other studies would be needed to eliminate other causes such as Eisenmenger physiology or repeated pulmonary emboli. The cyanosis most likely is caused by a right-to-left shunt through a foramen ovale.

HISTORY

The patient is a 32-year-old woman who has suddenly developed severe dyspnea. She indicates that she can hear a noise in her chest. She states a physician told her previously that she has a heart murmur, but she has not seen a physician in many years.

PHYSICAL EXAMINATION

She is extremely dyspneic.

Her systolic blood pressure is 144 mm Hg, and the diastolic blood pressure is 82 mm Hg. The heart rate is 115 beats per minute.

Coarse rales are heard in both lungs. The arterial pulse is normal except for tachycardia. Neck veins cannot be evaluated because of tachycardia and the tensing of neck muscles as she struggles to breathe. The apex impulse is located in the fifth intercostal space 1 to 2 cm to the left of the left midclavicular line.

Auscultation of the heart reveals the following (note figure on the right):

The grade 4 systolic murmur radiates laterally and can be heard over the cervical and thoracic vertebrae. The murmur is easily heard over the sacrum and is heard faintly on top of the head.

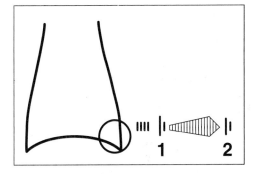

1, 2, First, second heart sounds.

CHEST X-RAY FILM

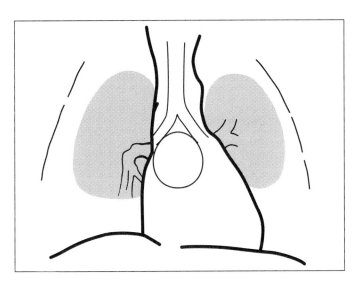

ELECTROCARDIOGRAM

There is sinus rhythm. The heart rate is 120 depolarizations per minute. The PR interval is 0.14 second. The QRS duration is 0.08 second. The QT interval is 0.34 second. The total 12-lead QRS amplitude is 170 mm.

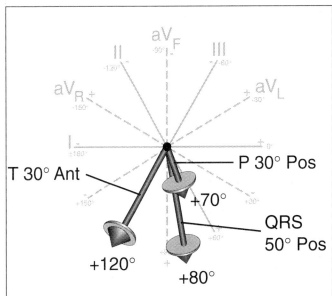

WHAT IS DIFFERENTIAL DIAGNOSIS?

WHAT IS FINAL DIAGNOSIS?

HISTORY

The sudden development of severe dyspnea should lead one to consider pulmonary embolism, pneumothorax, or acute pulmonary edema. Acute pulmonary edema could develop as the result of atrial fibrillation in a patient with mitral stenosis or aortic stenosis, the development of acute aortic valve regurgitation, a left atrial (LA) tumor, an acute myocardial infarction, or rupture of a chordae tendineae to the mitral valve. The patient states a heart murmur has been present before the present illness.

PHYSICAL EXAMINATION

The bilateral rales indicate the presence of acute alveolar pulmonary edema.

The location of the apical impulse indicates that there is slight cardiac enlargement.

An LA gallop sound is heard at the cardiac apex. Note that the loud systolic murmur radiates to the left and is easily heard over the spine and sacrum. It is even heard on top of the head. This type of murmur is almost always caused by ruptured chordae tendineae of the mitral valve.

No diastolic murmurs are heard. The diastolic rumble of mitral stenosis is not present. An LA tumor can produce a diastolic rumble at the apex because it blocks the mitral valve during diastole. No such murmur is heard. An LA tumor may produce the "wrecking ball" phenomenon and gradually destroy the mitral valve. When this occurs, it may produce a systolic murmur of mitral valve regurgitation, but the murmur does not radiate as described in this patient. The murmur is characteristic of ruptured chordae tendineae.

CHEST X-RAY FILM

Alveolar pulmonary edema is present, with only slight LV enlargement. The left atrium is slightly enlarged.

There is no sign of acute pneumothorax.

The cardiac contour associated with mitral stenosis is not evident.

Such a patient could have acute MI, LA tumor, or rupture of the chordae tendineae.

See Patient 1 for a normal chest x-ray film.

ELECTROCARDIOGRAM

The patient has sinus tachycardia. An LA abnormality is noted.

The direction of the mean QRS vector is normal. The 12-lead QRS amplitude is at the upper limit of the normal range. The mean T vector is directed +120 degrees in the frontal plane and 30 degrees anteriorly. The QRS-T angle is about 80 degrees, and the mean T vector is directed abnormally to the right of the vertical mean QRS vector. This indicates an abnormality of the repolarization process. The abnormalities suggest the presence of left ventricular (LV) hypertrophy.

See Patient 1 for a normal ECG.

DIFFERENTIAL DIAGNOSIS

Mitral stenosis with atrial fibrillation can be excluded because: (1) the rhythm is sinus tachycardia, (2) there is no diastolic rumble at the apex, and (3) there is the loud murmur of mitral valve regurgitation. The contour of the heart on the chest x-ray film does not suggest mitral stenosis.

There is no murmur of acute aortic valve regurgitation.

Pneumothorax is not present on the chest x-ray film.

MI is unlikely because she has had no chest pain and the ECG does not reveal the signs of MI. Rupture of a papillary muscle of the mitral valve could conceivably produce such a murmur, but such patients usually have other signs of infarction.

An LA tumor could produce the acute pulmonary edema but infrequently produces a murmur such as described in this patient.

Rupture of the chordae tendineae of the mitral valve is the most likely diagnosis. The patient had a murmur before the development of the unusual systolic murmur, atrial gallop sound at the apex, and acute pulmonary edema. This suggests that the ruptured chordae occurred in a patient with mitral valve prolapse in whom the heart was only slightly enlarged. Infective endocarditis should always be considered and ruled out in such a patient.

FINAL DIAGNOSIS

The patient undoubtedly has ruptured the chordae tendineae to the mitral valve. The etiology of the basic disease must now be considered.

Rupture of the chordae tendineae of the mitral valve may be caused by endocarditis, trauma, or rupture related to myxomatous degeneration of the chordae and mitral valve leaflets. The patient has no history of trauma, so this etiology can be eliminated.

There is no way to exclude endocarditis in this patient, who has a history of a heart murmur. Admittedly, there is no fever and no history of dental work or other source of bacteremia, but this is not adequate to eliminate the disease. Blood cultures should be obtained even though the most likely diagnosis is rupture of the chordae that are weakened by myxomatous degeneration. The chances are that the murmur she recalls was caused by mitral valve prolapse.

DIAGNOSTIC PRINCIPLES

This patient has been presented for two reasons.

First, it affords an opportunity to discuss the causes of acute pulmonary edema with a normal, or nearly normal, heart size. As stated earlier, this can occur as a result of MI, rupture of a chordae tendineae, LA myxoma, mitral valve or aortic valve stenosis with uncontrolled atrial fibrillation, and acute aortic valve regurgitation.

Second, it permits the discussion of the murmur caused by ruptured chordae tendineae. The murmur described here is said to occur when the chordae tendineae of the *anterior* leaflet of the mitral valve ruptures. Some believe that rupture of the chordae tendineae to the posterior leaflet of the mitral valve *produces* a murmur that simulates aortic valve stenosis. In my experience, the chords of both mitral leaflets have occurred whenever I have diagnosed rupture of the chordae tendineae of the mitral valve.

BIBLIOGRAPHY

Shaver JA, Salerni R: Auscultation of the heart. In Schlant RC, Alexander RW, editors: *Hurst's the heart*, ed 8, New York, 1994 McGraw-Hill, p 297.

HISTORY

The patient is a 28-year-old-man who has previously been asymptomatic. While lifting a heavy box, he developed severe chest pain and dyspnea.

PHYSICAL EXAMINATION

The body temperature is normal.

The systolic blood pressure is 150 mm Hg, and the diastolic blood pressure is 45 mm Hg.

The pulsation of the internal jugular venous pulse is illustrated in the diagram on the right.

Auscultation reveals the following:

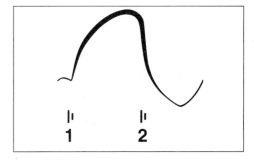

1, *2*, First, second heart sounds. See figure credits.

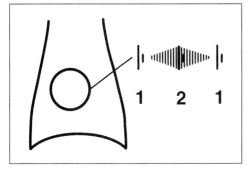

See figure credits.

CHEST X-RAY FILM

Pulmonary congestion is present.

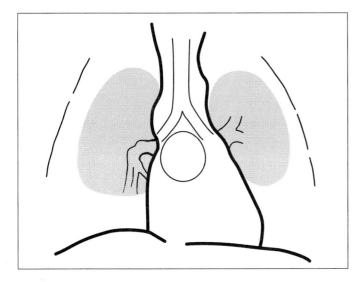

ELECTROCARDIOGRAM

Sinus tachycardia is present. The heart rate is 105 depolarizations per minute. The PR interval is 0.17 second. The QRS duration is 0.08 second. The QT interval is 0.34 second. The total 12-lead QRS amplitude is 178 mm.

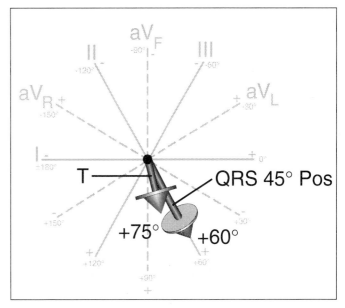

WHAT IS DIFFERENTIAL DIAGNOSIS?

WHAT IS FINAL DIAGNOSIS?

HISTORY

The patient's age and gender, plus the association of acute chest pain and dyspnea related to sudden effort, are almost diagnostic of rupture of a sinus of Valsalva. A pneumothorax could produce similar complaints.

PHYSICAL EXAMINATION

The arterial pulse pressure is wide. The prominent internal jugular venous pulse can be easily seen during systole. The pulsation may actually be an arterial pulse seen in the jugular veins. There is a continuous murmur heard in the third right intercostal space near the sternum. These abnormalities indicate that the posterior sinus of Valsalva has ruptured into the right atrium.

CHEST X-RAY FILM

The heart is normal size, but pulmonary congestion is present. The proximal part of the aorta is slightly enlarged. There is no sign of pneumothorax.

The differential diagnosis should include all the causes of heart failure in a patient with a normal-sized heart (see discussion of Patient 17).

See Patient 1 for a normal chest x-ray film.

ELECTROCARDIOGRAM

The ECG is normal. This forces one to consider all of the types of heart disease that can be associated with a normal ECG.

See Patient 1 for another normal ECG.

DIFFERENTIAL DIAGNOSIS

The symptoms related to effort plus the physical findings are diagnostic of rupture of a posterior sinus of Valsalva aneurysm into the right atrium.

A somewhat similar clinical picture could develop as the result of endocarditis of the aortic valve and its surrounding structures. An aortic valve ring abscess can tunnel into the right atrium. There are no other clues to support the diagnosis of endocarditis. Despite this, blood cultures should be obtained.

FINAL DIAGNOSIS

Rupture of a congenital aneurysm of the posterior sinus of Valsalva into the right atrium.

DIAGNOSTIC PRINCIPLE

Whenever one hears a continuous murmur on the front of the chest, it is wise to think of the following conditions: a patent ductus arteriosus produces a continuous murmur that is heard best just below the middle of the left clavicle. When the continuous murmur is heard best in other areas of the precordium, one should consider the possibility of an aorticopulmonary septal defect, rupture of an aneurysm of the sinus of Valsalva in which the rupture enters the right atrium or right ventricle, and a coronary arteriovenous fistula in which the coronary artery enters the right ventricle. When the murmur develops suddenly, as it did in this patient, it usually results from the rupture of a sinus of Valsalva.

BIBLIOGRAPHY

Nugent EW, Plauth WH, Edwards JE, Williams WH: The pathology, pathophysiology, recognition, and treatment of congenital heart disease. In Schlant RC, Alexander RW, editors: *Hurst's the heart*, ed 8, New York, 1994, McGraw-Hill, pp 1784-1785.

FIGURE CREDITS

Upper and *lower*, Modified and reproduced with permission from Hurst JW: The examination of the heart: the importance of initial screening, *Dis Mon* 36(5):280 (upper), 286 (lower), 1990.

HISTORY

The patient is a 38-year-old woman. She has noticed increasing dyspnea on effort for the last year. She has fainted on one occasion.

PHYSICAL EXAMINATION

The patient is slightly cyanotic and has slight clubbing of the fingers.

The systolic blood pressure is 110 mm Hg, and the diastolic blood pressure is 68 mm Hg.

The pulse rate is 88 beats per minute.

When the trunk is elevated 45 degrees, the jugular venous pulsations appear as shown in the top diagram.

The precordial pulsations are shown in the middle figure to the right.

The heart sounds are shown in the lower figure on the right.

CHEST X-RAY FILM

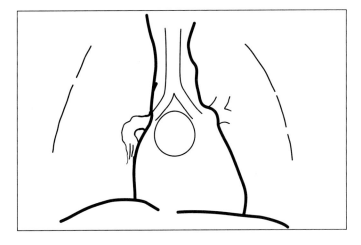

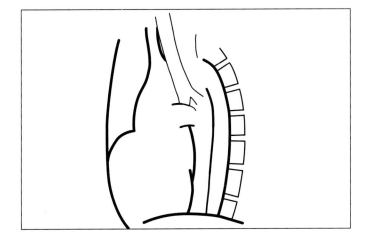

WHAT IS DIFFERENTIAL DIAGNOSIS?

WHAT IS FINAL DIAGNOSIS?

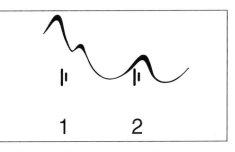

1, 2, First, second heart sounds. See figure credits.

The movements of the front of the chest are depicted as follows.

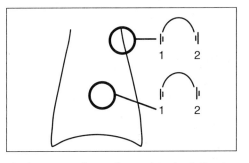

The heart sounds are depicted in the following diagram.

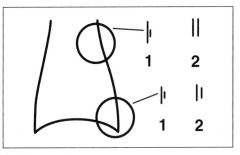

See figure credits.

ELECTROCARDIOGRAM

The heart rhythm is normal. There are 88 depolarizations per minute. The PR interval is 0.19 second. The amplitude of the P wave in lead II is 3 mm. The QRS duration is 0.10 second. The QT interval is 0.34 second.

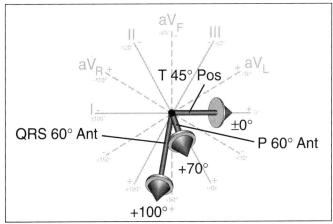

HISTORY

Increasing dyspnea on effort for a year could be caused by pulmonary disease, such as interstitial fibrosis; heart disease such as mitral or aortic valve disease, cardiomyopathy, or certain types of congenital heart disease, such as ostium secundum atrial septal defect; or primary pulmonary artery hypertension. Within this context the syncope leads one to consider mitral stenosis, aortic valve stenosis, hypertrophic subaortic stenosis, a cardiac dysrhythmia, left atrial tumor, pulmonary hypertension, or vasovagal syncope.

PHYSICAL EXAMINATION

The presence of cyanosis indicates that the patient may have severe chronic lung disease or a right-to-left cardiac shunt.

There is an abnormal prominent *a* wave in the jugular venous pulsation (see upper figure). This indicates poor compliance of the right ventricle.

A prominent prolonged systolic pulsation is felt in the second left intercostal space near the sternum (see middle figure). This indicates dilatation of the main pulmonary artery. Furthermore, the movement is typical of an increase in pressure rather than an increase in volume.

There is an abnormally prolonged anterior movement of the precordium, indicating right ventricular (RV) hypertrophy (see middle figure). The movement is typical of that caused by an increase in pressure rather than an increase in volume.

Auscultation in the second left intercostal area reveals that the pulmonary valve closure sound is abnormally loud (see lower figure). The pulmonary valve closure sound is easily heard at the apex and this is abnormal.

A grade 1 or 2 systolic murmur may be heard in the second left intercostal space adjacent to the sternum. This murmur is usually associated with a dilated pulmonary artery.

These abnormalities indicate the presence of RV hypertrophy and severe pulmonary arterial hypertension.

CHEST X-RAY FILM

On posteroanterior and lateral views, the lungs appear normal.

The right atrium is large, as is the main pulmonary artery. The right pulmonary artery is large and tapers promptly. There is evidence of RV hypertrophy in the lateral view.

The abnormalities indicate the presence of right ventricular hypertrophy and pulmonary artery hypertension. There is no evidence of lung disease. It follows that the heart disease is either caused by Eisenmenger physiology, primary pulmonary hypertension, or repeated pulmonary emboli.

See Patient 1 for a normal chest x-ray film.

ELECTROCARDIOGRAM

The amplitude of the P wave is abnormally large. The mean P vector is directed +70 degrees in the frontal plane and 60 degrees anteriorly. The abnormalities indicate a right atrial abnormality.

The mean QRS vector is directed +100 degrees to the right in the frontal plane and 60 degrees anteriorly. The QRS duration is 0.10 second. This indicates right ventricular hypertrophy.

The mean T vector is directed 0 degrees in the frontal plane and 45 degrees posteriorly. This abnormality is caused by RV hypertrophy and is related to systolic pressure overload of the right ventricle.

The abnormalities should lead one to consider all the causes of RV hypertrophy.

The ECG shown in Fig. 4-55 shows RV hypertrophy caused by subpulmonic stenosis. The RV hypertrophy shown in Fig. 4-55 is similar to that caused by primary pulmonary hypertension.

See Patient 1 for a normal ECG.

DIFFERENTIAL DIAGNOSIS

The patient could have Eisenmenger physiology, primary pulmonary hypertension, or repeated pulmonary emboli.

Eisenmenger physiology is excluded because there is no history of heart disease before a year ago and no evidence of left ventricular disease such as might be present when Eisenmenger physiology is caused by patent ductus or interventricular septal defect. The toes were not more cyanotic than the fingers, as they are with a patent ductus arteriosus with reversed shunt resulting from Eisenmenger physiology. The second heart sound is not characteristic of Eisenmenger physiology associated with an atrial septal defect.

There is no evidence for discrete episodes of pulmonary emboli.

It must be emphasized that these three diagnostic possibilities cannot always be separated using only low technology, because when the pulmonary artery pressure, RV pressure, and right atrial pressure reach certain levels, the shunts associated with them diminish. Accordingly, the heart murmurs become altered to the point they may not have diagnostic value. It also must be pointed out that patients can have small pulmonary emboli without experiencing discrete episodes of dyspnea.

FINAL DIAGNOSIS

Pulmonary hypertension. The most likely diagnosis is *primary pulmonary hypertension*, but other studies would be needed to eliminate other causes such as Eisenmenger physiology or repeated pulmonary emboli. The cyanosis most likely is caused by a right-to-left shunt through a foramen ovale.

DIAGNOSTIC PRINCIPLE

Systemic hypertension can be diagnosed with the use of the sphygmomanometer. Pulmonary artery hypertension should be suspected when the pulmonary valve closure sound is louder than normal and is heard at the cardiac apex. Patients with pulmonary hypertension have an abnormal systolic pulsation in the second left interspace near the sternum and an anterior systolic lift of the precordium caused by RV hypertrophy. The main pulmonary artery and the right branch of the pulmonary artery are larger than normal in the chest x-ray film. The right pulmonary artery and its branches taper quickly after leaving the right hilar area. The left branch of the pulmonary artery is also large and tapers promptly, but it is more difficult to see and study than the right branch.

When causes of Eisenmenger physiology or repeated pulmonary emboli are excluded, the diagnosis becomes primary pulmonary hypertension.

BIBLIOGRAPHY

Fishman AP: Pulmonary hypertension. In Schlant RC, Alexander RW, editors: *Hurst's the heart*, ed 8, New York, 1994, McGraw-Hill, pp. 1857-1874.

FIGURE CREDITS

Upper and *lower*, Modified and reproduced with permission from Hurst JW: The examination of the heart: the importance of initial screening, *Dis Mon* 36(5):280 (upper), 284 (lower), 1990.

HISTORY

The patient, a 67-year-old man, traveled to New York from Los Angeles. He was walking in the New York airport when he had acute dyspnea and slumped to the floor. He had no previous symptoms. He had a transurethral resection of the prostate gland eight months ago.

PHYSICAL EXAMINATION

The patient is slightly cyanotic. The heart rate is 120 beats per minute, and the respiratory rate is 32 per minute. The systolic blood pressure is 90 mm Hg, and the diastolic blood pressure is 60 mm Hg.

The external neck veins are distended when the trunk is elevated 45 degrees, but tachycardia makes the analysis of the internal jugular venous pulsations difficult.

An outward movement of the precordium occurs during systole.

There are no abnormal murmurs. The pulmonary valve closure sound is louder than normal.

CHEST X-RAY FILM

ELECTROCARDIOGRAM

Sinus tachycardia is present. There are 120 depolarizations per minute. The amplitude of the P wave in lead II is 3 mm. The PR interval is 0.18 second. The QRS duration is 0.08 second. The QT interval is 0.34 second. The 12-lead total QRS amplitude is 165 mm.

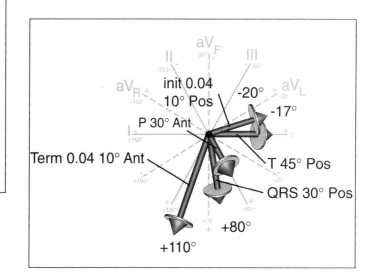

WHAT IS DIFFERENTIAL DIAGNOSIS?

WHAT IS FINAL DIAGNOSIS?

HISTORY

The history of a long plane trip followed by acute dyspnea and cardiovascular collapse should lead one to consider acute pulmonary embolism. A second choice would be acute myocardial infarction (MI).

The previous surgical procedure could have been followed by venous disease of the legs that set the stage for pulmonary embolism.

PHYSICAL EXAMINATION

Circulatory collapse plus cyanosis should lead one to consider the possibility of pulmonary embolism. A second choice would be acute MI or acute pneumothorax.

The abnormally loud pulmonary valve closure sound indicates the presence of pulmonary artery hypertension. The outward movement of the precordium during systole suggests the presence of right ventricular dilatation.

CHEST X-RAY FILM

The patient has no pulmonary edema. The left leaf of the diaphragm is abnormally elevated. This abnormality could be caused by atelectasis of the left lower lobe of the lung. The right atrium is slightly enlarged.

There is no sign of pneumothorax.

The subtle clues suggest the possibility of acute pulmonary embolism but do not exclude MI.

See Patient 1 for a normal chest x-ray film.

ELECTROCARDIOGRAM

Sinus tachycardia is present. A right atrial abnormality is present. The 12-lead total QRS amplitude is normal.

The mean initial 0.04-second vector is directed -17 degrees in the frontal plane and 10 degrees posterior, and the mean terminal 0.04-second vector is directed +110 degrees in the frontal plane and 10 degrees anteriorly. The mean QRS vector is directed +80 degrees in the frontal plane and 30 degrees posteriorly.

The mean T vector is directed 0 degrees in the frontal plane and 45 degrees posteriorly. It is directed away from the anterior region of the heart.

There are two possible explanations for the ECG:

• The ECG is classic for acute pulmonary embolism because there is sinus tachycardia, a right atrial abnormality, an initial 0.04-second vector directed to the left, and a terminal 0.04-second vector directed to the right, and the mean T vector is directed away from the right ventricle. These QRS abnormalities are caused by a unique type of conduction defect created by acute pulmonary embolism. The T wave abnormality results from a repolarization abnormality in the right ventricle.

• The ECG abnormalities could be caused by acute inferior MI. One could postulate that: (1) the initial 0.04-second abnormality is caused by an inferior MI; (2) the T wave abnormality results from inferoanterior myocardial epicardial ischemia; and (3) the left posterior inferior division block accounts for the abnormality in the terminal 0.04-second vector. Although this is possible and such a misinterpretation often occurs, it is not nearly as likely as assuming the abnormalities are caused by acute pulmonary embolism.

The ECG shown in Fig. 4-80 was recorded from a patient with acute pulmonary embolism.

See Patient 1 for a normal ECG.

DIFFERENTIAL DIAGNOSIS

The long plane trip, history of a surgical procedure, acute dyspnea, circulatory collapse, elevated left leaf of the diaphragm, and ECG abnormalities that favor pulmonary embolism over MI, lead one to diagnose acute pulmonary embolism to the left lung.

FINAL DIAGNOSIS

Acute pulmonary embolism to the left lung.

DIAGNOSTIC PRINCIPLE

This is not a typical example of the usual acute pulmonary embolism. Most acute pulmonary emboli do not produce the classic findings depicted here. Most pulmonary emboli are small and may produce little more than tachycardia and mild dyspnea. The ECG is often normal or may show only a T wave abnormality. Atrial fibrillation may be precipitated by pulmonary embolism.

BIBLIOGRAPHY

Newman JH, Ross JC: Chronic cor pulmonale. In Schlant RC, Alexander RW, editors: *Hurst's the heart*, ed 8, New York, 1994, McGraw-Hill, pp 1880-1889.

Weissman NJ, Fuster V: Diagnosis of pulmonary artery hypertension, *Heart Dis Stroke* 1:196-201, 1992.

HISTORY

The patient is a 41-year-old woman who is complaining of increasing dyspnea on effort. She gives a history of episodes of palpitation. She is taking digitalis.

PHYSICAL EXAMINATION

Regular rhythm is present. The heart rate is 80 beats per minute.

The systolic blood pressure is 124 mm Hg, and the diastolic blood pressure is 78 mm Hg.

The cardiac apical impulse, located in the fifth left intercostal space, is larger than normal, and the systolic movement lasts one half of systole.

Auscultation in the second left intercostal space near the sternum reveals that the second heart sound is widely split and remains fixed during inspiration and expiration. In fact, the gap between aortic valve closure and pulmonary valve closure is quite large. The pulmonary valve closure sound is slightly louder than normal.

A grade 3 holosystolic murmur is heard at the apex. The murmur radiates laterally.

CHEST X-RAY FILM

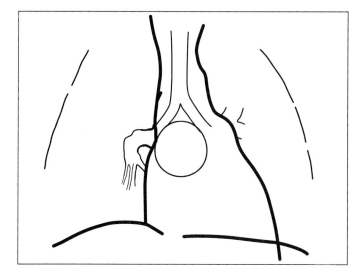

ELECTROCARDIOGRAM

The heart rhythm is normal. There are 78 depolarizations per minute. The PR interval is 0.21 second. The QRS duration is 0.12 second. The QT interval is 0.32 second. The 12-lead total QRS amplitude is 190 mm.

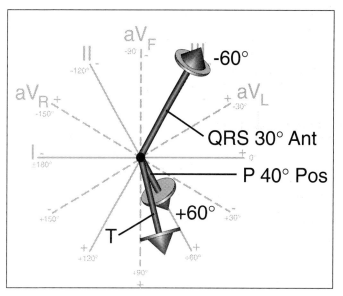

WHAT IS DIFFERENTIAL DIAGNOSIS?

WHAT IS FINAL DIAGNOSIS?

HISTORY

A 41-year-old woman who has increasing dyspnea with effort and palpitation could have lung disease, mitral stenosis, mitral valve prolapse with severe mitral regurgitation, or an atrial septal defect. She probably had episodes of atrial fibrillation or junctional tachycardia in the past.

PHYSICAL EXAMINATION

The size, strength, and duration of the apical impulse indicates left ventricular (LV) hypertrophy.

The second heart sound is widely split and remains fixed during inspiration and expiration. This abnormality suggests the presence of a left-to-right shunt at the atrial level. The second sound is so widely split and fixed that right bundle branch block (RBBB) plus a left-to-right shunt at the atrial level should be considered. The louder than normal pulmonary valve closure sound suggests pulmonary artery hypertension.

CHEST X-RAY FILM

The chest x-ray film reveals evidence of LV enlargement and an increase in pulmonary artery blood flow (note enlargement of the main pulmonary artery and its branches). The increased pulmonary arterial blood flow suggests a left-to-right intracardiac shunt. The left atrium is larger than normal. The large left atrium and left ventricle are against the diagnosis of ostium secundum atrial septal defect.

An ostium primum atrial septal defect, interventricular septal defect, or patent ductus arteriosus could produce the abnormalities. Mitral valve regurgitation from prolapse of the mitral valve or rheumatic heart disease could cause all the abnormalities except for the increase in pulmonary blood flow.

See Patient 1 for a normal chest x-ray film.

ELECTROCARDIOGRAM

The PR interval is prolonged at 0.21 second. The mean P vector is directed 60 degrees in the frontal plane and 40 degrees posteriorly; this is abnormal and indicates a left atrial (LA) abnormality. The QRS duration is 0.12 second. The mean QRS vector is directed -60 degrees to the left and 30 degrees anteriorly. RBBB plus left anterosuperior division block are present. The mean T vector is directed 135 degrees away from the mean QRS vector.

This type of ECG can be produced by an ostium primum atrial septal defect, multiple infarctions from coronary artery disease, cardiomyopathy, or primary conduction system disease.

See ECG in Fig. 4-63.

See Patient 1 for a normal ECG.

DIFFERENTIAL DIAGNOSIS

- Mitral valve regurgitation is definitely present. It could be caused by rheumatic heart disease or severe mitral valve prolapse. These conditions would not produce an increase in pulmonary blood flow, as is noted in this patient's chest x-ray film.
- Whenever pulmonary blood flow is increased, it is proper to consider an intracardiac left-to-right shunt. An ostium secundum atrial septal defect would not cause LA or LV enlargement. Also, the ECG is not characteristic of the ECG associated with an ostium secundum atrial septal defect.

The absence of the usual murmurs of a ventricular septal defect or patent ductus arteriosus rule against these conditions.
- All the clinical findings in this patient indicate an ostium primum atrial septal defect with a cleft mitral valve. In this clinical setting, the ECG abnormalities are diagnostic of ostium primum atrial septal defect.

FINAL DIAGNOSIS

Ostium primum atrial septal defect with a cleft mitral valve.

DIAGNOSTIC PRINCIPLE

RBBB (or right ventricular conduction delay) plus left anterosuperior division block can be caused by ostium primum atrial septal defect, cardiomyopathy, multiple infarcts from coronary heart disease, and primary disease of the conduction system.

The auscultatory abnormalities plus the radiographic findings plus the ECG abnormalities enable the physician to recognize patients with ostium primum atrial septal defects.

BIBLIOGRAPHY

Nugent EW, Plauth WH, Edwards JE, Williams WH: The pathology, pathophysiology, recognition, and treatment of congenital heart disease. In Schlant RC, Alexander RW, editors: *Hurst's the heart*, ed 8, New York, 1994, McGraw-Hill, pp 1778-1781.

HISTORY

The patient is a 73-year-old woman who is experiencing severe retrosternal chest pain and dyspnea. She has been well except for hypertension. The hypertension was first detected when she was 38 years old. She called an ambulance and arrived at the emergency clinic 22 minutes later. She is being admitted to the coronary care unit.

PHYSICAL EXAMINATION

The pulse is regular at a rate of 105 beats per minute. The systolic blood pressure is 110 mm Hg, and the diastolic pressure is 70 mm Hg.

All peripheral pulses could be felt.

Rales are present in both lungs. The patient preferred to sit upright because of severe dyspnea.

The external neck veins are distended, and the pulsation of the internal jugular veins are noted near the patient's ears. The wave form, however, is normal.

There are no heart murmurs.

The second heart sound is more widely split than normal. The duration of the split decreases on inspiration.

On the third hospital day, the physician heard a new grade 3 systolic murmur near the center of the sternum.

CHEST X-RAY FILM

Pulmonary edema is present.

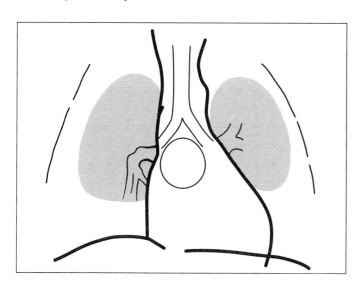

ELECTROCARDIOGRAM

Sinus tachycardia is present. There are 110 depolarizations per minute. The PR interval is 0.18 second. The QRS duration is 0.12 second. The QT interval is 0.36 second. The 12-lead total QRS amplitude is 170 mm.

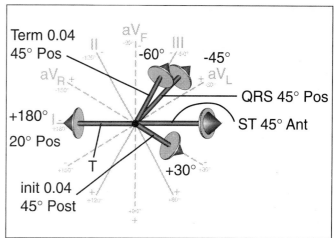

WHAT IS DIFFERENTIAL DIAGNOSIS?

WHAT IS FINAL DIAGNOSIS?

HISTORY

The patient's complaints are characteristic of acute myocardial infarction (MI) and pulmonary edema.

The history of hypertension since age 38 suggests that the patient most likely has essential hypertension.

PHYSICAL EXAMINATION

The peripheral arterial pulses are felt in the legs. This usually excludes coarctation of the aorta as a cause for hypertension.

When first seen, the patient had pulmonary congestion, hypotension, and tachycardia. The loud systolic murmur appeared on the third day. The murmur is characteristic of rupture of the ventricular septum. Paroxysmal splitting of the second sound is usually caused by left bundle branch block (LBBB).

CHEST X-RAY FILM

The heart is only slightly enlarged, but pulmonary congestion is present. This suggests MI, acute aortic or mitral valve regurgitation from endocarditis, rupture of a chordae tendinae to the mitral valve, mitral or aortic valve stenosis with acute atrial fibrillation, or left atrial myxoma.

No additional signs of mitral stenosis are present. There is no evidence of rib notching, as occurs with coarctation of the aorta.

See Patient 1 for a normal chest x-ray film.

ELECTROCARDIOGRAM

There is sinus tachycardia. The QRS duration indicates bundle branch block. The amplitude of the mean QRS vector is at the upper limit of normal, but when there is bundle branch block, it is difficult to determine whether or not this indicates left ventricular hypertrophy. The mean QRS vector is directed -45 degrees to the left and 45 degrees posteriorly. The mean initial 0.04-second vector is directed +30 degrees in the frontal plane and 45 degrees posteriorly. The mean terminal 0.04-second vector is directed -60 degrees in the frontal plane and 45 degrees posteriorly.

The direction of the mean QRS vector and mean terminal 0.04-second vector are typical of complicated LBBB plus left anterosuperior division block. The direction of the mean QRS vector when there is uncomplicated LBBB is rarely more than 30 to 60 degrees to the left of its preblock direction. Because the direction of the preblock mean QRS vector is usually +30 to +60 degrees, the postblock QRS direction is rarely more than -30 degrees to the left when there is uncomplicated LBBB.

The mean ST vector is directed 0 degrees in the frontal plane and 45 degrees anteriorly; it is produced by anteroseptolateral epicardial injury. Note that the mean ST vector is not directed parallel with the mean T vector as it is with uncomplicated LBBB.

The mean T vector is directed at +180 degrees in the frontal plane and 20 degrees posteriorly; it is produced by anteroseptolateral epicardial ischemia.

The ventricular gradient is abnormal.

The ECG is abnormal because of anterolateral MI and complicated LBBB plus left anterosuperior division block.

This ECG serves to point out that an abnormal mean initial 0.04-second vector caused by MI cannot develop when there is LBBB but that other signs of MI can develop with LBBB. This ECG also illustrates the difference in complicated and uncomplicated LBBB.

See Patient 1 for a normal ECG.

DIFFERENTIAL DIAGNOSIS

The abnormalities are diagnostic of anteroseptolateral MI with ruptured interventricular septum, pulmonary edema, complicated LBBB, plus left anterosuperior division block. No other conditions should be considered.

FINAL DIAGNOSIS

Acute anteroseptolateral MI with ruptured interventricular septum. The patient is a woman with essential hypertension who undoubtedly has an acute occlusion of an atheromatous lesion in the left anterior descending coronary artery.

DIAGNOSTIC PRINCIPLE

Rupture of the interventricular septum is usually recognized by hearing a systolic murmur in the midsternal area in a patient with other signs of an acute MI.

Whereas abnormal Q waves may not develop in patients with acute MI who have LBBB, other signs of acute infarction, including abnormal ST and T waves, are commonly observed.

BIBLIOGRAPHY

Roberts R, Morris DC, Pratt CM, Alexander RW: Pathophysiology, recognition, and treatment of acute myocardial infarction and its complications. In Schlant RC, Alexander RW, editors: *Hurst's the heart*, ed 8, New York, 1994, McGraw-Hill, p 1151.

HISTORY

The patient is a 63-year-old woman who has become increasingly dyspneic over 2 days. She has no previous history of heart or lung disease and has been examined yearly.

PHYSICAL EXAMINATION

The systolic blood pressure is 190 mm Hg, and the diastolic blood pressure is 40 mm Hg. The pulse rate is 90 beats per minute. The rhythm is normal.

Carotid artery pulsation is shown in the following diagram.

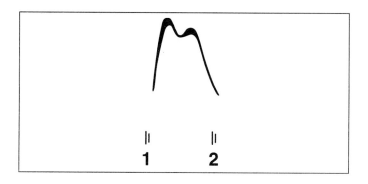

I, 2, First, second heart sounds. See figure credits.

The apical impulse is shown in the following diagram.

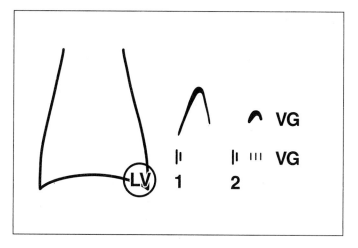

LV, left ventricle; *VG,* ventricular gallop. See figure credits.

The internal jugular venous pulse reveals the pulsation shown in the following diagram.

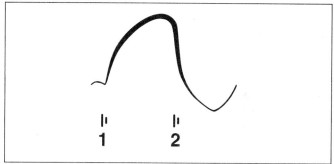

See figure credits.

Auscultation of the heart reveals the murmurs depicted in the following diagram.

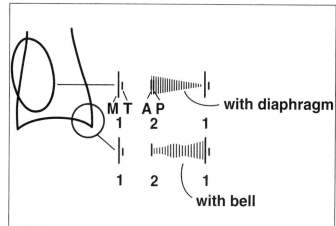

M, Mitral; *T,* tricuspid; *A,* aortic; and *P,* pulmonary valve closure sounds. See figure credits.

CHEST X-RAY FILM

Pulmonary congestion is present.

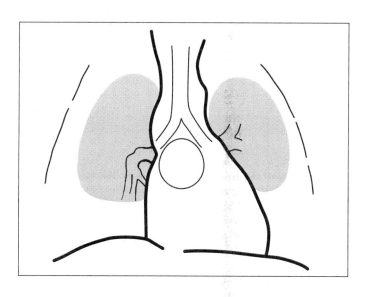

ELECTROCARDIOGRAM

The heart rhythm is normal. There are 88 depolarizations per minute. The PR interval is 0.18 second. The QRS duration is 0.10 second. The QT interval is 0.36 second. The total QRS amplitude is 175 mm.

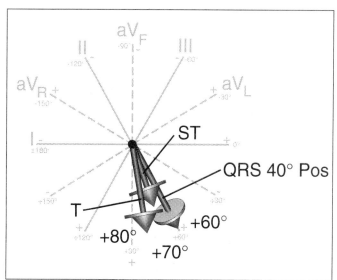

WHAT IS DIFFERENTIAL DIAGNOSIS?

WHAT IS FINAL DIAGNOSIS?

HISTORY

Many types of heart or lung disease could produce dyspnea that increases over 2 days. This symptom alone is not sufficient to determine the etiology of the dyspnea. One could consider two categories of possibilities: (1) the patient could have had long-standing heart or lung disease, and some new condition precipitated a worsening of the basic disease; or (2) the patient could have had no prior evidence of heart or lung disease, and the dyspnea was caused by a rather sudden event that led to the symptom.

The patient has no history of heart or lung disease and has been examined annually.

PHYSICAL EXAMINATION

There is an abnormally wide arterial pulse pressure. This suggests aortic valve regurgitation or peripheral arteriovenous fistula.

The contour of the deep jugular venous pulse indicates tricuspid valve regurgitation (upper right figure). It is usually caused by heart disease of the left side of the heart but can be caused by isolated disease of the right side of the heart, such as occurs with endocarditis of the tricuspid valve, carcinoid heart disease, or primary pulmonary hypertension. The tricuspid valve ring is a poorly developed structure, and less elevation of the right ventricular systolic pressure or volume is required to produce incompetence of the valve compared with the amount of elevation of left ventricular (LV) pressure or volume required to produce mitral valve incompetence. The abnormal jugular venous pulse indicates severe heart failure.

A pulsus bisferiens is felt in the carotid artery (upper left figure). This can be caused by aortic regurgitation or idiopathic hypertrophic subaortic stenosis.

The apical impulse is larger than normal and hyperdynamic (lower left figure). This suggests LV enlargement caused by volume overload, such as occurs with aortic or mitral valve regurgitation.

There is a high-pitched, diastolic murmur heard along the sternal border (lower right figure). It is louder on the right sternal border and is caused by severe aortic valve regurgitation. When the murmur of aortic regurgitation is louder along the right side of the sternum than it is along the left side of the sternum, it is commonly caused by disease of the aortic root. The diastolic rumble at the apex most likely results from an Austin Flint murmur, which is secondary to aortic regurgitation.

No evidence of lung disease is found on physical examination.

CHEST X-RAY FILM

Evidence of heart failure is seen.

The left ventricle is slightly enlarged. When heart failure caused by aortic valve regurgitation develops over a short time, but the heart size remains normal or is only slightly enlarged, it is wise to consider an acute cause of aortic regurgitation.

One must always look for a dilated aortic root in patients with acute aortic valve regurgitation. Regrettably, the aortic root can become significantly dilated but may not be detected on the routine chest film. The aortic root in this patient is abnormally dilated.

See Patient 1 for a normal chest x-ray film.

ELECTROCARDIOGRAM

The ECG could represent diastolic pressure overload of the left ventricle because the QRS amplitude is at the upper limits of normal and the mean ST segment vector is relatively parallel with the large mean T vector. The large mean T vector is normally directed. The ECG could be normal, and the mean ST segment vector could be caused by normal early repolarization.

Diastolic overload of the left ventricle can be caused by aortic or mitral valve regurgitation.

See Patient 1 for a normal ECG.

DIFFERENTIAL DIAGNOSIS

The patient has evidence of acute aortic valve regurgitation and severe heart failure.

Little evidence suggests aortic dissection. The patient has no chest pain, which occurs in 90% of patients with aortic dissection, and all peripheral pulses are hyperdynamic.

No evidence suggests Marfan syndrome.

Endocarditis of the aortic valve seems unlikely in the absence of fever or previous valve disease. Still, endocarditis cannot be excluded.

The patient could have a tear in a myxomatous aortic valve, but this occurs infrequently.

The patient could have annuloaortic ectasia, which is now being recognized as a cause of chronic and acute aortic valve regurgitation.

FINAL DIAGNOSIS

It is not always possible to separate annuloaortic ectasia from endocarditis of the aortic valve or a tear in a myxomatous aortic valve. Other studies, including an esophageal echocardiogram and blood cultures, are needed. The point is that the patient has *acute* aortic regurgitation, and the approach to the patient is quite different than with chronic aortic valve regurgitation.

DIAGNOSTIC PRINCIPLE

The heart may not be enlarged or may be enlarged only slightly when acute aortic valve regurgitation is the cause for heart failure.

Acute aortic regurgitation may be caused by annuloaortic ectasia, aortic dissection, endocarditis of the aortic valve, a tear in a myxomatous aortic valve, aortic root dilatation associated with Marfan disease, and trauma.

A routine chest x-ray film may not reveal evidence of a dilated aortic root.

BIBLIOGRAPHY

Hurst JW, Rackley CE, Becker AE, Wilcox BR: Valvular heart disease. In Hurst JW, editor-in-chief: *Atlas of the heart*, St Louis, 1988, Mosby, pp 4.17-4.24.
Rackley CE, Edwards JE, Wallace RB, Katz NM: Pulmonary valve disease. In Hurst JW, editor: *Hurst's the heart*, ed 8, New York, 1994, McGraw-Hill, pp 805-819.

FIGURE CREDITS

Upper right, reproduced with permission, and *upper left, lower left*, and *lower right*, modified and reproduced with permission, from Hurst JW: The examination of the heart: the importance of initial screening, *Dis Mon* 36(5):278 (upper right), 280 (upper left), 282 (lower left), 285 (lower right), 1990.

HISTORY

The patient is a 43-year-old woman. She had a left mastectomy for cancer of the breast 4 months ago and is being seen now for her complaint of dyspnea on effort.

PHYSICAL EXAMINATION

The systolic blood pressure is 110 mm Hg, and the diastolic blood pressure is 70 mm Hg.

Pulsus alternans is noted in the femoral artery.

The external jugular veins are distended, and a prominent V wave is noted in the internal jugular veins when the trunk of the patient is elevated 45 degrees.

The apical impulse is larger than normal and is located in the fifth intercostal space in the anterior axillary line. The characteristics of the apical impulse are shown in the diagram to the right.

An LV gallop sound is heard at the apex.

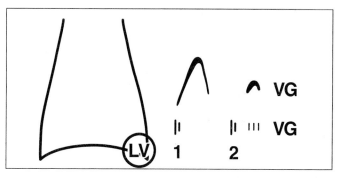

1, 2, First, second heart sounds; *LV,* left ventricle; *VG,* ventricular gallop. See figure credit.

CHEST X-RAY FILM

Pulmonary congestion is present.

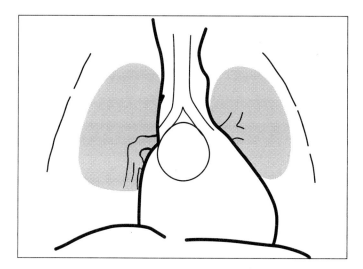

WHAT ADDITIONAL QUESTIONS WOULD YOU ASK PATIENT?

WHAT IS DIFFERENTIAL DIAGNOSIS?

WHAT IS FINAL DIAGNOSIS?

ELECTROCARDIOGRAM

Sinus tachycardia is present. There are 96 depolarizations per minute. The PR interval is 0.19 second. The second half of the P wave measures -0.06 mm·sec in lead V$_1$. The QRS duration is 0.10 second. The QT interval is 0.38 second. The total QRS amplitude is 100 mm.

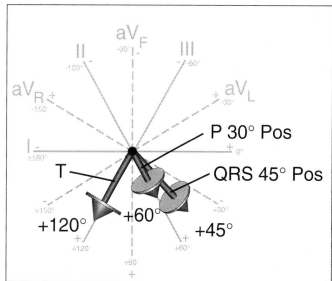

HISTORY

The history leads one to consider two possibilities. The patient could have neoplastic heart disease; that is, the breast cancer could cause pericardial effusion or could involve the heart muscle. Alternately, if the patient is receiving chemotherapy such as doxorubicin (Adriamycin), the patient could have cardiomyopathy because of the drug.

PHYSICAL EXAMINATION

The pulsus alternans indicates left ventricular (LV) dysfunction. The ejection fraction is usually less than 30% to 35% with a pulsus alternans. This indicates disease of the left ventricle. Pericardial effusion may also be present, but the pulsus alternans indicates that pericardial effusion is not the only abnormality present.

The external neck veins are abnormally distended, and the internal jugular veins pulsate at a level higher than normal. There is a large positive V wave indicating tricupsid valve regurgitation.

The apical impulse is larger than normal and displaced leftward. The positive systolic wave is abnormally prolonged, signifying LV dilatation. A ventricular gallop sound is felt.

There are no murmurs. An LV gallop sound indicates ventricular dysfunction.

Ample evidence indicates LV disease and heart failure.

CHEST X-RAY FILM

There is evidence of left atrial (LA) enlargement, LV enlargement, and heart failure. No evidence indicates pericardial fluid, although a little may be present as a part of heart failure.

See Patient 1 for a normal chest x-ray film.

ELECTROCARDIOGRAM

Sinus tachycardia is present. The mean P wave vector is abnormal and indicates an LA abnormality. Such an abnormality typically occurs when there is high diastolic pressure in the left ventricle (as with heart failure).

The total QRS amplitude is abnormally low.

The QRS–T angle is abnormal and indicates a repolarization abnormality.

The ECG abnormalities could result from myocardial disease, pericardial effusion, or both. The abnormal P wave favors myocardial disease.

See Patient 1 for a normal ECG.

ADDITIONAL QUESTION

The patient was asked if she was taking doxorubicin (Adriamycin). She responded that she did take the drug.

DIFFERENTIAL DIAGNOSIS

The differential diagnosis lies between pericardial effusion and dilated cardiomyopathy. The pulsus alternans, abnormal apical impulse, and LV gallop sound favor the latter but do not eliminate the presence of a little pericardial effusion.

In the clinical setting described here, dilated cardiomyopathy caused by doxorubicin is more common than neoplastic infiltration of the myocardium.

FINAL DIAGNOSIS

Dilated cardiomyopathy caused by doxorubicin (Adriamycin) toxicity.

DIAGNOSTIC PRINCIPLE

The heart is often involved with neoplastic disease. The neoplastic disease may be primary or secondary. Dilated cardiomyopathy may be produced by cancer chemotherapy, such as with doxorubicin. The clues to the diagnosis of myocardial disease are different from the clues to the diagnosis of pericardial effusion.

BIBLIOGRAPHY

Crawley IS, Schlant RC: Effect of noncardiac drugs, electricity, poisons, and radiation on the heart. In Schlant RC, Alexander RW, editors: *Hurst's the heart*, ed 8, New York, 1994, McGraw-Hill, pp 1991-1992.

FIGURE CREDIT

Modified and reproduced with permission from Hurst JW: The examination of the heart: the importance of initial screening, *Dis Mon* 36(5):282, 1990.

HISTORY

The patient is a 58-year-old man who has severe retrosternal pain and marked dyspnea. This is his first illness. He calls an ambulance and arrives at the emergency clinic 35 minutes later.

PHYSICAL EXAMINATION

He is pale, sweating profusely, and severely dyspneic even in the sitting position. The arterial pulse rate is 80 beats per minute. The systolic blood pressure is 90 mm Hg, and the diastolic pressure is 50 mm Hg.

Rales are heard throughout both lungs.

The external jugular veins are distended. The internal jugular venous wave form is normal but the A C V waves are noted above the clavicle when the patient's trunk is elevated to 45 degrees.

The apical impulse is larger than normal.

The first heart sound is faint. The second sound is more widely split than normal, and the duration of the split increases with inspiration.

A grade 3 systolic murmur is heard at the apex.

CHEST X-RAY FILM

Pulmonary edema is present.

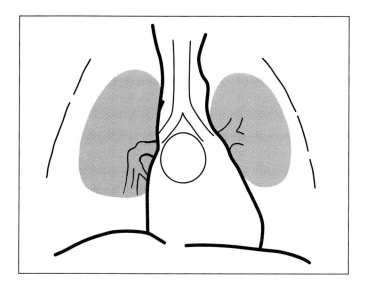

ELECTROCARDIOGRAM

The heart rhythm is normal. There are 70 depolarizations per minute. The PR interval is 0.20 second. The QRS duration is 0.12 second. The QT interval is 0.34 second.

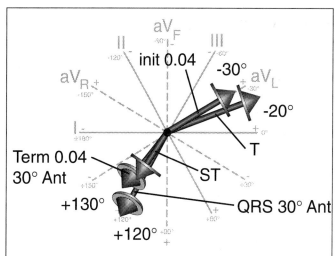

WHAT IS DIFFERENTIAL DIAGNOSIS?

WHAT IS FINAL DIAGNOSIS?

HISTORY

This patient's history is characteristic of myocardial infarction (MI) and acute pulmonary congestion.

PHYSICAL EXAMINATION

Pulmonary edema is evident. Pulmonary rales indicate that the infarct is located in the left ventricle.

The slow pulse, especially when the systemic blood pressure is low, favors an acute inferior MI.

The abnormal splitting of the second heart sound suggests right bundle branch block (RBBB).

The systolic murmur at the apex suggests the possibility of rupture of a papillary muscle to the mitral valve. A systolic murmur at the apex can also be caused by papillary muscle dysfunction and, rarely, rupture of the interventricular septum near the apex. The murmur also indicates that the infarction is located in the left ventricle.

CHEST X-RAY FILM

Pulmonary edema is present, but the heart size is normal. This always suggests an acute event such as MI, acute aortic or mitral valve regurgitation from endocarditis, acute rupture of the chordae tendineae to the mitral valve, or mitral stenosis with acute atrial fibrillation. No other signs of mitral stenosis appear on the x-ray film.

See Patient 1 for a normal chest x-ray film.

ELECTROCARDIOGRAM

The ECG reveals 70 depolarizations per minute. The duration of the QRS complex is 0.12 second, indicating bundle branch block. The mean QRS vector is directed +120 degrees and 30 degrees anteriorly. A mean initial 0.04-second vector is directed -30 degrees to the left, indicating an inferior dead zone. The mean terminal 0.04-second vector is directed +130 degrees and 30 degrees anteriorly. This indicates RBBB. The mean QRS vector and the mean terminal 0.04-second vector are directed farther to the right than usual for uncomplicated RBBB. Accordingly, a good possibility exists that there is RBBB plus left posteroinferior division block.

The direction of the mean ST vector indicates inferoanterior epicardial injury. The direction of the mean ST vector could also be caused by an inferoseptal infarction that also involves the lower portion of the right ventricle. The direction of the mean T vector indicates inferior epicardial ischemia.

The constellation of abnormalities indicates acute inferior infarction with RBBB block plus left posteroinferior division block.

This example illustrates that RBBB does not mask the abnormalities caused by MI and that left posteroinferior division block is likely when the mean QRS vector is directed more than +120 degrees to the right. Involvement of the lower part of the right ventricle *may* be involved when the ST vector is directed inferiorly slightly to the right and parallel with the frontal plane.

See the ECG in Fig. 4-62, which is similar to the ECG discussed here.

See Patient 1 for a normal ECG.

DIFFERENTIAL DIAGNOSIS

This patient has an acute inferior MI. The hypotension and slow pulse are often associated with such an infarct. The pulmonary edema and systolic murmur at the apex suggest the possibility of papillary muscle dysfunction or rupture.

The direction of the mean ST vector in the ECG should lead one to consider the *possibility* of right ventricular infarction in addition to the inferoseptal infarction. An electrocardiographic diagnosis of right ventricular infarction becomes more likely when the mean ST vector is directed more to the right and anteriorly. The pulmonary rales and apical systolic murmur indicate that the left ventricle has been severely damaged.

FINAL DIAGNOSIS

Atherosclerotic coronary heart disease with acute inferior MI with papillary muscle rupture or dysfunction. There were no clinical signs of right ventricular infarction.

DIAGNOSTIC PRINCIPLE

When a new systolic murmur develops at the cardiac apex of a patient with MI, it may be caused by papillary muscle dysfunction or papillary muscle rupture. An echocardiogram may be needed to separate the two conditions.

When the QRS duration is 0.12 second and the mean QRS vector is directed farther to the right than 120 degrees, RBBB plus left posteroinferior division block may be present.

One should consider involvement of the right ventricle when the ST vector is directed inferiorly, slightly to the right and parallel with the frontal plane. There were no clinical signs of right ventricular infarction in this patient.

All the signs of MI can occur when there is RBBB.

BIBLIOGRAPHY

Gaasch WH, O'Rourke RA, Cohn LH, Rackley CE: Mitral valve disease. In Schlant RC, Alexander RW, editors: *Hurst's the heart*, ed 8, New York, 1994, McGraw-Hill, pp 1492-1493.

HISTORY

The patient, a 47-year-old woman, is complaining of slight dyspnea on effort and fatigue.

PHYSICAL EXAMINATION

The patient is obese.

The arterial pulse rate is 70 beats per minute. The systolic blood pressure is 126 mm Hg, and the diastolic blood pressure is 84 mm Hg.

The neck veins and arterial pulsations are normal.

The apical impulse is not felt because she is obese.

The heart sounds are normal, and no murmurs or gallop sounds are heard.

CHEST X-RAY FILM

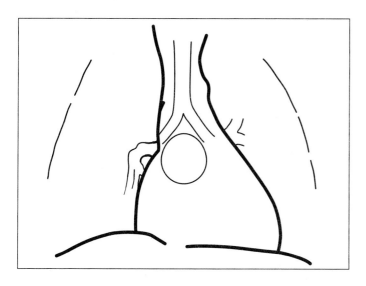

ELECTROCARDIOGRAM

The heart rhythm is normal. There are 75 depolarizations per minute. The PR interval is 0.16 second. The QRS duration is 0.09 second. The QT interval is 0.34 second. The 12-lead QRS amplitude is 75 mm.

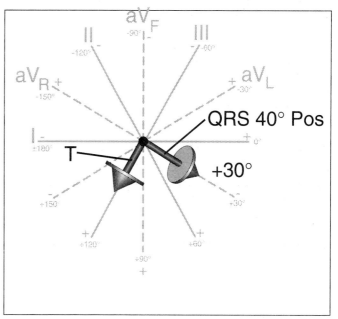

WHAT IS DIFFERENTIAL DIAGNOSIS?

WHAT IS FINAL DIAGNOSIS?

HISTORY

The history yields few clues. The patient could have heart disease, lung disease, myxedema, or anemia, or perhaps obesity alone could cause the symptoms.

PHYSICAL EXAMINATION

The examination of the lungs and heart yields no abnormalities. Her obesity could prevent an adequate examination of precordial movements.

CHEST X-RAY FILM

The cardiac silhouette is abnormal. The heart is large, and the left border irons out the slight prominence normally produced by the main pulmonary artery. The lungs are not congested.

The shape of the cardiac silhouette and absence of pulmonary congestion suggests a moderate-sized pericardial effusion. A second choice would be dilated cardiomyopathy.

See Patient 1 for a normal chest x-ray film.

See Fig. 3-2, *A* and *B*.

ELECTROCARDIOGRAM

The ECG shows an abnormally low QRS amplitude. The total 12-lead QRS amplitude is 75 mm (normal range, 80 to 185). The mean QRS vector is directed +30 degrees in the frontal plane and 40 degrees posteriorly. The mean T vector is directed at +120 degrees in the frontal plane and is parallel with the frontal plane. The QRS-ST angle is 90 degrees.

Low amplitude of the QRS complexes can be caused by pericardial effusion, myocarditis, cardiomyopathy, myxedema, obesity, or anasarca. There is no bradycardia as there would be with myxedema, and no evidence of anasarca on physical examination.

See Patient 1 for a normal ECG.

See Fig. 4-77.

DIFFERENTIAL DIAGNOSIS

Only three possibilities exist: pericardial effusion, myocarditis, or dilated cardiomyopathy. Pericardial effusion is favored because the neck veins are normal, excluding tricuspid valve regurgitation, which would likely be present with dilated cardiomyopathy of this degree. In addition, there is no pulsus alternans, gallop sounds, or pulmonary congestion, which would probably occur with myocarditis or cardiomyopathy.

The normal neck veins exclude cardiac tamponade.

FINAL DIAGNOSIS

Pericardial effusion, etiology to be determined. Myxedema must be excluded.

DIAGNOSTIC PRINCIPLE

Pericardial effusion can be present, and the physical examination, including the examination of the neck veins, may be normal. The neck veins become abnormal only when there is cardiac tamponade or pericardial constriction. The clues to the diagnosis are usually found in the ECG and chest x-ray film.

Pericardial effusion does not always cause the heart sounds to be fainter than normal and pericardial effusion may not eliminate the presence of a pericardial rub.

BIBLIOGRAPHY

Shabetai R: Diseases of the pericardium. In Schlant RC, Alexander RW, editors: *Hurst's the heart*, ed 8, New York, 1994, McGraw-Hill, pp 1652-1662.

HISTORY

This 2-month-old infant seems to be in pain during the time he sucks on his bottle. He quits sucking and cries as his respiratory rate increases.

PHYSICAL EXAMINATION

The heart rate is 120 beats per minute. The patient has no cyanosis. No murmurs are present.

It is not possible to determine the size of the heart.

CHEST X-RAY FILM

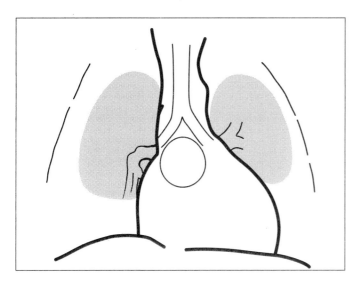

ELECTROCARDIOGRAM

Sinus rhythm is present. There are 130 depolarizations per minute. The PR interval is 0.13 second. The QRS duration is 0.05 second. The QT interval is 0.28 second.

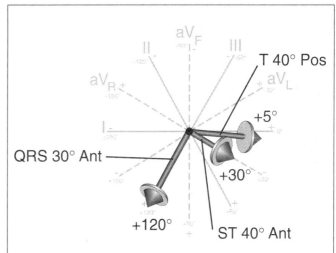

WHAT IS DIFFERENTIAL DIAGNOSIS?

WHAT IS FINAL DIAGNOSIS?

HISTORY

Apparent discomfort during the effort of sucking on the bottle should lead one to consider the possibility of myocardial ischemia caused by an anomalous origin of a coronary artery.

PHYSICAL EXAMINATION

There are no murmurs. This rules out the types of congenital heart disease that produce murmurs.

CHEST X-RAY FILM

The chest x-ray film shows that the heart is slightly large and severe pulmonary congestion caused by heart failure.

ELECTROCARDIOGRAM

The mean QRS vector is directed normally in this 2-month-old infant. Note that the mean ST vector is directed at 30 degrees in the frontal plane and 40 degrees anteriorly. The mean ST vector suggests epicardial injury, as might occur when the left coronary artery originates from the pulmonary artery. The mean T vector is directed at +5 degrees and 40 degrees posteriorly. This is normal for an infant.

DIFFERENTIAL DIAGNOSIS

The symptoms during sucking the bottle plus the epicardial injury in the ECG lead one to suspect that the left main coronary artery originates from the pulmonary artery and that fibroelastosis of the left ventricle is present.

Myocarditis is a less likely possibility.

FINAL DIAGNOSIS

Left main coronary artery originating from the pulmonary artery with fibroelastosis of the left ventricle. These abnormalities have produced severe heart failure.

DIAGNOSTIC PRINCIPLE

Congenital heart disease is typically recognized by the presence of heart murmurs.

An anomaly of the coronary arteries may be present without a heart murmur. The ECG abnormalities shown here indicate that the left main coronary artery arises from the pulmonary artery.

Fibroelastosis of the left ventricle is apparently related to hypoxia of the subendocardial area of the left ventricle.

BIBLIOGRAPHY

Waller BF: Nonatherosclerotic coronary heart disease. In Schlant RC, Alexander RW, editors: *Hurst's the heart*, ed 8, New York, 1994, McGraw-Hill, p 1244.

HISTORY

The patient is an 8-month-old boy who has failed to gain weight.

PHYSICAL EXAMINATION

The femoral arterial pulses can be felt.

The patient is cyanotic and the respiratory rate is slightly increased. The heart rate is 120 beats per minute.

The neck veins appear to be abnormal, but the rapid heart rate prevents an accurate analysis of the movements.

There is an abnormal hyperdynamic anterior lift of the precordial area.

The second heart sound seems to be split, but the heart rate is too rapid for accurate analysis.

A grade 2 systolic murmur is heard in the second and third intercostal spaces near the sternum.

The liver is enlarged.

CHEST X-RAY FILM

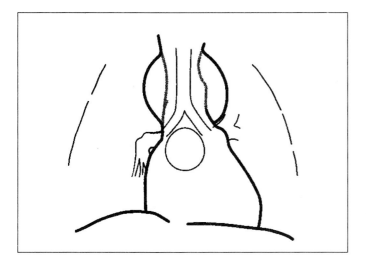

ELECTROCARDIOGRAM

Sinus tachycardia is present. There are 140 depolarizations per minute. The PR interval is 0.12 second. The QRS duration is 0.06 second. The QT interval is 0.28 second.

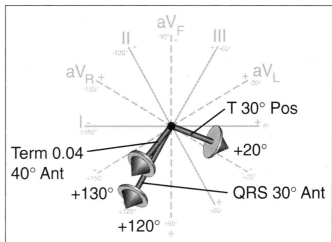

WHAT IS DIFFERENTIAL DIAGNOSIS?

WHAT IS FINAL DIAGNOSIS?

HISTORY

The failure to gain weight could be caused by any of many cardiac or noncardiac conditions. It is of little help in making a diagnosis but does imply that a serious condition is present.

PHYSICAL EXAMINATION

The patient is cyanotic, indicating that a right-to-left shunt is probably present. The abnormal hyperdynamic movement of the anterior portion of the chest suggests that there is volume overload of the right ventricle.

Regrettably, the heart rate is so rapid that it is not possible to study the neck veins or analyze the second heart sound except to note that it is split.

The murmur may be from an interventricular septal defect or rapid flow in the pulmonary artery. However, an isolated ventricular septal defect would not cause cyanosis.

The liver is large, most likely because of heart failure.

All the causes of cyanosis must be considered except for type 4 truncus arteriosus. Truncus is ruled out because the second sound is split.

CHEST X-RAY FILM

The x-ray film is diagnostic of the type of congenital heart disease present in this patient. In this patient, the abnormalities noted on the chest x-ray film are much more useful in establishing the diagnosis than clues gleaned from the history, physical examination, and ECG.

Note the increase in the size of the main pulmonary artery and its right and left branches. The right atrium and right ventricle are enlarged. The round structure located in the superior portion of the chest is caused by total anomalous pulmonary venous drainage. This gives the appearance of a "snowman."

The x-ray film is diagnostic of total anomalous pulmonary venous connection plus an ostium secundum atrial septal defect.

ELECTROCARDIOGRAM

The ECG shown here reveals right ventricular dominance, which may be normal for an 8-month-old infant.

DIFFERENTIAL DIAGNOSIS

The chest x-ray film is diagnostic of total anomalous pulmonary venous connection. No other condition produces the "snowman."

FINAL DIAGNOSIS

Total anomalous pulmonary venous connection plus an ostium secundum atrial septal defect. Further studies are needed to delineate the exact venous connection.

Pulmonary congestion may develop because pulmonary venous obstruction may occur in patients with this condition. Cyanosis may develop because pulmonary arteriolar resistance may increase or because obstruction of the pulmonary veins may produce a right-to-left-shunt.

The anomalous veins may enter the right atrium, the left innominate vein, the coronary sinus, the superior vena cava, the azygos vein, portal vein, or gastric vein.

DIAGNOSTIC PRINCIPLES

A "snowman" type shadow in the chest x-ray film suggests the presence of total anomalous pulmonary venous connection plus an ostium secundum atrial septal defect.

BIBLIOGRAPHY

Nugent EW, Plauth WH, Edwards JE, Williams WH: The pathology, pathophysiology, recognition, and treatment of congenital heart disease. In Schlant RC, Alexander RW, editors: *Hurst's the heart*, ed 8, New York, 1994, McGraw-Hill, pp 1804-1806.

HISTORY

The patient is a 68-year-old man who complains that he has had increasing dyspnea on effort and orthopnea for 2 weeks. He has also noted slight swelling of the lower portion of his legs. He denies chest discomfort.

He gives no history of rheumatic fever. In fact, he had been quite well all his life except for a laminectomy performed for a painful herniated intervertebral disk.

PHYSICAL EXAMINATION

The systolic blood pressure is 170 mm Hg, and the diastolic blood pressure is 50 mm Hg.

The carotid pulse is abnormal (see diagram on the right).

The apical impulse is hyperdynamic and larger than normal. It is located in the fifth intercostal space in the anterior axillary line (see diagram below).

There are no cardiac murmurs. A left ventricular (LV) gallop sound is heard.

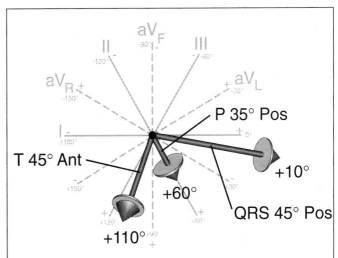

I, 2, First, second heart sounds. See figure credits.

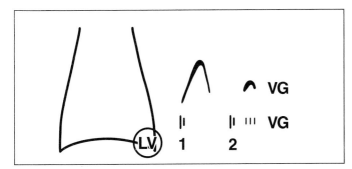

LV, Left ventricle; *VG*, ventricular gallop. See figure credits.

CHEST X-RAY FILM

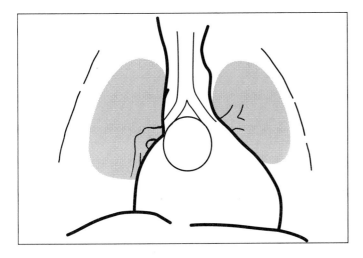

WHAT IS DIFFERENTIAL DIAGNOSIS?

WHAT LOW-TECHNOLOGY PROCEDURE WOULD YOU PERFORM?

WHAT IS FINAL DIAGNOSIS?

ELECTROCARDIOGRAM

The rhythm is normal. There are 92 depolarizations per minute. The PR interval is 0.16 second. The QRS duration is 0.10 second. The QT interval is 0.34 second. The total 12-lead QRS amplitude is 200 mm.

155

HISTORY

The history indicates the presence of severe heart failure. The cause must be determined.

PHYSICAL EXAMINATION

The wide pulse pressure is abnormal and should prompt a careful search for aortic valve regurgitation, but none is found. The carotid pulse reveals a pulsus bisferiens, and the apical impulse reveals a large hyperdynamic left ventricle. An LV gallop sound is present, which indicates LV dysfunction.

These abnormalities could be caused by severe anemia, thyrotoxicosis, a peripheral arteriovenous (AV) fistula, and possibly idiopathic hypertrophic subaortic stenosis (IHSS), although cardiac murmurs and atrial gallop sounds are often heard in patients with IHSS.

CHEST X-RAY FILM

There is evidence of heart failure and a large heart. All chambers appear to be enlarged. No valvular calcification can be seen. The abnormalities should stimulate the observer to look for a cause of generalized cardiac enlargement, including dilated cardiomyopathy, or chronic circulatory overload. Aortic root dilatation is absent, which is a point against chronic aortic valve regurgitation.

See Patient 1 for a normal chest x-ray film.

ELECTROCARDIOGRAM

Sinus tachycardia is present. The PR interval, QRS duration, and QT interval are normal. The mean P vector reveals a left atrial abnormality. The mean QRS vector is larger than normal. It is directed at +10 degrees in the frontal plane and 45 degrees posteriorly. The mean T vector is directed at +110 degrees in the frontal plane and 45 degrees anteriorly.

The electrocardiographic abnormalities suggest LV preponderance.

Dilated cardiomyopathy, secondary to many conditions including ischemic cardiomyopathy, could cause the ECG abnormalities. Aortic stenosis, aortic or mitral valve regurgitation, and hypertension could also cause the abnormalities. Remotely, patent ductus arteriosus or interventricular septal defect could produce the abnormalities. Severe anemia, thyrotoxicosis, or peripheral AV fistula could be responsible for the abnormalities.

See Patient 1 for a normal ECG.

DIFFERENTIAL DIAGNOSIS

• Aortic valve regurgitation as a cause of the hyperdynamic circulation is ruled out because there is no murmur. In fact, valvular heart disease and congenital heart disease, including patent ductus arteriosus or interventricular septal defect, are excluded because no murmurs are present.
• Dilated cardiomyopathy is possible, but the hyperdynamic circulation rules against it.
• The hyperdynamic circulation could be caused by anemia, thyrotoxicosis, or an AV fistula. There are no other clues to thyrotoxicosis, and the mucous membranes appear normal.

LOW-TECHNOLOGY PROCEDURE

Place the stethoscope on the laminectomy scar. You will hear a continuous murmur there. The patient has an acquired peripheral AV fistula.

FINAL DIAGNOSIS

Peripheral AV fistula, which is producing severe heart failure.

DIAGNOSTIC PRINCIPLE

When there is a hyperdynamic circulation, a large heart, and heart failure and when no cardiac murmurs are heard, it is wise to look for the continuous murmur of a peripheral AV fistula.

"So, don't look so very far until you listen over every scar."

A pulsus bisferiens can be produced by aortic valve regurgitation or IHSS or may accompany a hyperdynamic circulation, such as occurs with peripheral AV fistula.

BIBLIOGRAPHY

Fowler NO: High-cardiac output states. In Schlant RC, Alexander RW, editors: *Hurst's the heart*, ed 8, New York, 1994, McGraw-Hill, pp 508-509.

FIGURE CREDITS

Upper, reproduced with permission, and *lower*, modified and reproduced with permission from Hurst JW: The examination of the heart: the importance of initial screening, *Dis Mon* 36(5):278 (upper), 282 (lower), 1990.

HISTORY

The patient is a 23-year-old man without complaints. He states that he has always had a very slow heart rate and a heart murmur. He is being examined because he wishes to procure a $100,000 life insurance policy.

PHYSICAL EXAMINATION

The systolic blood pressure is 160 mm Hg, and the diastolic blood pressure is 75 mm Hg.

The pulse rate is 60 beats per minute.

A cannon wave is observed in the neck veins, and a cannon sound is heard at the cardiac apex.

A grade 3 systolic murmur is heard in the third left intercostal space adjacent to the sternum.

CHEST X-RAY FILM

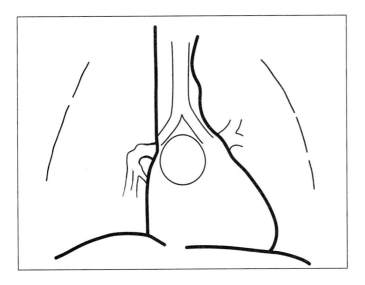

ELECTROCARDIOGRAM

There is complete heart block. The atrial rate is 70 depolarizations per minute, and the ventricular rate is 60 depolarizations per minute. The QRS duration is 0.09 second. The QT interval is 0.40 second. The 12-lead total QRS amplitude is 190 mm.

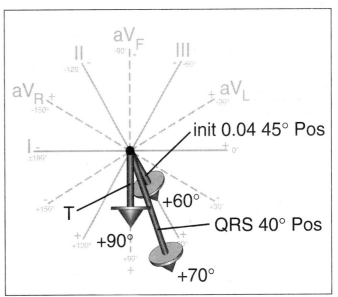

WHAT IS DIFFERENTIAL DIAGNOSIS?

WHAT IS FINAL DIAGNOSIS?

HISTORY

The patient could have congenital complete heart block. The murmur could be produced by an interventricular septal defect. One should not speculate further with the data presented in the history.

PHYSICAL EXAMINATION

The pulse rate is 60 beats per minute. The wide pulse pressure is caused by a higher-than-normal systolic pressure and normal diastolic pressure. This suggests that the wide pulse pressure is not caused by aortic valve regurgitation but is related to a greater-than-normal cardiac stroke output associated with bradycardia.

The cannon wave noted in the internal jugular venous pulse appears when the right atrium contracts against a closed tricuspid valve, which occurs throughout ventricular systole. This is diagnostic of complete atrioventricular (A-V) block.

The heart sounds are abnormal because about twice each minute the first sound is louder than it is with the remainder of the beats. The loud first sound occurs when the atrium contracts immediately before the ventricle contracts. This is called a *cannon sound* and occurs several times each minute when there is complete A-V block.

The murmur indicates the presence of an interventricular septal defect.

CHEST X-RAY FILM

The pulmonary blood flow is normal.

One might suspect that something is wrong with the aorta; it is either larger than normal or displaced a little to the right. The left ventricle may be larger than normal, and the rounded apex suggests the shape of the right ventricle may be abnormal.

See Patient 1 for a normal chest x-ray film.

ELECTROCARDIOGRAM

Complete A-V block is present. The QRS duration is normal, indicating that the ventricular focus is located in the upper part of the muscular portion of the interventricular septum.

The initial 0.04-second vector is directed more posteriorly than normal, and the 12-lead total QRS amplitude is larger than usual. The initial 0.04-second vector is abnormal and could indicate anterior myocardial infarction. This patient's young age is against this possibility and indicates some type of congenital heart disease.

The increased 12-lead total QRS amplitude suggests left ventricular hypertrophy.

See Patient 1 for a normal ECG.

DIFFERENTIAL DIAGNOSIS

The complete A-V block, murmur suggesting interventricular septal defect, aorta shifted to the right, and ECG abnormalities are diagnostic of congenitally corrected transposition of the great arteries with an interventricular septal defect. The heart rate is not 60-70 beats per minute because the ventricular impulse originates high in the ventricular septum.

FINAL DIAGNOSIS

Congenitally corrected transposition of the great arteries with interventricular septal defect.

DIAGNOSTIC PRINCIPLE

This interesting and unusual type of congenital heart disease should be considered in every young patient with complete A-V heart block. This condition occurs when the anatomic left ventricle and aorta delivers blood to the periphery but the left ventricle has the morphology of the right ventricle, and when the pulmonary artery and anatomic right ventricle delivers blood to the lungs but the right ventricle has the morphology of the left ventricle. The mitral valve remains with the left ventricle, and the tricuspid valve remains with the right ventricle. Such patients typically have an interventricular septal defect and complete A-V block.

This is another example of an ECG abnormality that may be misinterpreted as being caused by myocardial infarction.

BIBLIOGRAPHY

Nugent EW, Plauth WH, Edwards JE, Williams WH: The pathology, pathophysiology, recognition, and treatment of congenital heart disease. In Schlant RC, Alexander RW, editors: *Hurst's the heart*, ed 8, New York, 1994, McGraw-Hill, pp 1813-1815.

HISTORY

The patient, a 36-year-old female, is complaining of increasing dyspnea on effort and episodes of palpitation.

PHYSICAL EXAMINATION

Withheld for now; see **Discussion and Answers**, *Heart Sounds and Murmurs*, for related questions.

CHEST X-RAY FILM

ELECTROCARDIOGRAM

Atrial fibrillation is present, with a ventricular rate of 120 depolarizations per minute. The QRS duration is 0.09 second. The QT interval is 0.34 second. The 12-lead QRS amplitude is 158 mm.

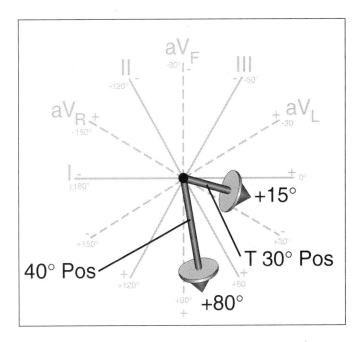

WHAT IS DIFFERENTIAL DIAGNOSIS?

DIAGRAM HEART SOUNDS AND MURMURS

WHAT IS FINAL DIAGNOSIS?

HISTORY

Whenever a young adult female complains of dyspnea on effort and palpitation, it is wise to consider the diagnosis of mitral stenosis caused by rheumatic heart disease, mitral valve prolapse with severe mitral valve regurgitation, or an ostium secundum atrial septal defect or primary pulmonary hypertension.

PHYSICAL EXAMINATION

See *Heart Sounds and Murmurs* below.

CHEST X-RAY FILM

The diagram illustrates several clues to the diagnosis of mitral stenosis. Note the four "bumps" along the left heart border. They are, from above downward, the aortic knob, the larger-than-normal pulmonary artery, the left atrial (LA) appendage, and the border of the left ventricle. Also note the larger-than-normal pulmonary arteries and the quickly tapering right pulmonary artery, which suggests pulmonary artery hypertension. The left atrium is enlarged; note the horizontal position of the left bronchus. The size of the right ventricle cannot be determined in the postero-anterior view.

The superior veins are prominent, indicating elevation of the LA pressure.

These abnormalities indicate the presence of mitral stenosis with pulmonary hypertension.

See Patient 1 for a normal chest x-ray film.

See Fig. 3-4.

ELECTROCARDIOGRAM

The ECG shows atrial fibrillation, a vertical mean QRS vector that is directed slightly posteriorly, and a mean T vector that is directed at +15 degrees and posteriorly away from the right ventricle. These abnormalities should lead one to suspect the presence of mitral stenosis.

See Patient 1 for a normal ECG.

See Fig. 4-51 for an ECG showing normal rhythm and other clues to the diagnosis of mitral stenosis.

DIFFERENTIAL DIAGNOSIS

The constellation of clues just discussed supports the diagnosis of mitral valve blockade. The most common cause for such a condition is *rheumatic mitral stenosis*. In very young persons, it could be caused by congenital mitral stenosis. *Ergot toxicity* can cause mitral stenosis. A *left atrial myxoma* can also cause mitral valve blockade. A tumor plop can imitate an opening snap of mitral stenosis, but the first heart sound is not unusually loud as it is with mitral stenosis.

HEART SOUNDS AND MURMURS

The heart sounds heard in the second right and left intercostal spaces adjacent to the sternum might sound as illustrated in the following diagram. The heart sounds and murmurs heard at the cardiac apex are also illustrated in the following diagram.

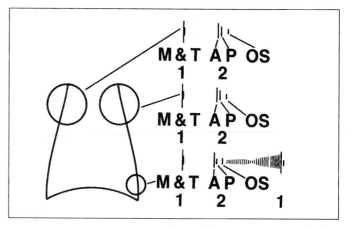

Opening snap (OS), as well as other auscultatory features, of mitral stenosis. *Upper diagram*, Note the abnormally loud mitral (M) component of the first heart sound when one is listening in the second right intercostal space. It is louder than the second sound. The pulmonary valve closure sound (P) may be heard. OS of the mitral valve is also heard in this area. *Middle diagram*, The first heart sound is louder than normal, and an OS is heard when one is listening in the second left intercostal space. The P is often heard. *Lower diagram*, The first sound is loud. An OS is heard. A low-pitched, rumbling murmur of mitral stenosis also is heard. Note that the diastolic rumble of mitral stenosis is heard only at the cardiac apex, whereas the loud first sound and OS are widely transmitted. T, Tricuspid; A, aortic valve closure. See figure credits.

FINAL DIAGNOSIS

Rheumatic heart disease with mitral stenosis, pulmonary artery hypertension, and atrial fibrillation.

DIAGNOSTIC PRINCIPLE

Mitral stenosis can be recognized by hearing the abnormal heart sounds and murmurs, identifying the abnormalities in the chest x-ray film, and identifying the characteristic abnormalities on the ECG, including an LA abnormality when there is normal rhythm. Whenever the first heart sound is equal to or louder than the second sound in intensity in the second right intercostal space near the sternum, the physician should consider mitral stenosis.

The enlarged and visible LA appendage is usually caused by rheumatic mitral valve stenosis or rheumatic mitral regurgitation. It is rarely, if ever, seen with nonrheumatic mitral valve disease.

One must always consider the likelihood of an LA tumor as a cause for the mitral valve blockade. An echocardiogram may be needed to differentiate between the two conditions.

BIBLIOGRAPHY

Gaasch WH, O'Rourke RA, Cohn LH, Rackley CE: Mitral valve disease. In Schlant RC, Alexander RW, editors: *Hurst's the heart,* ed 8, New York, 1994, McGraw-Hill, pp 1483-1491.
Hall RJ, Cooley DA, McAllister HA, Frazier OH: Neoplastic heart disease. In Schlant RC, Alexander RW, editors: *Hurst's the heart,* ed 8, New York, 1994, McGraw-Hill, pp 2010-2012.

FIGURE CREDIT

Reproduced with permission from Hurst JW: The examination of the heart: the importance of initial screening, *Dis Mon* 36(5):284, 1990.

HISTORY

The patient is a 38-year-old woman who is complaining of episodes of severe palpitation, during which she almost faints. She has experienced the episodes for many years, but they have become more frequent and last longer. The usual episode lasts about 45 minutes.

An ECG made on arrival in the emergency clinic during a previous episode revealed an irregular, wide QRS complex rhythm with a ventricular rate of 220 depolarizations per minute. The rhythm spontaneously reverted to normal 10 minutes later.

PHYSICAL EXAMINATION

The physical examination is normal. The heart rhythm is regular, and the heart rate is 86 beats per minute.

CHEST X-RAY FILM

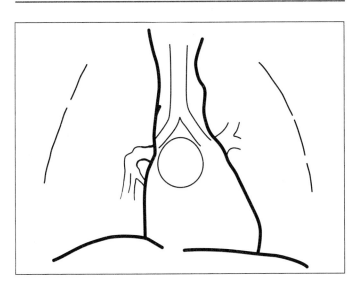

ELECTROCARDIOGRAM

Normal sinus rhythm is present. There are 86 depolarizations per minute. The PR interval is 0.12 second. The QRS duration is 0.14 second. The initial portion of the QRS complex is slurred. The 12-lead QRS amplitude is 170 mm.

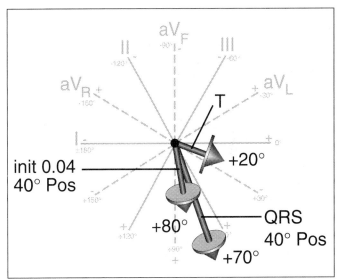

WHAT IS DIFFERENTIAL DIAGNOSIS?

WHAT IS FINAL DIAGNOSIS?

HISTORY

The patient has episodes of atrial fibrillation. Whenever this is known to occur, the physician should search for mitral stenosis, mitral valve regurgitation, atherosclerotic coronary heart disease, apathetic thyrotoxicosis, sick-sinus syndrome, any severe heart disease, atrial septal defect, tricuspid atresia, Ebstein anomaly, Wolff-Parkinson-White syndrome, and lone atrial fibrillation.

PHYSICAL EXAMINATION

The normal physical examination excludes all the conditions just listed except sick-sinus syndrome, coronary disease, apathetic thyrotoxicosis, Wolff-Parkinson-White syndrome, and lone atrial fibrillation.

CHEST X-RAY FILM

The chest x-ray film is normal. This excludes all the conditions listed in **History** except apathetic thyrotoxicosis, sick-sinus syndrome, coronary disease, Wolff-Parkinson-White syndrome, and lone atrial fibrillation.

See Patient 1 for a normal chest x-ray film.

ELECTROCARDIOGRAM

The ECG shows preexcitation of the ventricles. The short PR interval, slurred initial portion of the QRS complex (called a delta wave), and wide QRS complexes are characteristic of ventricular preexcitation and leads one to diagnose Wolff-Parkinson-White syndrome. The initial 0.04 second of the QRS complex, when viewed as a vector, can create abnormal Q waves that may lead unwary physicians (and many computers) to misdiagnose myocardial infarction.

The ECG made in the emergency clinic showed atrial fibrillation with a ventricular rate of 220 depolarizations per minute. Such a rapid ventricular rate in patients with atrial fibrillation implies that there is a bypass tract around the atrioventricular node.

See Patient 1 for a normal ECG.

See Fig. 4-78.

DIFFERENTIAL DIAGNOSIS

The normal physical examination excludes valvular heart disease, tricuspid atresia, Ebstein anomaly, and atrial septal defect.

It would be unlikely for the sick-sinus syndrome or coronary disease to be present for many years before the age of 38 in a woman.

Thyrotoxicosis should always be considered in a patient with atrial fibrillation, but the ventricular rate of 220 depolarizations per minute is faster than it usually is in patients with thyrotoxicosis.

Lone atrial fibrillation is excluded by the ECG abnormalities.

The ECG abnormalities are diagnostic of the Wolff-Parkinson-White syndrome.

FINAL DIAGNOSIS

Wolff-Parkinson-White syndrome with atrial fibrillation.

DIAGNOSTIC PRINCIPLE

First, when atrial fibrillation occurs with a ventricular rate of 220 (or more) depolarizations per minute, one should consider the possibility of preexcitation of the ventricles via a bypass tract.

Second, remember that when preexcitation of the ventricles occurs, there may be abnormal Q waves that can, and often are, mistaken as being caused by myocardial infarction.

Third, whenever preexcitation of the ventricles is diagnosed, the physician should search for clues to the presence of Ebstein anomaly, idiopathic hypertrophic suboartic stenosis, and ostium secundum atrial septal defect because the condition can occur with these anomalies. Most often, however, the anomaly occurs as an isolated condition. It does not, however, prevent additional coronary disease or dilated cardiomyopathy from occurring. This is emphasized because further diagnostic thinking often ceases once preexcitation of the ventricles is identified.

BIBLIOGRAPHY

Myerburg RJ, Kessler KM, Castellanos A: Recognition, clinical assessment, and management of arrhythmias and conduction disturbances. In Schlant RC, Alexander RW, editors: *Hurst's the heart*, ed 8, New York, 1994, McGraw-Hill, pp 717-720.

PUZZLE 33

The smart medical resident, who was also a marathon runner, asked me to take the following test. He planned to give the test to the house staff and wanted to know if the electrocardiograms were good examples of the abnormalities he wanted to discuss.

NO. 1

Heart rate: 70 depolarizations per minute

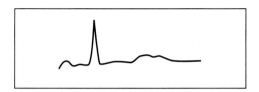

NO. 2

Heart rate: 70 depolarizations per minute

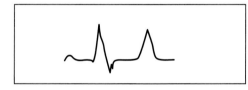

NO. 3

Heart rate: 70 depolarizations per minute

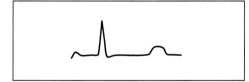

NO. 4

Heart rate: 40 depolarizations per minute

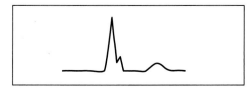

NO. 5

Heart rate: 70 depolarizations per minute

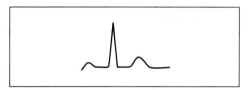

NO. 6

Heart rate: 50 depolarizations per minute; 12-lead QRS amplitude: 190 mm

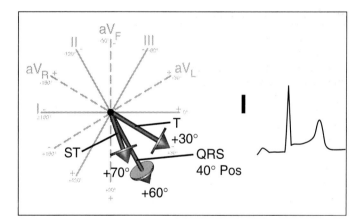

NO. 7

Heart rate: 75 depolarizations per minute

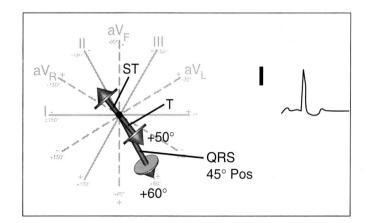

NO. 1

This ECG is typical of hypokalemia. The apparent long QT interval is created because the U wave (see second hump) joins the low-amplitude T wave.

This patient has essential hypertension and is receiving hydrochlorothiazide.

NO. 2

This ECG is characteristic of hyperkalemia. The QRS duration is slightly increased (any type of QRS conduction disturbance can occur). The T wave is large and tent shaped, and the ascending limb is similar to the descending limb.

This patient has hyperkalemia secondary to renal failure from lupus erythematous.

NO. 3

The long QT interval is caused by a long ST segment, which is characteristic of hypocalcemia.

This patient has hypoparathyroidism.

NO. 4

The notch and bump on the descending limb of the QRS complex is an Osborn wave.

This homeless patient almost froze to death.

The Osborn wave is related to hypothermia but may rarely be seen under other circumstances.

NO. 5

This ECG shows a short QT interval, and the ST segment is short. This may occur normally but may result from hypercalcemia.

This patient has hyperparathyroidism caused by adenoma of the parathyroid gland.

NO. 6

There are 50 depolarizations per minute. The mean QRS vector is larger than normal because the total 12-lead QRS amplitude is 190 mm. The mean ST vector is relatively parallel with the mean QRS vector, which is directed normally. The mean T vector is large and is only a few degrees away from the mean QRS vector. The ascending limb of the T wave ascends gradually, whereas the descending limb of the T wave descends rapidly.

The ST segment vector and large T wave suggest early repolarization, which can occur normally.

The abnormally large QRS amplitude suggests left ventricular hypertrophy.

The slow heart rate and increase in QRS amplitude, plus the signs of early repolarization, can occur in athletes without other evidence of heart disease.

The tracing was made on a resident, who, please remember, was a marathon runner.

NO. 7

The QT interval is 0.28 second. The mean QRS vector is directed normally. The mean ST segment vector is directed opposite to the mean T vector. The short mean T vector is almost parallel with the mean QRS vector.

These abnormalities are characteristic of digitalis effect. Digitalis does not alter the size or direction of the mean QRS vector unless it produces ventricular dysrhythmia. The mean T vector becomes shorter (and may disappear) as a result of digitalis, but the direction of the mean T vector does not change as long as the wave can be seen. The new vector, the vector representing the ST segment displacement, results from extremely early repolarization forces; it is directed opposite to the terminal mean T vector.

This patient has a normal heart but experiences episodes of supraventricular tachycardia. She is taking digoxin in an effort to prevent the episodes.

HISTORY

The patient, a 22-year-old man, has no symptoms and is applying for a life insurance policy.

PHYSICAL EXAMINATION

The systolic blood pressure is 115 mm Hg, and the diastolic blood pressure is 60 mm Hg.

The femoral pulsations are graded as 4. The heart rate is 82 beats per minute. Auscultation of the heart reveals the murmur depicted in the diagram shown on the right.

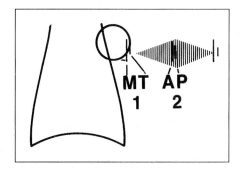

1, 2, First, second heart sounds; *M,* mitral, *T,* tricuspid, *P,* pulmonary, and *A,* aortic valve closure sounds. See figure credits.

CHEST X-RAY FILM

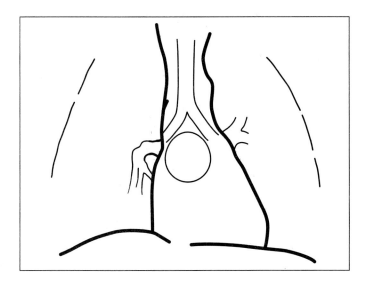

ELECTROCARDIOGRAM

The heart rhythm is normal. There are 78 depolarizations per minute. The PR interval is 0.14 second. The QRS duration is 0.08 second. The QT interval is 0.32 second.

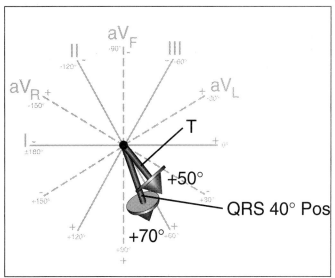

WHAT IS DIFFERENTIAL DIAGNOSIS?

WHAT IS FINAL DIAGNOSIS?

HISTORY

This 22-year-old asymptomatic man could have a normal heart. He might have coarctation of the aorta, a bicuspid aortic valve, mitral valve prolapse, an ostium secundum atrial septal defect, a small ventricular septal defect, or a patent ductus arteriosus.

PHYSICAL EXAMINATION

The absence of hypertension and the prominent femoral pulsation exclude coarctation of the aorta.

The murmur is continuous. Note how it builds up in systole, encompasses the second heart sound, and continues into diastole. This type of murmur, heard in the second intercostal space near the sternum, is characteristic of patent ductus arteriosus. No other murmurs or abnormal heart sounds are heard, which excludes ostium secundum atrial septal defect, aortic valve stenosis (bicuspid valve), a ventricular septal defect, or mitral valve prolapse.

CHEST X-RAY FILM

The x-ray film is normal.

The heart could be normal. Rib notching from coarctation of the aorta is not seen.

A bicuspid aortic valve with mild stenosis (or regurgitation) could be present, as could a small interventricular septal defect, patent ductus arteriosus, or slight mitral valve prolapse.

See Patient 1 for a normal chest x-ray film.

ELECTROCARDIOGRAM

The ECG is normal.

The heart could be normal. The 22-year-old patient could have coarctation of the aorta, a bicuspid aortic valve, mitral valve prolapse, patent ductus arteriosus, or a small interventricular septal defect.

See Patient 1 for a normal ECG.

DIFFERENTIAL DIAGNOSIS

The murmur is characteristic of a patent ductus arteriosus.

The continuous murmur produced by an aortic-pulmonary artery window, a coronary arteriovenous fistula, or a rupture of the sinus of Valsalva is almost never heard in this area of the chest.

A normal venous hum can occasionally be heard in this location. Such a murmur is commonly heard in children but is uncommon in adults.

FINAL DIAGNOSIS

Patent ductus arteriosus.

DIAGNOSTIC PRINCIPLE

Patent ductus arteriosus with a left-to-right shunt and normal pulmonary artery pressure produces a continuous murmur that is heard best just beneath the middle of the left clavicle. Should pulmonary arteriolar disease develop, the pulmonary artery pressure becomes elevated, and the shunt may become right-to-left. Should this occur the toes will be more cyanotic than the fingers, and the continuous murmur may disappear.

A small patent ductus arteriosus may not produce an abnormal chest x-ray film or abnormal ECG.

A continuous murmur may be due to the rupture of the sinus of Valsalva, coronary arteriovenous fistula, or aortopulmonary window. Murmurs due to these causes are not heard just beneath the middle of the left clavicle and should not be confused with the murmur of patent ductus arteriosus.

BIBLIOGRAPHY

Nugent EW, Plauth WH, Edwards JE, Williams WH: The pathology, pathophysiology, recognition, and treatment of congenital heart disease. In Schlant RC, Alexander RW, editors: *Hurst's the heart*, ed 8, New York, 1994, McGraw-Hill, pp 1781-1784.

FIGURE CREDIT

Reproduced with permission from Hurst JW: The examination of the heart: the importance of initial screening, *Dis Mon* 36(5):286, 1990.

HISTORY

The patient is a 44-year-old man. He is complaining of weakness, constant mild retrosternal chest tightness, and slight dyspnea. The chest pain began 3 hours before he came to the emergency clinic.

PHYSICAL EXAMINATION

The heart rhythm is regular. The heart rate is 92 beats per minute.

The systolic blood pressure is 120 mm Hg, and the diastolic blood pressure is 72 mm Hg.

The physical examination is normal.

CHEST X-RAY FILM

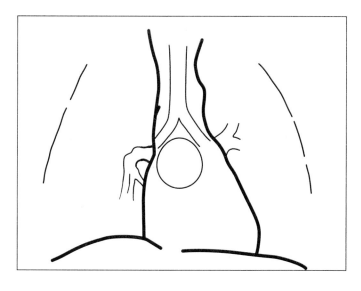

ELECTROCARDIOGRAM

The rhythm is normal. There are 88 depolarizations per minute. The PR interval is 0.18 second. The QRS duration is 0.10 second. The QT interval is 0.36 second. The 12-lead QRS amplitude is 155 mm.

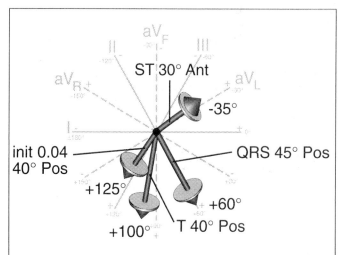

WHAT IS DIFFERENTIAL DIAGNOSIS?

WHAT IS FINAL DIAGNOSIS?

HISTORY

The history is typical of myocardial infarction (MI). The usual cause of MI is coronary atherosclerotic heart disease, but there are other causes of abrupt obstruction to coronary artery blood flow.

Dissection of the aorta could cause the chest discomfort, but this disease usually produces severe chest and upper back pain.

The chest discomfort is not characteristic of the pain associated with pericarditis, which is usually aggravated by inspiration.

PHYSICAL EXAMINATION

The blood pressure, heart rhythm, neck veins, arterial pulsations, precordial movements, and auscultation of the heart are normal.

One can conclude that valvular heart disease, hypertensive heart disease, and cardiomyopathy are not present and that dissection of the aorta and acute pericarditis are not present.

Based on the results of the physical examination, the patient could have no heart disease or coronary atherosclerotic heart disease.

CHEST X-RAY FILM

The x-ray film is normal. Based on this finding alone, the heart could be normal or the patient could have coronary atherosclerotic heart disease, mild valvular heart disease, mild hypertension, hypertrophic cardiomyopathy, restrictive cardiomyopathy, pericarditis, or cardiac dysrhythmias.

There are no signs of dissection of the aorta.

See Patient 1 for a normal chest x-ray film.

ELECTROCARDIOGRAM

The heart rhythm and rate are normal.

The direction and amplitude of the mean QRS vector are normal. The mean initial 0.04-second QRS vector is directed inferiorly and posteriorly (away from an anterior dead zone); it is directed posterior to the mean QRS vector. This indicates an anterior myocardial dead zone.

The mean ST vector is directed anteriorly and laterally. It is caused by epicardial myocardial injury of the anterior portion of the myocardium.

The mean T vector is directed inferiorly to the right and posteriorly. It is caused by epicardial ischemia of the anterolateral portion of the myocardium.

The abnormal initial 0.04-second QRS vector (making abnormal Q waves), abnormal ST segment vector, and abnormal T vector indicate the presence of an anterolateral MI.

See Patient 1 for a normal ECG.

See Fig. 4-70.

DIFFERENTIAL DIAGNOSIS

The diagnosis is acute anterior MI, which is most likely caused by coronary atherosclerotic heart disease.

The mild pain, normal peripheral arterial pulsations, and normal chest x-ray film of the heart and aorta make dissection of the aorta unlikely.

Acute pericarditis can be ruled out: the chest pain is not consistent with pericarditis, there is no pericardial friction rub, and the ECG is diagnostic of MI.

FINAL DIAGNOSIS

Anterolateral MI caused by coronary atherosclerotic heart disease.

DIAGNOSTIC PRINCIPLE

The history of retrosternal tightness and ECG signs of MI make it possible to diagnose MI. Because these abnormalities are often the *only* clues discovered initially, each of us must become highly skilled at recognizing them. Failure to do so can lead to inadequate use of thrombolytic therapy.

BIBLIOGRAPHY

Hurst JW: *Cardiovascular diagnosis: the initial examination of the heart*, St Louis, 1993, Mosby, pp 353-371.

HISTORY

The patient, a 5-year-old asymptomatic boy, is being seen by the physician before going to summer camp.

PHYSICAL EXAMINATION

The systolic blood pressure is 115 mm Hg, and the diastolic blood pressure is 70 mm Hg. The femoral artery pulsation is normal.

There is a continuous murmur heard in the neck when the patient is sitting. The murmur disappears when he is lying down. The first and second heart sounds are normal. A third sound is heard in early diastole at the apex. A faint (Grade 1) systolic murmur is heard in the second left intercostal space near the sternum.

CHEST X-RAY FILM

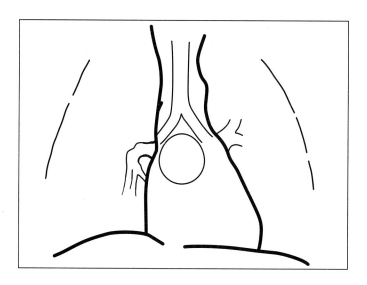

ELECTROCARDIOGRAM

Sinus tachycardia is present. There are 105 depolarizations per minute. The PR interval is 0.14 second. The QRS duration is 0.06 second. The QT interval is 0.32 second.

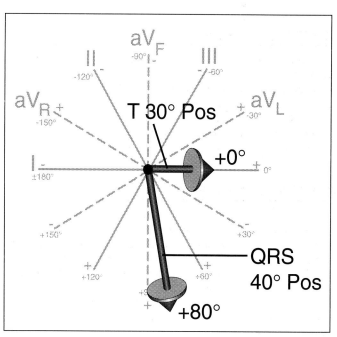

WHAT IS FINAL DIAGNOSIS?

HISTORY

The patient is an asymptomatic boy. The heart could be normal, or he could have a bicuspid aortic valve, an ostium secundum atrial septal defect, a small interventricular septal defect, a patent ductus arteriosus, coarctation of the aorta, or mitral valve prolapse.

PHYSICAL EXAMINATION

The continuous murmur in the neck heard when the patient is sitting but not heard when he is lying down is caused by the rapid flow of blood in the cervical veins. It is called a *venous hum*. It is a normal finding in children.

The faint systolic murmur heard in the second left intercostal space near the sternum is a normal finding in children.

A third heart sound heard in early diastole at the cardiac apex is normal in children.

The normal blood pressure with normal femoral artery pulsation excludes coarctation of the aorta.

The absence of other murmurs excludes other types of congenital heart disease. Occasionally, a young patient may have a bicuspid aortic valve that does not produce a significant murmur.

CHEST X-RAY FILM

The x-ray film is normal.

The heart itself could be normal. The absence of rib notching does not exclude coarctation of the aorta because rib notching may not occur in patients until they are 10 to 12 years of age. A normal chest film could be seen in patients with a bicuspid aortic valve, small interventricular septal defect, or small patent ductus arteriosus.

ELECTROCARDIOGRAM

The ECG is normal. The vertical and slightly posterior direction of the mean QRS vector is normal. Remember that the mean QRS vector in the newborn is directed to the right and anteriorly; it gradually shifts to the vertical position, then to the leftward and posterior position as the child grows older. The mean QRS vector attains the normal adult position by about age 16. The mean T vector is directed to the left and posteriorly; this, as well as the QRS-T angle of 80 degrees, is normal for a 5-year-old boy. The mean T vector does not attain its adult position until about age 16.

See Fig. 4-8.

FINAL DIAGNOSIS

Normal venous hum in the neck. This finding must not be confused with a patent ductus arteriosus, even when it is heard below the left clavicle.

DIAGNOSTIC PRINCIPLE

A continuous murmur may be heard in the neck of normal children. The murmur is heard when the child is sitting. It disappears with pressure on the neck veins or when the child lies down.

Be careful: just because you hear a normal venous hum in a patient does not exclude heart disease. There could also be a separate continuous murmur caused by a patent ductus arteriosus in the same patient.

BIBLIOGRAPHY

Hurst JW: *Cardiovascular diagnosis: the initial examination of the heart*, St Louis, 1993, Mosby, pp 182, 183.

HISTORY

The patient, a 2-year-old boy, has not gained weight. The parents state they have detected slight cyanosis and an increase in respiratory rate.

PHYSICAL EXAMINATION

The patient is slightly cyanotic.

The femoral arterial pulses are bounding.

A systolic anterior movement of the sternal area is detected, and the apical impulse is displaced laterally.

Only one component of the second heart sound can be heard. A systolic click is noted near the cardiac apex, and a high-pitched diastolic murmur is heard along the sternal border. A systolic murmur is heard near the center of the sternum, and a continuous murmur is heard in the back.

CHEST X-RAY FILM

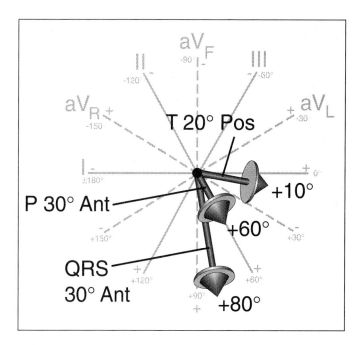

ELECTROCARDIOGRAM

Sinus tachycardia is present. There are 125 beats per minute. The PR interval is 0.14 second. The QRS duration is 0.07 second. The QRS complexes are larger than normal.

WHAT IS DIFFERENTIAL DIAGNOSIS?

WHAT IS FINAL DIAGNOSIS?

HISTORY

The history of cyanosis and difficulty breathing leads one to consider a right-to-left intracardiac shunt such as tetralogy of Fallot, transposition of the great arteries, tricuspid atresia, and truncus arteriosus.

PHYSICAL EXAMINATION

The single second heart sound is an important clue and leads one to consider truncus arteriosus, although the pulmonary valve closure sound may be difficult to hear when there is tetralogy of Fallot or tricuspid atresia.

The systolic click heard near the apex suggests a dilated aorta or a common trunk.

The systolic murmur is characteristic of an interventricular septal defect. The high-pitched diastolic murmur is caused by either aortic or truncal regurgitation. The continuous murmur heard in the back suggests torrential pulmonary blood flow. This excludes tetralogy of Fallot, tricuspid atresia, and transposition of the great arteries.

CHEST X-RAY FILM

The heart is enlarged; note the rounded contour of the left heart borders.

The "aortic arch" is on the right side. This always leads one to consider tetralogy of Fallot or truncus arteriosus.

Pulmonary blood flow is increased. This excludes tetralogy of Fallot, tricuspid atresia, and type 4 truncus arteriosus.

The large "aorta" or "trunk" rules out transposition of the great arteries.

The abnormalities suggest the presence of type 1, 2, or 3 truncus arteriosus.

ELECTROCARDIOGRAM

A right atrial abnormality is present.

Note that the mean QRS vector is large and directed +80 degrees in the frontal plane and 30 degrees anteriorly. This suggests left and right ventricular hypertrophy.

The abnormalities are not typical of those seen in tetralogy of Fallot, tricuspid atresia, or transposition of the great arteries. This tracing could be associated with type 1, 2, or 3 truncus arteriosus.

DIFFERENTIAL DIAGNOSIS

The slight cyanosis, a single second heart sound, a murmur suggesting interventricular septal defect, the continuous murmur heard in the back, the diastolic murmur heard along the left sternal border, the systolic click, a right-sided "aorta" or "trunk," increased pulmonary blood flow, and ECG evidence of right and left ventricular hypertrophy indicate the presence of type 1, 2, or 3 truncus arteriosus.

The increase in pulmonary blood flow and biventricular hypertrophy exclude tetralogy of Fallot or tricuspid atresia.

The broad "aorta" or "trunk" excludes transposition of the great arteries.

FINAL DIAGNOSIS

Type 1, 2, or 3 truncus arteriosus. The pulmonary arteries arise from the aorta in types 1, 2, and 3 truncus. Such patients may develop severe heart failure. Type 4 truncus is very different; there are no pulmonary arteries. Therefore, the patient is extremely cyanotic and succumbs from hypoxia.

DIAGNOSTIC PRINCIPLE

Once again, the study of the second heart sound is important. A major clue to the diagnosis of truncus arteriosus is the single second heart sound noted during inspiration. A split second sound excludes truncus arteriosus. The right-sided trunk and increase in pulmonary blood flow are also major clues to the diagnosis.

BIBLIOGRAPHY

Hurst JW, Nugent EW, Anderson RH, Wilcox BR: Congenital heart disease. In Hurst JW, editor-in-chief: *Atlas of the heart*, New York, 1988, Gower, pp 3.95-3.97.

HISTORY

The patient is a 64-year-old man who is having increasing dyspnea associated with effort. Ankylosing spondylitis has gradually developed over the last 20 years.

PHYSICAL EXAMINATION

Severe ankylosing spondylitis is obvious.

The heart rate is 50 beats per minute; it is regular.

The systolic blood pressure is 180 mm Hg, and the diastolic blood pressure is 50 mm Hg.

The first heart sound varies in intensity during the period of auscultation.

The jugular venous pulsation is shown in the following diagram.

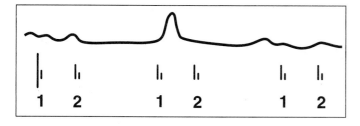

1, 2, First, second heart sounds. See figure credits.

The apical impulse is larger than normal and displaced to the left (see diagram).

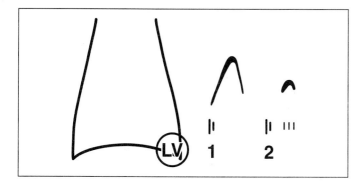

LV, Left ventricle. See figure credits.

The heart sounds and murmurs are illustrated in the following diagram.

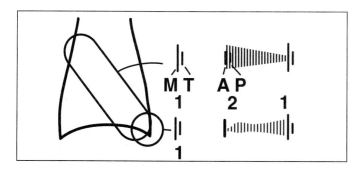

M, Mitral, *T,* tricuspid, *A,* aortic, and *P,* pulmonary valve closure sounds. See figure credits.

CHEST X-RAY FILM

The chest film reveals ankylosing spondylitis and mild pulmonary congestion. The early portion of the aorta appears to be larger than normal, but the bony abnormality makes interpretation of the cardiac silhouette difficult. The left ventricle appears to be enlarged.

Pulmonary congestion is present.

ELECTROCARDIOGRAM

Complete heart block is present. The atrial rate is 84 depolarizations per minute, and the ventricular rate is 40 depolarizations per minute. The QRS duration is 0.10 second. The QT interval is 0.38 second. The 12-lead QRS amplitude is 200 mm.

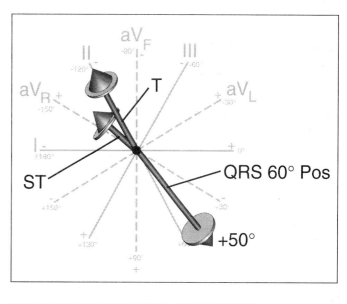

WHAT IS DIFFERENTIAL DIAGNOSIS?

WHAT IS FINAL DIAGNOSIS?

HISTORY

The history of ankylosing spondylitis should lead the physician to consider the complications of this condition, which include aortic valve regurgitation, complete heart block, and heart failure.

Also, this patient serves to emphasize that at times the physician cannot avoid performing a physical examination while he or she is taking the history.

PHYSICAL EXAMINATION

Ankylosing spondylitis is obvious. The wide pulse pressure with diastolic blood pressure of 50 mm Hg should prompt one to consider aortic valve regurgitation.

Cannon waves are seen in the neck veins when the right atrium contracts against a closed tricuspid valve that occurs during ventricular systole (upper figure). When cannon waves are seen in a patient with an abnormally slow and regular heart rate, they are diagnostic of complete atrioventricular (A-V) heart block.

The apical impulse is abnormal. Its shape indicates left ventricular (LV) hypertrophy caused by volume overload of the left ventricle (middle figure).

When complete heart block is present, the PR interval varies from beat to beat so that the intensity of the first heart sound varies. When the PR interval is short (0.14 to 0.16 second) the first heart sound is loud. This is called a *cannon sound*.

The murmur of aortic valve regurgitation is obvious (lower figure). An Austin Flint rumbling murmur is heard at the cardiac apex.

CHEST X-RAY FILM

Ankylosing spondylitis is present, as is pulmonary congestion.

The left ventricle is thought to be enlarged, as is the aortic root. The chest deformity makes interpretation of the chest film difficult.

One should suspect aortic valve regurgitation in a patient with ankylosing spondylitis.

See Patient 1 for a normal chest x-ray film.

ELECTROCARDIOGRAM

Complete heart block is present. The QRS duration is normal, so one can assume that the ventricular focus is located high in the septum.

The mean QRS vector is larger than normal and is directed +50 degrees in the frontal plane and 60 degrees posteriorly. The chest deformity may be responsible for the increased amplitude of the QRS complexes, but LV hypertrophy is also a possible cause for the abnormality. The mean T and ST vectors are directed opposite to the mean QRS vector.

The ECG shows LV hypertrophy. It is characteristic of systolic pressure overload of the left ventricle. Such a tracing occurs in patients with aortic valve stenosis, hypertension, primary hypertrophy, and *late in the course* of aortic or mitral valve regurgitation.

See Patient 1 for a normal ECG.

DIFFERENTIAL DIAGNOSIS

The triad of ankylosing spondylitis, complete heart block, and aortic valve regurgitation is accepted as an entity.

FINAL DIAGNOSIS

The heart disease, including aortic valve regurgitation, complete heart block, and heart failure, is related to the ankylosing spondylitis.

DIAGNOSTIC PRINCIPLE

This patient serves as an example of the numerous types of heart disease that should be considered when there are skin lesions, bony abnormalities, neurologic abnormalities, or other external features that can be identified at a glance.

For example, blue sclerae should lead one to suspect osteogenesis imperfecta, which is often associated with aortic or mitral valve regurgitation; a "fingerized" thumb should identify the Holt-Oran syndrome, in which an ostium secundum atrial septal defect often occurs; the skin lesions of lupus erythematosus should lead one to consider complications such as pericarditis, aortic valve regurgitation, or coronary thrombosis or arteritis; and scleroderma may be associated with pulmonary hypertension and cardiomyopathy. Also, Friedreich ataxia may be accompanied by myocardial disease and conduction disturbances; deafness and syncope in a child may be indicative of Jervell and Lange-Nielsen syndrome (long QT interval); large submaxillary glands may be a clue to amyloid heart disease; xanthelasma of the eyelids may suggest coronary atherosclerotic heart disease; and the Emery-Dreifuss type of neuromuscular disease may be associated with atrial standstill and sudden death.

The list is endless, but the diagnostic point is clear: the external clues to the presence of heart disease are abundant. Our challenge is to know them and search for them.

BIBLIOGRAPHY

Healy BP, Schlant RC, Gonzalez EB: The heart and connective tissue disease. In Schlant RC, Alexander RW, editors: *Hurst's the heart*, ed 8, New York, 1994, McGraw-Hill, p 1928.

FIGURE CREDITS

Upper, Modified and reproduced with permission from Hurst JW: *Cardiovascular diagnosis: The initial examination of the heart*, St Louis, 1993, Mosby, p 137.
Middle and lower, Modified and reproduced with permission from Hurst JW: The examination of the heart: the importance of initial screening, *Dis Mon* 36(5):282 (middle), 285 (lower), 1990.

HISTORY

The patient, a 46-year-old man, complains of severe chest pain. The pain is felt with equal intensity in the front of the chest and in the interscapular area. He also complains of inability to move his legs.

PHYSICAL EXAMINATION

The systolic blood pressure in the right arm is 170 mm Hg, and the diastolic blood pressure is 96 mm Hg. The systolic blood pressure in the left arm is 130 mm Hg, and the diastolic blood pressure is 78 mm Hg.

The femoral arterial pulsation seems to be less than normal in both legs.

There are no abnormal venous pulsations of the internal jugular veins. The right sternoclavicular joint moved during systole.

The apical impulse is located in the fifth intercostal space but is felt 2 cm to the left of the anterior axillary line.

A grade 2 murmur of aortic valve regurgitation is heard along the left sternal border.

The patient cannot move his legs.

CHEST X-RAY FILM

ELECTROCARDIOGRAM

The heart rhythm is normal. There are 88 depolarizations per minute. The PR interval is 0.18 second. The QRS duration is 0.10 second. The QT interval is 0.38 second. The total 12-lead QRS amplitude is 200 mm.

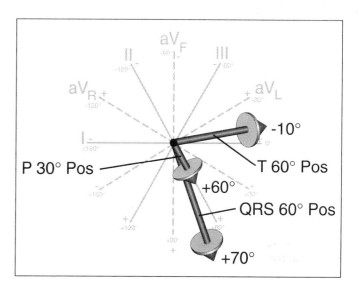

WHAT IS DIFFERENTIAL DIAGNOSIS?

WHAT IS FINAL DIAGNOSIS?

HISTORY

The chest pain was felt in the interscapular area. This should lead the physician to consider the diagnosis of aortic dissection. Whenever a patient has chest pain and simultaneously has an acute neurologic deficit, the physician should strongly consider dissection of the aorta. Whenever a patient has chest pain but develops a neurologic deficit several days later, the physician should suspect myocardial infarction followed by a cerebral embolus from a mural thrombus in the left ventricle.

PHYSICAL EXAMINATION

The systolic and diastolic blood pressures are elevated above normal in the right arm. These pressures are normal in the left arm. The femoral arterial pulsations are less than normal in both legs. These abnormalities, along with the right sternoclavicular joint pulsation, aortic valve regurgitation, abnormal apical impulse, and paralysis of the legs, indicate dissection of the aorta with involvement of the spinal arteries in a hypertensive patient.

CHEST X-RAY FILM

There is no rib notching, which tends to exclude coarctation of the aorta.

The root of the aorta is larger than normal. This could be caused by hypertension, aortic valve stenosis or regurgitation, dissection of the aorta, annuloaortic ectasia, atherosclerotic or luetic (syphilitic) aneurysm of the aortic root, or arteritis of the proximal portion of the aorta.

The left ventricle is enlarged.

See Patient 1 for a normal chest x-ray film.

ELECTROCARDIOGRAM

There is a left atrial abnormality, which is usually associated with left ventricular (LV) disease or mitral valve disease.

The mean QRS vector is directed at +70 degrees in the frontal plane and 60 degrees posteriorly. The total QRS amplitude is larger than normal, indicating LV hypertrophy.

The mean T vector is directed -10 degrees in the frontal plane and 60 degrees posteriorly, indicating anterior epicardial ischemia. The mean T vector is not directed as it should be with LV hypertrophy. One is forced to postulate that the T wave abnormality is caused by a condition other than LV hypertrophy. The abnormality could be caused by non-Q wave infarction in a hypertensive patient who also has coronary disease, a non-Q wave infarction in a patient with aortic valve stenosis who also has coronary disease, or a non-Q wave infarction caused by dissection of the aorta that also involves dissection of the left coronary artery.

See Patient 1 for a normal ECG.

DIFFERENTIAL DIAGNOSIS

The location of the chest pain and simultaneous paralysis of the legs are diagnostic of dissection of the aorta. In addition, other clues to dissection of the aorta include: pulsation of the right sternoclavicular joint, unequal blood pressure in the arms, diminished femoral artery pulsation, aortic valve regurgitation, and a dilated aortic root.

The mean T vector in the ECG is not related to the apparent LV hypertrophy. The mean T vector most likely represents a non-Q wave infarction, which is probably caused by dissection of the left coronary artery.

The patient probably had essential hypertension for many years.

FINAL DIAGNOSIS

Dissection of the entire aorta with dissection of the left coronary artery plus dissection of the spinal arteries.

DIAGNOSTIC PRINCIPLE

Dissection of the aorta is usually caused by cystic medial necrosis of the aorta and other arteries. It usually occurs in hypertensive patients. It is important to remember that a neurologic deficit occurring at the time of chest pain indicates dissection of the aorta until proved otherwise.

The mean T vector should not be directed posteriorly when there are ECG signs of LV hypertrophy. When it is, one must consider the likelihood that the abnormality is caused by anterior myocardial ischemia from some type of coronary disease.

BIBLIOGRAPHY

Lindsay J Jr, DeBakey ME, Beall AC: Diagnosis and treatment of diseases of the aorta. In Schlant RC, Alexander RW, editors: *Hurst's the heart*, ed 8, New York, 1994, McGraw-Hill, pp 2170-2175.

HISTORY

The patient is a 64-year-old male. He has always had an annual physical examination and has always been pronounced "normal." He is returning for his yearly examination.

PHYSICAL EXAMINATION

The pulse rate is 82 beats per minute.

The systolic blood pressure is 220 mm Hg and the diastolic blood pressure is 100 mm Hg. The systolic blood pressure in the legs is 260 mm Hg.

The carotid arterial pulsation is prominent. The venous pulsations are normal in the neck.

The systolic apical impulse is a little prominent, and an atrial gallop sound is heard at the cardiac apex.

A bruit is heard over the left renal area.

CHEST X-RAY FILM

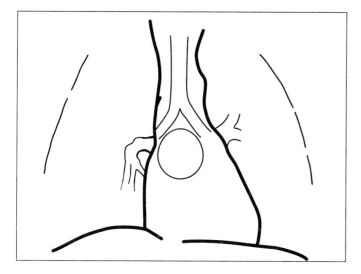

ELECTROCARDIOGRAM

The heart rhythm is normal. There are 80 depolarizations per minute. The PR interval is 0.18 second. The QRS duration is 0.09 second. The QT interval is 0.36 second. The total 12-lead QRS amplitude is 175 mm. The 12-lead QRS amplitude was 150 mm in the ECG made 1 year ago.

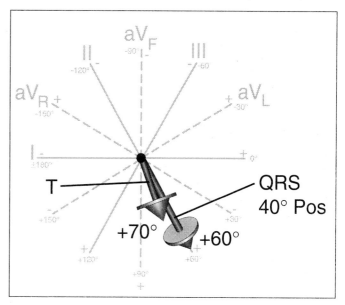

WHAT IS DIFFERENTIAL DIAGNOSIS?

WHAT IS FINAL DIAGNOSIS?

HISTORY

There is no past history of disease. Such a patient could have developed asymptomatic coronary atherosclerotic heart disease or hypertension within the preceding year.

PHYSICAL EXAMINATION

The patient has marked elevation of systolic and diastolic blood pressure. The blood pressure has not been elevated previously and has been checked annually for many years. A bruit can be heard over the left renal area of the upper abdomen.

Whenever a patient develops hypertension for the first time beyond the age of 50 years, one must consider the possibility of secondary hypertension rather than essential (or primary) hypertension.

It is likely that this patient has renovascular disease caused by obstructive atherosclerosis of the renal arteries.

Pheochromocytoma and aldosteroma are not likely but must be excluded.

Coarctation of the aorta can be ruled out because the systolic pressure in the legs is higher than in the arms, and also because this patient has new onset hypertension at age 64.

No evidence indicates cardiac valvular disease in this patient.

CHEST X-RAY FILM

The chest film is normal.

The patient could have a normal heart or could have hypertension, coronary atherosclerotic heart disease, mild valvular disease, hypertrophic cardiomyopathy, or congenital heart disease, such as a small ductus arteriosus or a small ventricular septal defect.

The patient has hypertension of recent onset, and the heart has not had time to react with the development of left ventricular (LV) hypertrophy.

ELECTROCARDIOGRAM

The ECG, viewed in isolation, could be normal.

The total QRS amplitude is 170 mm; 1 year ago the total QRS amplitude was 150 mm Hg. The change could be caused by LV hypertrophy.

See Patient 1 for a normal ECG.

DIFFERENTIAL DIAGNOSIS

This 64-year-old man developed hypertension during the last year. He has secondary hypertension. No other cardiac diseases are apparent. The most likely cause of the hypertension is atherosclerotic renovascular disease.

FINAL DIAGNOSIS

Secondary hypertension caused by renovascular disease.

DIAGNOSTIC PRINCIPLE

This patient is presented because, despite recent advances in the understanding of hypertension, its etiology is often ignored.

A basic diagnostic principle is that the *cause* of symptoms, abnormal physical findings, abnormal physiological derangements, abnormal radiographic findings, ECG abnormalities, and abnormal laboratory findings must be determined. It is alarming that in 1994 the cause of chest pain, of heart failure, of a murmur, of a stroke, or of other conditions is often ignored. *Cardiovascular disease of ignored etiology is not the same as cardiovascular disease of unknown etiology.*

BIBLIOGRAPHY

Hall WD, Wollam GL, Tuttle EP Jr: Diagnostic evaluation of the patient with systemic arterial hypertension. In Schlant RC, Alexander RW, editors: *Hurst's the heart,* ed 8, New York, 1994, McGraw-Hill, pp 1411-1425.

HISTORY

The patient, a 53-year-old man, has no cardiovascular symptoms. He is being seen in consultation before the surgical repair of a left inguinal hernia.

PHYSICAL EXAMINATION

The pulse rate is 75 beats per minute.

The systolic blood pressure is 132 mm Hg and the diastolic blood pressure is 78 mm Hg.

The pulsations in the neck veins are normal, as are the pulsations of the peripheral arteries.

Auscultation of the heart reveals the abnormality shown in the diagram to the right.

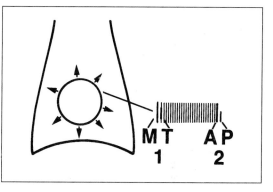

1, 2, First, second heart sounds; *M*, mitral, *T*, tricuspid, *A*, aortic, and *P*, pulmonary valve closure sounds. See figure credit.

CHEST X-RAY FILM

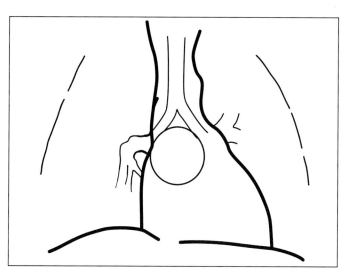

ELECTROCARDIOGRAM

The heart rhythm is normal. There are 82 depolarizations per minute. The PR interval is 0.14 second. The QRS duration is 0.09 second. The QT interval is 0.36 second. The total 12-lead QRS amplitude is 160 mm.

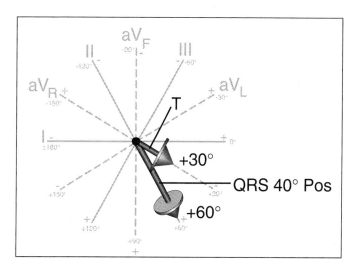

WHAT IS DIFFERENTIAL DIAGNOSIS?

WHAT OTHER QUESTION WOULD YOU ASK?

WHAT LOW-TECHNOLOGY PROCEDURE WOULD YOU PERFORM?

WHAT IS FINAL DIAGNOSIS?

HISTORY

The history as given offers no diagnostic clues. The patient could have a normal heart, a secundum atrial septal defect, a ventricular septal defect, aortic valve stenosis or regurgitation, mitral valve prolapse, or symptomless atherosclerotic coronary heart disease.

PHYSICAL EXAMINATION

The only cardiovascular abnormality noted is the heart murmur. The location of the murmur suggests the possibility of aortic valve stenosis (bicuspid aortic valve), idiopathic hypertrophic subaortic stenosis (IHSS), or an interventricular septal defect. The shape of the murmur and second heart sound are characteristic of interventricular septal defect. Note that it is holosystolic and that the second heart sound is normal.

CHEST X-RAY FILM

The left ventricle is slightly large, as is the left atrium and main pulmonary artery and its branches. Pulmonary blood flow is increased.

See Patient 1 for a normal chest x-ray film.

ELECTROCARDIOGRAM

The total 12-lead QRS amplitude is within the normal range. The direction of the mean QRS vector and T vector is normal.

See Patient 1 for a normal ECG.

DIFFERENTIAL DIAGNOSIS

An ostium secundum atrial septal defect is excluded because (1) the murmur is louder than is usually heard with an ostium secundum atrial septal defect; (2) the second heart sound is not widely split and fixed; (3) the ECG does not show a right ventricular conduction delay; and (4) the chest x-ray film shows a slightly large left atrium and left ventricle, which are not characteristic of an ostium secundum atrial septal defect.

The radiographic findings and ECG could be caused by aortic valve stenosis (bicuspid aortic valve). The shape of the murmur, however, is holosystolic; this is not characteristic of the murmur of aortic valve stenosis, which is usually more diamond shaped. Also, there is no systolic ejection sound, as occurs with a bicuspid aortic valve, and the second sound is normal.

The shape of the murmur is not characteristic of IHSS. The ECG of this patient is normal, whereas the ECG of most patients with IHSS shows left ventricular hypertrophy, an initial 0.04-second abnormality, or an ST segment or T wave abnormality.

Although symptomless coronary disease may be present, the murmur indicates the presence of either valvular or congenital heart disease.

The location and shape of the murmur are characteristic of congenital interventricular septal defect.

The radiologic and ECG findings are consistent with a small interventricular septal defect.

OTHER QUESTION

The patient, when specifically queried, stated he had the heart murmur all his life.

LOW-TECHNOLOGY PROCEDURE

The patient is asked to perform isometric exercise (handgrip). He does so, and the murmur does not change in intensity. This result is against the diagnosis of IHSS, in which the murmur would become fainter with handgrip.

FINAL DIAGNOSIS

Congenital interventricular septal defect.

DIAGNOSTIC PRINCIPLE

It is useful to study the effect of isometric exercise, or the Valsalva maneuver, or abrupt standing from a squatting position as a means of identifying the etiology of a systolic murmur.

BIBLIOGRAPHY

Nugent EW, Plauth WH, Edwards JE, Williams WH: The pathology, pathophysiology, recognition, and treatment of congenital heart disease. In Schlant RC, Alexander RW, editors: *Hurst's the heart*, ed 8, New York, 1994, McGraw-Hill, pp 1768-1773.

FIGURE CREDIT

Reproduced with permission from Hurst JW: The examination of the heart: the importance of initial screening, *Dis Mon* 36(5):285, 1990.

HISTORY

The patient is a 54-year-old woman complaining of episodes of palpitation. She was told that she had a heart murmur when she was 10 years of age.

PHYSICAL EXAMINATION

The heart rhythm is regular, with 82 beats per minute.

The systolic blood pressure is 138 mm Hg and the diastolic blood pressure is 72 mm Hg.

The pulsation of the neck veins is normal, as are the pulsations of the peripheral arteries.

There is a rapid systolic anterior lift of the precordium. The apical impulse is identified in the fifth left intercostal space but is located several centimeters to the left midclavicular line. The apical impulse itself is 4 cm in diameter and is hyperdynamic (see diagram on the right).

Auscultation of the heart reveals the following abnormalities:

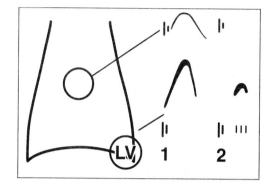

I, 2, First, second heart sounds; *LV,* left ventricle. See figure credits.

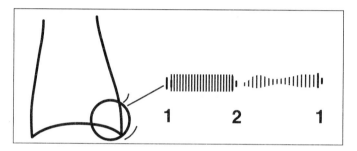

See figure credits.

CHEST X-RAY FILM

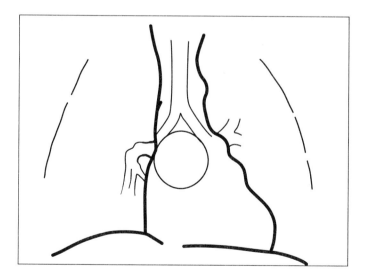

ELECTROCARDIOGRAM

The heart rhythm is normal. There are 80 depolarizations per minute. The last half of the P wave in lead V_1 measures -0.06 mm•second. The PR interval is 0.20 second. The QRS duration is 0.09 second. The QT interval is 0.36 second. The total 12-lead QRS amplitude is 190 mm.

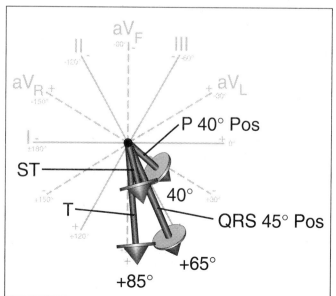

WHAT IS DIFFERENTIAL DIAGNOSIS?

WHAT IS FINAL DIAGNOSIS?

HISTORY

From the history alone, one might deduce that the murmur was produced by congenital heart disease, such as patent ductus arteriosus, interventricular septal defect, ostium primum atrial septal defect, a large ostium secundum atrial septal defect, or aortic valve stenosis or regurgitation from a bicuspid aortic valve. The murmur could also be produced by mitral valve regurgitation caused by rheumatic fever. Mitral stenosis is unlikely because the murmur was heard at age 10. Finally, the murmur could be produced by mitral valve prolapse.

PHYSICAL EXAMINATION

See upper figure. There is an abnormal systolic movement of the anterior precordium. This could be caused by right ventricular hypertrophy or mitral valve regurgitation. The latter occurs when the left atrium, which is located posteriorly between the heart and spine, expands as a result of moderately severe mitral regurgitation. The apical impulse is characteristic of diastolic overload of the left ventricle. The apical movement felt one-third into diastole is caused by a rapid diastolic filling. There is a palpable left ventricular gallop.

See lower figure. There is a loud systolic murmur heard at the cardiac apex caused by mitral valve regurgitation. No systolic click or clicks are heard. The murmur radiates laterally but does not radiate up and down the spine. There is an apical diastolic rumble heard at the apex. The first part of the rumble is a left ventricular gallop sound. It is undoubtedly caused by the torrential blood flow into the left ventricle during diastole, which consists of the normal blood volume from the left atrium, plus the volume of blood in the left atrium that resulted from mitral regurgitation.

These murmurs could be caused by rheumatic mitral valve disease with predominant mitral regurgitation, or by an ostium primum atrial septal defect. The latter is not likely because the second heart sound was not widely split. Mitral valve prolapse is not likely because there is no systolic click or clicks, and the murmur had been heard since age 10.

All the other conditions listed in *History* are excluded because the characteristic murmurs associated with them are not present.

CHEST X-RAY FILM

The contour of the left side of the heart, from above downward, results from the aortic knob, a larger-than-normal pulmonary artery, a large left atrial appendage, and a large left ventricle. This is known as a four-bump heart. The border-forming left atrial appendage is almost always caused by rheumatic mitral valve stenosis or regurgitation.

See Patient 1 for a normal chest x-ray film.

ELECTROCARDIOGRAM

The ECG shows a left atrial abnormality and diastolic overload of the left ventricle. Note the larger-than-normal QRS vector. The mean T vector is large and is located about 45 degrees from the mean QRS vector. The ST vector is parallel with the mean T vector.

This could be the result of mitral or aortic valve regurgitation, patent ductus arteriosus, or interventricular septal defect. The ECG is not typical of an ostium primum atrial septal defect, an ostium secundum atrial septal defect, or tetralogy of Fallot.

See Patient 1 for a normal ECG.

DIFFERENTIAL DIAGNOSIS

It is highly likely that the patient has moderately severe rheumatic mitral valve regurgitation and is having episodes of uncontrolled atrial fibrillation. Mitral valve prolapse is possible, but there is no systolic click and the patient knows the murmur has been present since age 10.

Ostium primum atrial septal defect with a cleft mitral valve is excluded because the ECG does not show right bundle branch block plus left anterosuperior division block.

The other possible conditions are excluded because the murmurs, the ECG, and chest film are not characteristic of them and because all the data favor mitral valve regurgitation, most likely as the result of rheumatic fever that was unrecognized.

FINAL DIAGNOSIS

Moderately severe mitral valve regurgitation caused by rheumatic heart disease. The patient was probably having episodes of atrial fibrillation.

DIAGNOSTIC PRINCIPLE

The apical impulse and murmur are characteristic of mitral valve regurgitation. The diagnostic rumble at the apex is caused by an increase in blood flow across the mitral valve during diastole.

The diagnostic value of the enlarged left atrial appendage as seen on the chest x-ray film must be emphasized. Whenever the left atrial appendage is seen, it is diagnostic of mitral valve stenosis or regurgitation. Furthermore, it usually implies that the mitral valve disease is caused by rheumatic heart disease. It rarely, if ever, occurs as a result of mitral regurgitation from other causes. Perhaps acute rheumatic myocarditis damages the atria, including the atrial appendages, so that an increase in pressure within the left atrium causes the left atrial appendage to enlarge.

BIBLIOGRAPHY

Gaasch WH, O'Rourke RA, Cohn LH, Rackley CE: Mitral valve disease. In Schlant RC, Alexander RW, editors: *Hurst's the heart*, ed 8, New York, 1994, McGraw-Hill, pp 1491-1502.

FIGURE CREDITS

Upper and *lower*, Modified and reproduced with permission from Hurst JW: The examination of the heart: the importance of initial screening, *Dis Mon* 36(5):282 (upper), 285 (lower), 1990.

HISTORY

The patient is a 64-year-old woman complaining of dyspnea on effort for the past month.

PHYSICAL EXAMINATION

The pulse rate is 90 beats per minute.

The systolic blood pressure is 116 mm Hg, and the diastolic blood pressure is 72 mm Hg.

The external jugular veins are abnormally distended when the patient's trunk is elevated 45 degrees. The *a* wave is prominent in the internal jugular pulse.

Pulsus alternans is noted in the femoral artery.

The apex impulse is larger than normal and is located 2 cm to the left of the midclavicular line.

Atrial and ventricular gallop sounds are heard at the apex.

No murmurs are heard.

CHEST X-RAY FILM

Pulmonary congestion is apparent.

ELECTROCARDIOGRAM

The heart rhythm is normal. There are 105 depolarizations per minute. The PR interval is 0.18 second. The QRS duration is 0.10 second. The QT interval is 0.38 second. The total QRS amplitude is 60 mm.

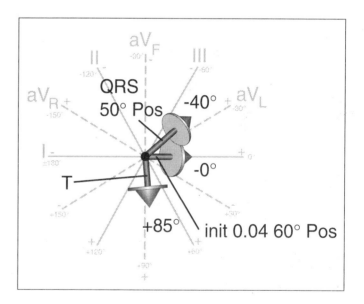

WHAT IS DIFFERENTIAL DIAGNOSIS?

WHAT IS FINAL DIAGNOSIS?

HISTORY

The history of dyspnea on effort for 1 month indicates a high probability of heart or lung disease. The lung disease could be caused by interstitial fibrosis or repeated pulmonary emboli. Heart disease probabilities include mitral stenosis, mitral valve prolapse, dilated cardiomyopathy, and painless myocardial ischemia from coronary atherosclerotic heart disease (angina equivalent).

PHYSICAL EXAMINATION

The prominent *a* wave in the internal jugular venous pulse suggests poor right ventricular (RV) compliance, and the abnormal external jugular distension suggests the presence of heart failure.

The pulsus alternans indicates left ventricular (LV) dysfunction.

The heart is slightly enlarged.

The atrial gallop heard at the apex indicates poor LV compliance, and the ventricular gallop sound indicates LV dysfunction.

The normal blood pressure, absence of murmurs, evidence of poor RV compliance, LV dysfunction, and cardiac enlargement suggest cardiomyopathy. The cause is to be determined.

CHEST X-RAY FILM

Heart failure is evident, and the heart is slightly enlarged. The contour of the heart is not characteristic of pericardial effusion.

These abnormalities suggest cardiomyopathy (etiology to be determined).

See Patient 1 for a normal chest x-ray film.

ELECTROCARDIOGRAM

The QRS amplitude is abnormally low. The mean QRS vector is directed about -40 degrees to the left and 50 degrees posteriorly. This represents left anterosuperior division block. The low QRS amplitude suggests several diseases, including myxedema or cardiomyopathy (especially amyloid involvement of the heart). The heart rate of 105 is against a diagnosis of myxedema. Pericardial effusion, which could cause low amplitude of the QRS complexes, would not produce the left anterosuperior division block.

The mean initial 0.04-second vector is directed 0 degrees in the frontal plane and 60 degrees posteriorly. It is directed more posteriorly than the mean QRS vector. This suggests an anterior "dead zone" effect. The dead zone could be caused by myocardial infarction from atherosclerotic heart disease, or could be related to cardiomyopathy from a condition such as amyloid disease.

See Patient 1 for a normal ECG.

DIFFERENTIAL DIAGNOSIS

The patient has heart failure, but the heart is only slightly enlarged.

Valvular heart disease can be ruled out because there are no murmurs.

Pulsus alternans and an apical ventricular gallop are clues to left ventricular dysfunction, whereas the prominent *a* wave suggests poor compliance of the right ventricle. These clues indicate cardiac muscle disease rather than pericardial effusion that could produce low-amplitude QRS complexes.

The patient could have diastolic dysfunction caused by painless myocardial ischemia secondary to coronary disease, but the QRS amplitude would not be abnormally low.

The abnormalities suggest restrictive cardiomyopathy caused by amyloid disease. This is another cause of ECG signs of pseudomyocardial infarction.

Constrictive pericarditis is excluded because of the prominent apical impulse and pulsus alternans.

FINAL DIAGNOSIS

Restrictive cardiomyopathy. It is most likely caused by amyloid infiltration of the myocardium, but there could be other causes.

DIAGNOSTIC PRINCIPLE

When heart failure occurs in a patient who has no history of chest discomfort from myocardial ischemia and whose heart is only slightly enlarged, has no signs of heart valve disease, has an ECG that shows low QRS voltage and signs of a "dead zone," and exhibits no evidence of pericardial disease, it is wise to consider the likelihood of restrictive cardiomyopathy. Amyloid disease of the heart is a common cause of these abnormalities.

REFERENCES

O'Connell JB, Renlund DG: Myocarditis and specific myocardial diseases. In Schlant RC, Alexander RW, editors: *Hurst's the heart*, ed 8, New York, 1994, McGraw-Hill, pp 1601-1602.

Shabetai R: Diseases of the pericardium. In Schlant RC, Alexander RW, editors: *Hurst's the heart*, ed 8, New York, 1994, McGraw-Hill, pp 1637-1646.

HISTORY

The patient, a 33-year-old female, has been cyanotic since birth. She has been able to work at a desk job. She refused surgical intervention for her heart disease.

PHYSICAL EXAMINATION

The pulse rate is 78 beats per minute.

The systolic blood pressure is 128 mm Hg and the diastolic blood pressure is 72 mm Hg.

The fingers and toes are equally cyanosed and clubbed.

There is a large *a* wave in the internal jugular venous pulsation.

The apical impulse is easily felt. It is displaced laterally.

The pulmonary valve closure sound is diminished in intensity. There is a loud systolic murmur heard with maximum intensity at the center of the left sternal border.

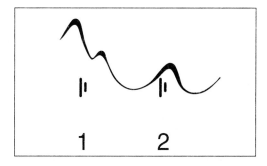

1, 2, First, second heart sounds. See figure credit.

CHEST X-RAY FILM

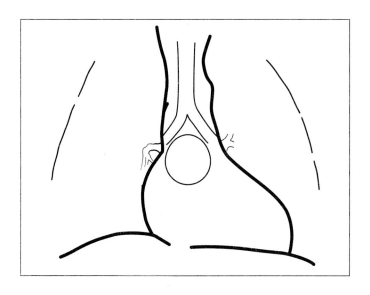

ELECTROCARDIOGRAM

The heart rhythm is normal. The heart rate is 86 depolarizations per minute. The amplitude of the P wave is 3 mm in lead II. The PR interval is 0.18 second. The QRS duration is 0.09 second. The QT interval is 0.36 second.

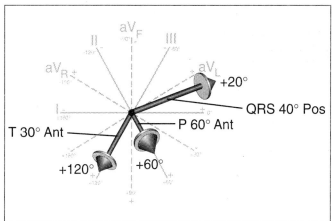

WHAT IS DIFFERENTIAL DIAGNOSIS?

WHAT IS FINAL DIAGNOSIS?

HISTORY

The patient gave a history of cyanosis since birth. She is now 33 years old. The most common type of heart disease that produces cyanosis and permits life until this age (or older) is tetralogy of Fallot. Patients with Eisenmenger physiology, tricuspid atresia, and Ebstein's anomaly with a patent foramen ovale who may also achieve this age or older.

PHYSICAL EXAMINATION

The fingers and toes are equally cyanotic and clubbed. It is always important to make this determination because, when the toes are more cyanosed and more clubbed than the fingers, it is virtually diagnostic of Eisenmenger physiology caused by a patent ductus arteriosus (with reversed blood flow in the ductus from pulmonary hypertension).

The prominent *a* wave noted in the jugular pulse suggests poor compliance of the right ventricle or tricuspid atresia.

The systolic murmur with diminished intensity of the pulmonary closure sound suggests pulmonary valve stenosis. The murmur could also be caused by an interventricular septal defect.

CHEST X-RAY FILM

There are three abnormalities: (1) the main pulmonary artery and its branches are small; (2) the pulmonary blood flow is diminished; and (3) the left ventricle and right atrium are large.

The abnormalities listed last rule against tetralogy of Fallot, Eisenmenger physiology, and transposition of the great vessels. The abnormalities could be caused by tricuspid atresia.

See Patient 1 for a normal chest x-ray film.

ELECTROCARDIOGRAM

The rate and intervals are normal.

There is a right atrial abnormality; note that the mean P vector is directed too far anteriorly, and the amplitude of the P wave in lead II is 3 mm.

The mean QRS vector is large and is directed abnormally to the left and posteriorly, suggesting left ventricular (LV) hypertrophy, and possibly left anterosuperior division block.

The mean T vector is directed abnormally to the right and anteriorly.

These abnormalities occur infrequently. When they are considered without other data, one could suspect diseases of the left ventricle plus a condition causing a right atrial abnormality. They are characteristic of the abnormalities seen with tricuspid atresia.

See Patient 1 for a normal ECG.

DIFFERENTIAL DIAGNOSIS

Tetralogy of Fallot must always be considered when a patient has been cyanotic since birth. The ECG of this patient did not show right ventricular (RV) hypertrophy; this excludes tetralogy of Fallot.

Eisenmenger physiology is ruled out because the ECG does not show RV hypertrophy or right bundle branch block (RBBB) and the x-ray film does not reveal large pulmonary arteries.

Ebstein anomaly with patent foramen ovale can be excluded because the shape of the heart on the x-ray film is not typical of this anomaly (which often resembles a pericardial effusion) and the ECG does not show a QRS conduction abnormality (e.g., RBBB).

Tricuspid stenosis is likely because there is cyanosis, a large *a* wave in the jugular pulse, LV hypertrophy (or RV smallness) in the ECG, and decreased pulmonary blood flow.

FINAL DIAGNOSIS

Congenital tricuspid atresia, patent foramen ovale, rudimentary right ventricle with pulmonary valve stenosis, and an interventricular septal defect.

DIAGNOSTIC PRINCIPLE

Most congenital heart diseases that produce cyanosis also produce RV hypertrophy in the ECG. Whenever one observes cyanosis and LV hypertrophy in the ECG of a patient with decreased pulmonary blood flow, tricuspid atresia should be diagnosed.

BIBLIOGRAPHY

Hurst JW, Nugent EW, Anderson RH, Wilcox BR: Congenital heart disease. In Hurst JW, editor-in-chief: *Atlas of the heart*, St Louis, 1988, Mosby, pp 3.66-3.69.

FIGURE CREDIT

Modified and reproduced with permission from Hurst JW: The examination of the heart: the importance of initial screening, *Dis Mon* 36(5):280, 1990.

HISTORY

The patient is a 58-year-old man who is complaining of chest tightness. The brief episodes of discomfort have been present for about 6 months. The discomfort has not changed in frequency, duration, or precipitating causes during this time. On questioning, the patient indicated that the discomfort was located in the retrosternal area and was about the size of his fist or larger. He feels the discomfort when he walks up an incline to his home after getting his newspaper. He never has the discomfort walking down the incline. The discomfort lasts about 1 minute if he discontinues walking.

He states that none of his family members died at a young age. He also states that he does not smoke. He recalls that his serum cholesterol level is 205 mg/dl.

PHYSICAL EXAMINATION

The pulse rate is 78 beats per minute.

The systolic blood pressure is 120 mm Hg, and the diastolic blood pressure is 80 mm Hg.

The remainder of the physical examination is normal.

CHEST X-RAY FILM

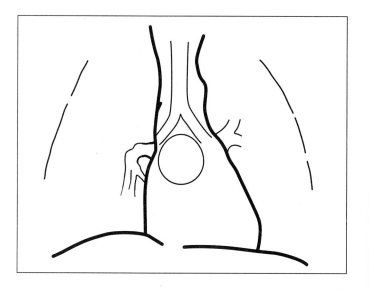

ELECTROCARDIOGRAM

The heart rhythm is normal. There are 82 depolarizations per minute. The PR interval is 0.15 second. The QRS duration is 0.08 second. The QT interval is 0.36 second. The 12-lead QRS amplitude is 172 mm.

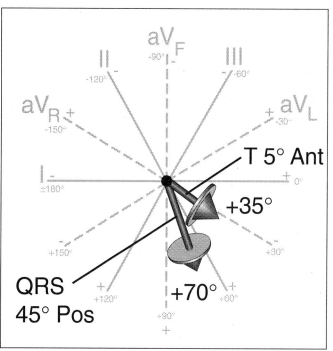

WHAT IS DIFFERENTIAL DIAGNOSIS?

WHAT IS FINAL DIAGNOSIS?

HISTORY

The patient is a 58-year-old man. The history of chest tightness produced by effort is clear and definite. The discomfort has been noted for 6 months and has not changed during that time. He has stable angina pectoris.

PHYSICAL EXAMINATION

The physical examination is normal. This excludes valvular disease, hypertension, and in most instances, cardiomyopathy.

A normal physical examination in a man of this age indicates that the patient may have a normal heart, or if heart disease is present, it is most likely atherosclerotic coronary heart disease.

CHEST X-RAY FILM

The chest film is normal. This implies that the heart may be normal, or if disease is present, it may be atherosclerotic coronary heart disease, mild valvular disease, cardiomyopathy, especially the hypertrophic type, or the patient could have a history of pericarditis or dysrhythmia.

ELECTROCARDIOGRAM

The resting ECG is normal. This indicates that the heart may be normal, or if disease is present, it may be atherosclerotic coronary heart disease, mild valvular heart disease, or previous pericarditis. The patient could have had a dysrhythmia in the past that was not present when the ECG was made.

DIFFERENTIAL DIAGNOSIS

The patient has stable angina pectoris. The absence of clues to the diagnosis of aortic valvular disease or cardiomyopathy, which can produce angina pectoris, indicates that the patient has obstructive coronary atherosclerosis as a cause of the angina.

The angina is classified as stable, because there has been no change in the frequency, duration, or precipitating causes for more than 60 days.

FINAL DIAGNOSIS

Stable angina pectoris caused by atherosclerotic coronary heart disease.

DIAGNOSTIC PRINCIPLE

How certain is the diagnosis of angina pectoris? The predictive value of this particular history indicating angina pectoris caused by myocardial ischemia is 90%.

The angina is most likely caused by obstructive coronary atherosclerosis, although rare causes may be found on coronary arteriography.

The angina pectoris is labeled as being *stable* because it has not changed within the last 60 days. This implies that the episodes of angina result from an increase in myocardial oxygen demand produced by effort rather than a change in the obstructing atherosclerotic lesions themselves.

This patient is presented to emphasize that the vascular biology, pathophysiology, symptoms, and treatment of stable angina pectoris is different than those of unstable angina pectoris.

The patient should not have a stress test for diagnostic purposes because it is not possible to improve the predictive value of the history, which is 90%.

This patient is also presented to indicate the value of the history and to point out that when the resting ECG is normal and there are no risk factors, such a history has considerable diagnostic value and must never be ignored.

BIBLIOGRAPHY

Schlant RC, Alexander RW: Diagnosis and management of chronic ischemic heart disease. In Schlant RC, Alexander RW, editors: *Hurst's the heart*, ed 8, New York, 1994, McGraw-Hill, pp 1056-1074.

HISTORY

The patient is a 46-year-old man who smokes at least a pack of cigarettes daily.

During the last year, he has complained of episodes of retrosternal discomfort that lasted 5 or 6 minutes. The pain is unrelated to meals or activity. He has occasionally detected the discomfort while smoking. Also, he noticed recently that his heart rate occasionally slowed during the episode of discomfort. The chest discomfort seemed to appear during the afternoon.

While in the physician's office, the patient experiences an episode of discomfort during which the physician is able to examine the patient and record an ECG (see *Physical Examination* and *Electrocardiogram* under **Clues and Questions**).

PHYSICAL EXAMINATION

During the episode, the systolic blood pressure is 136 mm Hg and the diastolic blood pressure is 76 mm Hg. The blood pressure remains the same during and after the episode of chest discomfort, but the pulse rate slows to 45 beats per minute during the episode.

The physician notes the patient's circumoral pallor and sweating during the episode of chest discomfort.

The examination of the heart is normal, as is the remainder of the examination.

CHEST X-RAY FILM

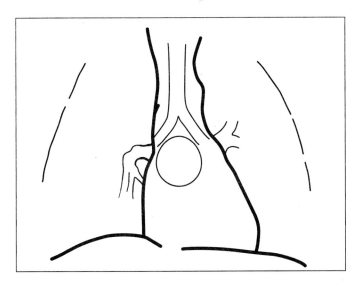

ELECTROCARDIOGRAM

There is 2:1 atrioventricular (A-V) block. The atrial rate is 90 depolarizations per minute. The ventricular rate is 45 per minute. The QRS duration is 0.10 second. The ECG returned to normal in about 10 minutes.

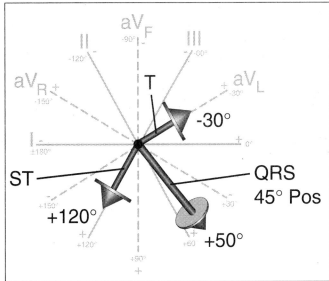

WHAT IS DIFFERENTIAL DIAGNOSIS?

WHAT IS FINAL DIAGNOSIS?

HISTORY

The episodes of retrosternal tightness were not related to effort, but the location of the discomfort forces one to consider that it may be caused by myocardial ischemia. The predictive value of this symptom is less than it is with stable angina related to effort (see Patient 45). The episodes were unrelated to eating, which makes esophageal reflux unlikely. The chest discomfort was occasionally caused by smoking; this suggests coronary artery spasm.

PHYSICAL EXAMINATION

The physician has the opportunity to observe the patient during an episode of discomfort. The circumoral pallor, sweating, and bradycardia that occurred during an episode of retrosternal tightness suggest myocardial ischemia.

CHEST X-RAY FILM

The chest film is normal. This does not rule out coronary disease, mild valvular disease, pericarditis, dysrhythmias, or hypertrophic cardiomyopathy.

See Patient 1 for a normal chest x-ray film.

ELECTROCARDIOGRAM

The ECG made during the episode of chest tightness shows 2:1 A-V block, an ST vector that is caused by inferior myocardial epicardial injury, and a mean T vector directed away from inferior myocardial ischemia. The QRS-T angle is about 80 degrees. The ECG made a few minutes after the chest tightness subsides is normal.

The transient ECG abnormalities are virtually diagnostic of coronary artery spasm. In fact, the location of the ST vector and 2:1 A-V block indicate that the spasm is located in the right coronary artery.

See Patient 1 for a normal ECG.

DIFFERENTIAL DIAGNOSIS

Esophageal reflux is ruled out because the chest tightness is unrelated to eating, and because diagnostic ECG abnormalities were recorded during an episode of discomfort.

The location and duration of the episodes of chest tightness suggest, but do not prove, that the discomfort is caused by myocardial ischemia. The ECG, however, is diagnostic of coronary artery spasm of the right coronary artery.

FINAL DIAGNOSIS

Variant angina pectoris (Prinzmetal's angina).

DIAGNOSTIC PRINCIPLE

This type of angina, first reported by Wilson and Johnston[1] in 1941, is different from ordinary angina. The episodes are not usually precipitated by effort. The chest discomfort in Wilson and Johnston's patient was precipitated by smoking a cigarette. They recorded an ECG during the time the patient smoked and identified the ST segment abnormality that is characteristic of the disorder. They postulated that the condition was caused by vasospasm of the epicardial arteries because the rate-pressure product did not change during the episode.

Prinzmetal, et al.,[2] in 1959 described the entire syndrome and initially labeled the condition as "reversed angina." He later called the symptoms *variant angina*. He also believed the condition was caused by coronary artery spasm.

Most patients with variant angina pectoris have coronary atherosclerosis plus coronary artery spasm, but a few patients have isolated coronary spasm.[3] A coronary arteriogram is needed to determine the exact status of the coronary arteries. Even this procedure, with ergonovine challenge, does not always clarify the problem.

Every effort should be made to record an ECG during an episode of discomfort in a patient with suspected Prinzmetal angina. The abnormalities occurring in the ECG may be diagnostic of the condition.

REFERENCES

1. Wilson FN, Johnston FD: The occurrence in angina pectoris of electrocardiographic changes similar in magnitude and in kind to those produced by myocardial infarction, *Am Heart J* 22:64-74, 1941.
2. Prinzmetal M, et al: Angina pectoris. I. A variant form of angina pectoris, *Am J Med* 27:375-388, 1959.
3. Theroux P, Waters D: Diagnosis and management of patients with unstable angina. In Schlant RC, Alexander RW, editors: *Hurst's the heart*, ed 8, New York, 1994, McGraw-Hill, pp 1097-1106.

HISTORY

The patient is a 50-year-old male who is being seen by a physician for the first time. He has no symptoms.

PHYSICAL EXAMINATION

The pulse rate is 78 beats per minute.

The systolic blood pressure is 165 mm Hg, and the diastolic blood pressure is 95 mm Hg in the right arm.

Auscultation of the heart reveals the following (note diagram on the right):

See *Low-Technology Procedures* under **Discussion and Answers.**

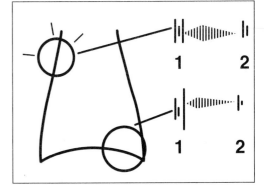

1, 2, First, second heart sounds. See figure credit.

CHEST X-RAY FILM

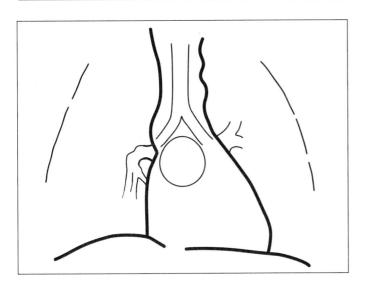

WHAT IS DIFFERENTIAL DIAGNOSIS?

WHAT LOW-TECHNOLOGY PROCEDURES WOULD YOU PERFORM?

WHAT IS FINAL DIAGNOSIS?

ELECTROCARDIOGRAM

The heart rhythm is normal. There are 70 depolarizations per minute. The PR interval is 0.15 second. The QRS duration is 0.09 second. The QT interval is 0.38 second. The total 12-lead QRS amplitude is 195 mm.

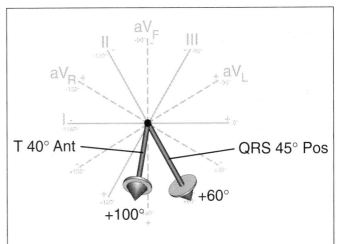

HISTORY

The history is noncontributory. The patient has no history of angina, dyspnea, palpitation, or syncope, but this does not eliminate heart disease.

PHYSICAL EXAMINATION

The systolic and diastolic blood pressures are elevated above normal.

See figure in *Physical Examination* under **Clues and Questions**. The loud ejection sound and diamond-shaped murmur heard in the second right intercostal space next to the sternum are characteristic of aortic valve stenosis caused by a congenital bicuspid valve. The ejection sound is often louder at the apex than it is in the second right intercostal space near the sternum.

CHEST X-RAY FILM

The upper portion of the left border of the aorta shows the "figure 3" sign of coarctation of the aorta. The upper part of the 3 is produced by a dilated left subclavian artery above the coarcted area, and the lower part of the 3 results from dilatation of the subclavian artery.

The root of the aorta is dilated, which suggests the possibility of aortic stenosis caused by a bicuspid aortic valve.

Rib notching could also be seen.

See Fig. 3-14.

See Patient 1 for a normal chest x-ray film.

ELECTROCARDIOGRAM

The rhythm, rate, and intervals are normal. The mean QRS vector is directed at +60 degrees in the frontal plane and 45 degrees posteriorly. It is larger than normal, suggesting the possibility of left ventricular (LV) hypertrophy.

The mean T vector is directed at +100 degrees in the frontal plane and 40 degrees anteriorly. The QRS-T angle is larger than normal, which also suggests LV hypertrophy.

See Patient 1 for a normal ECG.

DIFFERENTIAL DIAGNOSIS

The wise physician always asks the question, "Is the hypertension secondary to some as yet undiagnosed condition, or is it essential?"

The abnormalities noted on the chest x-ray film is diagnostic of coarctation of the aorta. The heart murmur and the enlargement of the proximal portion of the aorta suggest aortic stenosis caused by a congenital bicuspid aortic valve, which often occurs in patients with coarctation of the aorta.

LOW-TECHNOLOGY PROCEDURES

The femoral artery pulsation should be assessed. In most patients with coarctation of the aorta, the femoral artery pulsation is diminished and arrives shortly after the radial artery pulsation. Also, the blood pressure in the legs should be measured, which is lower than in the arms when there is coarctation of the aorta.

Auscultation of the back may be useful. The systolic murmur produced by the coarctation is usually heard in the interscapular area. Systolic bruits, a result of large intercostal arteries, may be heard over the back.

FINAL DIAGNOSIS

Coarctation of the aorta and congenital bicuspid aortic valve stenosis.

DIAGNOSTIC PRINCIPLE

Whenever the blood pressure is elevated above normal in the arms, the physician should ask, "Is the elevation of blood pressure caused by essential hypertension, or is it secondary to some other condition?"

The physician should always record a higher blood pressure in the legs than in the arms or be satisfied that the femoral artery pulsation is normal to exclude coarctation of the aorta.

A bicuspid aortic valve often occurs in patients with coarctation of the aorta.

BIBLIOGRAPHY

Nugent EW, Plauth WH, Edwards JE, Williams WH: The pathology, pathophysiology, recognition, and treatment of congenital heart disease. In Schlant RC, Alexander RW, editors: *Hurst's the heart*, ed 8, New York, 1994, McGraw-Hill, pp 1785-1790.

FIGURE CREDIT

Modified and reproduced with permission from Hurst JW: The examination of the heart: the importance of initial screening, *Dis Mon*, 36(5):285, 1990.

HISTORY

The patient is a 58-year-old man with a long history of dyspnea on effort. He has noted an increase in dyspnea during the last few days and has detected an increase in temperature. He has also noted an increase in sputum production and wheezing.

He has smoked one pack of cigarettes daily for 40 years.

PHYSICAL EXAMINATION

The temperature is elevated 1°F above normal.

There is an increase in the anteroposterior diameter of the chest.

His pulse rate is 115 beats per minute.

The systolic blood pressure is 142 mm Hg, and the diastolic blood pressure is 84 mm Hg. Pulsus paradoxus is present.

The patient is slightly cyanotic, and the face is ruddy in appearance.

The external neck veins are abnormally distended when the trunk is elevated 45 degrees. The internal jugular vein pulsation is shown in the diagram on the right.

The heart sounds are difficult to hear, and there are no murmurs.

Expiratory wheezing is noted throughout the lung fields, and an area of consolidation is detected in the base of the left lung.

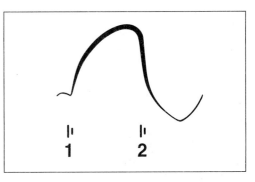

1, 2, First, second heart sounds. See figure credit.

CHEST X-RAY FILM

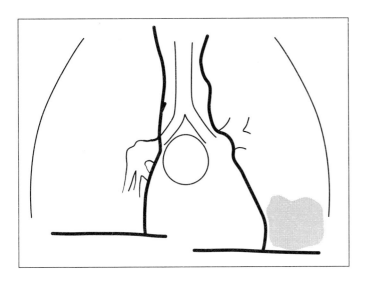

ELECTROCARDIOGRAM

Sinus tachycardia is present. There are 110 depolarizations per minute. The duration of the P wave in lead II is 0.12 second, and its amplitude is 3 mm. The PR interval is 0.17 second. The QRS duration is 0.09 second. The QT interval is 0.36 second. The total QRS amplitude is 80 mm.

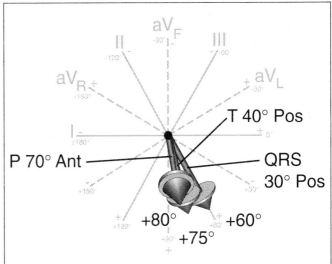

WHAT IS DIFFERENTIAL DIAGNOSIS?

WHAT IS FINAL DIAGNOSIS?

HISTORY

The history of dyspnea and wheezing for years plus excessive cigarette smoking indicate the strong likelihood that the patient has chronic obstructive pulmonary disease (COPD). The recent increase in dyspnea with fever and increase in sputum production suggest a superimposed pulmonary infection.

PHYSICAL EXAMINATION

The elevated body temperature, wheezing, and signs of consolidation in the left lower lung indicate pneumonia.

The cyanosis and ruddy appearance suggest chronic lung disease with erythrocytosis. Pulsus paradoxus may occur with cardiac tamponade, constrictive pericarditis, or COPD. In this patient, it is most likely caused by COPD.

There is evidence of tricuspid valve regurgitation (see figure in *Physical Examination* under **Clues and Questions**).

The wheezing makes auscultation difficult. One should be wary of this clinical setting because important auscultatory events such as the murmurs of aortic stenosis, aortic regurgitation, and mitral stenosis can be missed.

The clues thus far indicate the presence of COPD with heart failure precipitated by acute infection of the lung.

CHEST X-RAY FILM

The lungs appear hyperinflated, the anteroposterior diameter of the chest is increased, and each leaf of the diaphragm is flat. The pulmonary infiltrate is noted in the left lower lung base.

The heart is not large, but the pulmonary artery and its branches are larger than normal.

The x-ray film is characteristic of COPD and acute pulmonary infection. The large pulmonary artery suggests pulmonary artery hypertension in this clinical setting.

See Patient 1 for a normal chest x-ray film.

ELECTROCARDIOGRAM

The amplitude of the P waves is abnormal. The mean P vector is directed +80 degrees and 70 degrees anteriorly. This indicates a right atrial abnormality.

The 12-lead total QRS amplitude is abnormally low. The mean QRS vector is directed +60 degrees and 30 degrees posteriorly. The mean T vector is directed +75 degrees in the frontal plane and 40 degrees posteriorly, suggesting a repolarization abnormality in the right ventricle or anterior epicardial ischemia.

The right atrial abnormality in the setting of low QRS amplitude and a vertical mean QRS vector with a T vector that is directed posteriorly are typical of ECG changes seen in COPD.

See Fig. 4-79.

See Patient 1 for a normal ECG.

DIFFERENTIAL DIAGNOSIS

The patient clearly has COPD, with signs of abnormalities on the right side of the heart, and heart failure precipitated by acute pulmonary infection.

One must be careful in this setting because the features of COPD can mask the signs of other types of heart disease.

FINAL DIAGNOSIS

Cor pulmonale caused by COPD with heart failure precipitated by an acute pulmonary infection.

DIAGNOSTIC PRINCIPLE

Cor pulmonale is now defined as heart disease caused by respiratory system disease because abnormalities of the right side of the heart can be the result of disease of *any* part of the respiratory system. The cause of the condition is not limited to diseases of the lungs.

The other point to emphasize here is that the presence of COPD can make other types of heart disease difficult to recognize.

Finally, most patients with cor pulmonale caused by COPD and heart failure have arterial hypoxemia.

BIBLIOGRAPHY

Newman JH, Ross JC: Chronic cor pulmonale. In Schlant RC, Alexander RW, editors: *Hurst's the heart*, ed 8, New York, 1994, McGraw-Hill, pp 1895-1903.

FIGURE CREDIT

Modified and reproduced with permission from Hurst JW: The examination of the heart: the importance of initial screening, *Dis Mon* 36(5):280, 1990.

HISTORY

The patient is a 12-year-old boy.

After analyzing the following data, describe the history that the boy and his parents might give.

PHYSICAL EXAMINATION

Describe the most likely physical findings after analyzing the following data.

CHEST X-RAY FILM

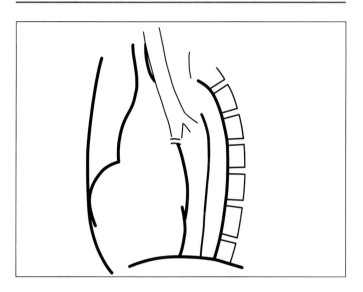

LEFT

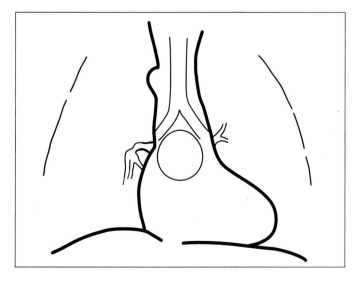

RIGHT

ELECTROCARDIOGRAM

The heart rhythm is normal. The heart rate is 88 depolarizations per minute. The amplitude of the P wave is 3 mm in lead II. The PR interval is 0.14 second. The QRS duration is 0.09 second. The QT interval is 0.34 second.

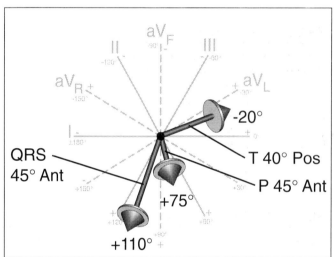

WHAT IS DIFFERENTIAL DIAGNOSIS?

WHAT IS FINAL DIAGNOSIS?

HISTORY

This 12-year-old boy and his parents may give a history of dyspnea on effort. The patient may also give a history of squatting after exercise. He may have noticed that his lips and fingernails are blue when compared with his 10-year-old sister.

PHYSICAL EXAMINATION

The patient has equal cyanosis and clubbing of the fingers and toes.

The blood pressure is normal.

The carotid artery pulsations are vigorous.

A prominent *a* wave is noted in the jugular venous pulse.

There is a prominent anterior precordial systolic movement caused by right ventricular (RV) hypertrophy.

A loud systolic murmur is heard in the second and third left intercostal spaces near the sternum. The pulmonary valve closure sound could not be heard.

CHEST X-RAY FILM

There are three important abnormalities illustrated here: (1) a decrease in pulmonary blood flow (note the small pulmonary arteries), (2) a right-sided aortic arch, and (3) RV hypertrophy (see left lateral view). These abnormalities suggest the presence of tetralogy of Fallot.

See Patient 1 for a normal chest x-ray film.

See Fig. 3-11.

ELECTROCARDIOGRAM

A right atrial abnormality is present. The QRS duration is normal. The mean QRS vector is directed abnormally to the right and anteriorly, and the mean T vector is directed to the left and posteriorly. These abnormalities indicate RV hypertrophy.

These abnormalities could be caused by any of several diseases that cause abnormally high pressure in the right ventricle.

See Patient 1 for a normal ECG.

DIFFERENTIAL DIAGNOSIS

Pulmonary valve stenosis is excluded because the main pulmonary artery and its left branch are small rather than large.

Eisenmenger physiology can be ruled out because the main pulmonary artery and its branches are small in this patient, whereas they are always large in patients with Eisenmenger physiology.

Primary pulmonary hypertension is excluded because the main pulmonary artery and its branches are small rather than large.

Tricuspid atresia can be excluded because the ECG does not show left ventricular hypertrophy.

The RV hypertrophy, decrease in pulmonary blood flow, and right-sided aortic arch suggest the presence of tetralogy of Fallot.

FINAL DIAGNOSIS

Tetralogy of Fallot with right-sided aortic arch.

DIAGNOSTIC PRINCIPLE

A right-sided aortic arch occurs often in patients with tetralogy of Fallot. The common trunk may be on the right side in patients with truncus arteriosus. Finally, a right-sided aortic arch can occur as an isolated abnormality. When an older child has a right-sided aortic arch, RV hypertrophy in the ECG, and decreased pulmonary blood flow, the diagnosis is almost always tetralogy of Fallot. This is true because patients with type 4 truncus arteriosus do not usually live to become adolescents, and those with types 1, 2, and 3 truncus have an increase in pulmonary blood flow.

BIBLIOGRAPHY

Nugent EW, Plauth WH, Edwards JE, Williams WH: The pathology, pathophysiology, recognition, and treatment of congenital heart disease. In Schlant RC, Alexander RW, editors: *Hurst's the heart*, ed 8, New York, 1994, McGraw-Hill, pp 1799-1802.

HISTORY

The patient is a 32-year-old muscular male. He complains of retrosternal discomfort produced by effort. He has noted this unpleasant sensation for about 6 months. The discomfort lasts about 3 minutes. He had an episode of syncope while in bed after he used a nasal decongestant.

His father died suddenly at age 41.

PHYSICAL EXAMINATION

The pulse rate is 88 beats per minute.

The systolic blood pressure is 128 mm Hg, and the diastolic blood pressure is 74 mm Hg.

There are no abnormal pulsations of the neck veins.

The carotid artery pulsation is shown in the diagram on the right.

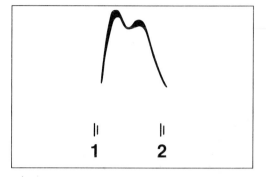

1, 2, First, second heart sounds. See figure credits.

The apex impulse is shown in the following diagram:

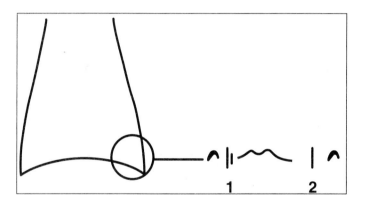

Auscultation of the heart reveals the following:

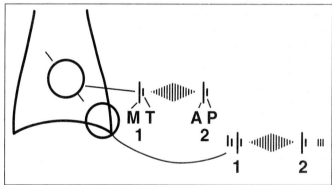

M, Mitral, *T,* tricuspid, *A,* aortic, and *P,* pulmonary valve closure sound. See figure credits.

CHEST X-RAY FILM

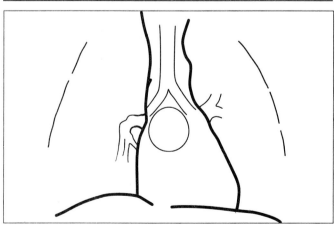

ELECTROCARDIOGRAM

The rhythm is normal. There are 84 depolarizations per minute. The second half of the P wave in V_1 measures -0.04 mm•second. The PR interval is 0.18 second. The QT interval is 0.36 second. The QRS amplitude is 230 mm.

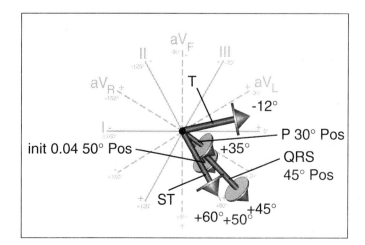

WHAT ADDITIONAL LOW-TECHNOLOGY PROCEDURES WOULD YOU PERFORM?

WHAT IS DIFFERENTIAL DIAGNOSIS?

WHAT IS FINAL DIAGNOSIS?

197

HISTORY

The young man has stable angina pectoris produced by effort and syncope precipitated by an inhalation of a nasal decongestant. His father died suddenly at age 41.

The history strongly suggests that the patient has idiopathic hypertrophic subaortic stenosis (IHSS). A less likely diagnosis is valvular aortic stenosis, coronary atherosclerosis, or a congenital anomaly of the coronary arteries.

PHYSICAL EXAMINATION

The examination of the neck veins reveals no abnormalities.

The carotid pulsation reveals a pulsus bisferiens. This type of pulsation occurs in patients with aortic valve regurgitation, IHSS, anemia, thyrotoxicosis, and catecholamine excess (see upper figure in *Physical Examination* under **Clues and Questions**).

The apical impulse is abnormal. An atrial gallop movement is felt, the abnormally prolonged systolic movement is strong and bifid, and a ventricular gallop movement also is felt (see middle figure in *Physical Examination* under **Clues and Questions**). This type of movement is characteristic of IHSS. It could be caused by aortic valve regurgitation.

A grade 2 systolic murmur is heard halfway between the "aortic area" located in the second right intercostal space and the "mitral area" located at the apex. The second heart sound is normal (see lower figure in *Physical Examination* under **Clues and Questions**). It is difficult to determine if there is predominant left ventricular (LV) outflow tract obstruction or mitral valve regurgitation.

Atrial and ventricular gallop sounds are heard at the cardiac apex (see lower figure in *Physical Examination* under **Clues and Questions**).

CHEST X-RAY FILM

The chest film shows no abnormality. This does not exclude IHSS, aortic valve stenosis, mild valvular disease of any type, or coronary disease, including anomalies of the coronary arteries, cardiac dysrhythmias, or pericarditis.

See Patient 1 for a normal chest x-ray film.

ELECTROCARDIOGRAM

There is a left atrial abnormality, which always suggests the presence of LV disease or mitral valve disease.

The total QRS amplitude is greater than normal. The QRS duration is normal, and the mean QRS vector is directed 45 degrees in the frontal plane and 45 degrees posteriorly. This abnormality indicates LV hypertrophy.

The initial mean 0.04-second vector is directed more posteriorly than the subsequent QRS forces. This produces abnormal Q waves in leads V_1, V_2, and a QRS wave in lead V_3. This indicates an initial QRS depolarization defect.

The mean ST vector is directed about +60 degrees in the frontal plane and is parallel with the frontal plane. This indicates predominant epicardial injury.

The mean T vector is directed superiorly -12 degrees in the frontal plane; it is parallel with the frontal plane.

The cluster of abnormalities suggests the presence of an acute myocardial infarction (MI) except for one factor: the total QRS amplitude is huge. This occurs infrequently with isolated MI. Whenever there is an increase in QRS amplitude and abnormal initial 0.04-second, ST, and T vectors suggesting infarction, it is wise to consider (1) aortic valve stenosis plus MI caused by coronary disease, (2) systemic hypertension plus coronary disease, or (3) IHSS.

See Fig. 4-74.

ADDITIONAL LOW-TECHNOLOGY PROCEDURES

Ask the patient to perform a Valsalva maneuver. The murmur should become louder during the test when it is caused by IHSS. This response occurred in this patient.

Ask the patient to grip your hand while you listen to the heart. The murmur should decrease in intensity during the test when it is caused by IHSS. This response occurred in this patient.

DIFFERENTIAL DIAGNOSIS

The history of sudden death in his father, stable angina, and syncope from exogenous catecholamines in a normotensive patient, plus pulsus bisferiens, plus the systolic murmur that becomes louder during the Valsalva maneuver and fainter during isometric exercise, plus the absence of aortic valve regurgitation, plus the normal-sized heart on the chest x-ray film, plus huge QRS amplitude with the initial 0.04-second vector of the QRS complexes suggesting infarction, indicate the presence of IHSS.

Aortic valve stenosis plus MI are excluded because of the change in murmur produced by the Valsalva maneuver and with isometric exercise.

FINAL DIAGNOSIS

Idiopathic hypertrophic subaortic stenosis.

DIAGNOSTIC PRINCIPLE

Once again, the signs of LV hypertrophy imply a condition other than, or in addition to, coronary atherosclerosis as a cause of angina or MI.

Patients with IHSS may have angina pectoris even though the epicardial coronary arteries are normal. Such patients also have syncope, which is always an ominous symptom. In this patient, syncope occurred, even though he was in bed, when he sniffed a nasal membrane decongestant that undoubtedly contained a catecholamine.

This genetically determined disease is much more common than was previously suspected and is often misdiagnosed in elderly patients. It is also frequently misdiagnosed as atherosclerotic coronary heart disease with angina and MI or as valvular aortic stenosis.

BIBLIOGRAPHY

Maron BJ, Roberts WC: Hypertrophy cardiomyopathy. In Schlant RC, Alexander RW, editors: *Hurst's the heart*, ed 8, New York, 1994, McGraw-Hill, pp 1621-1635.

FIGURE CREDITS

Upper, Reproduced with permission and *lower*, modified and reproduced with permission from Hurst JW: The examination of the heart: the importance of initial screening, *Dis Mon*, 36(5):278, 285, 1990.

INDEX